I0038127

Biomechanics for Today's World

Biomechanics for Today's World

First Edition

Jeff Bauer

SUNY – Cortland

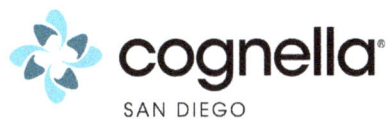

cognella®

SAN DIEGO

Bassim Hamadeh, CEO and Publisher
John Remington, Executive Editor
Danielle Gradisher, Project Editor
Casey Hands, Production Editor
Susana Christie, Developmental Editor
Emely Villavicencio, Senior Graphic Designer
Kylie Bartolome, Licensing Specialist
Natalie Piccotti, Director of Marketing
Kassie Graves, Senior Vice President, Editorial
Jamie Giganti, Director of Academic Publishing

Copyright © 2024 by Cognella, Inc. All rights reserved. No part of this publication may be reprinted, reproduced, transmitted, or utilized in any form or by any electronic, mechanical, or other means, now known or hereafter invented, including photocopying, microfilming, and recording, or in any information retrieval system without the written permission of Cognella, Inc. For inquiries regarding permissions, translations, foreign rights, audio rights, and any other forms of reproduction, please contact the Cognella Licensing Department at rights@cognella.com.

Trademark Notice: Product or corporate names may be trademarks or registered trademarks and are used only for identification and explanation without intent to infringe.

Cover image: Copyright © 2022 iStockphoto LP/kentoh.

Printed in the United States of America.

Contents

Contents

Chapter 1

Introduction to Biomechanics

Preparing to Learn: *Watch*

Biomechanics is the study of human and animal movement. It allows us to better understand our movement capabilities and often the mechanisms that lead to injury. From birth to death, movement is central to the human experience, and by combining an understanding of anatomy, physics, and instrumentation we are able to better appreciate the amazing machines we are gifted with.

This text was conceived with the notion of offering a wide variety of examples and applications of biomechanical knowledge to showcase the benefit of understanding the complexity of biological movement. From elite athletes to newborn babies, to those struggling with severe orthopedic injuries or dealing with a degenerative motor disease, biomechanists work to improve or maintain function while decreasing the occurrence and rate of injuries for all of us.

I hope as you go through this text you will find many examples of biomechanical activity that will surprise you and some that match your own personal experiences related to movement.

The following short video clips provide examples of biomechanics in the main areas of biomechanical research: sport, daily life, and medicine. Each video highlights just one case of many in which biomechanics makes a difference for those involved.

Sport: Javelin Throwing

One or more interactive elements has been excluded from this version of the text. You can view them online here: https://pb.cognella.com/83647-1b/?p=25#oembed-1

Please refer to the interactive ebook in Cognella Active Learning for interactive/media content.

Daily Life: Workplace Biomechanics Is Often Called Ergonomics

---

One or more interactive elements has been excluded from this version of the text. You can view them online here: https://pb.cognella.com/83647-1b/?p=25#oembed-2

Please refer to the interactive ebook in Cognella Active Learning for interactive/media content.

Medicine: Biomechanics at the Human Performance Lab – KU Medical Center

---

One or more interactive elements has been excluded from this version of the text. You can view them online here: https://pb.cognella.com/83647-1b/?p=25#oembed-3

Please refer to the interactive ebook in Cognella Active Learning for interactive/media content.

Preparing to Learn: *Respond*

Directions: Based on what you saw in the videos, respond to the following questions:

1. What was the purpose of the markers placed on the track athlete? What were the goals of the athlete and biomechanist for this study?
2. What is ergonomics? Are the goals of ergonomics and biomechanics the same? When is the term biomechanics first heard in the video, and what is the major area of injury discussed shortly thereafter? Can you think of other areas in which biomechanics shows up under a different name?
3. What types of instruments are discussed in this video to capture biomechanically relevant values? What groups of individuals can benefit from the use of biomechanical research highlighted in this short video?

Introduction to the Chapter

What is biomechanics? Where did it come from, and why should I care?

Biomechanics is a hybrid scientific discipline that helps explain the movement potential of living or once living organisms. The bio in biomechanics refers to the necessity of understanding the basic biology of the organism being studied. If that organism is a person, that biological and anatomical knowledge provides a basic blueprint of the human machine and its capabilities. Such knowledge allows for a better understanding of how internal and external forces can be used to accurately predict the movement and/or injury potential of the person at any given time or in any situation they may find themselves.

The mechanics portion of biomechanics refers to the static and dynamic branches of engineering mechanics that provide the equations and formulas to accurately analyze both moving and nonmoving mechanical systems. If we look at the human musculoskeletal system as a machine composed of simple machines (levers, pulleys, etc.) that is powered by chemical factories (muscles) with information regarding how these talk to one another (nervous system), then you have the human machine that we all live in.

Learning Objectives

After completing this chapter, students should be able to do the following:

- Define biomechanics
- List the main areas of biomechanical research
- List the goals of biomechanics
- Name the "fathers of biomechanics" and the three areas in which they contributed to the field of biomechanics
- Point out examples of applied biomechanics in everyday life situations

What Is Biomechanics?

Biomechanics is a hybrid science that uses information from musculoskeletal anatomy, mechanical physics, and advanced motion technologies to help us better understand how and why we move.

Movement is basic to our survival, and gaining a deeper understanding of what it takes to move safely and efficiently is necessary for anyone, but especially for those interested in becoming human motion specialists like those studying exercise science, physical education, physical therapy, athletic training, coaching, occupational therapy, or a host of other human performance–related disciplines.

What makes biomechanics unique is that it models the human or other movement system as something that can be better understood when viewing it through the lens of basic mechanical physics. That does not mean that biomechanics is "just" physics hidden behind a curtain of human examples and applications. Biomechanics is much more than that. It is method of objectively seeing, discovering, and predicting a wide spectrum of human and animal movement in a way not done through any of the other science courses typically offered to students.

The Goals of Biomechanics

The goals of biomechanics are to increase or maintain people's movement ability while at the same time working to decrease the likelihood and severity of movement-related injury. At times those goals conflict as pushing a body to its movement limits makes it more likely to suffer injury. That is a conundrum faced by biomechanists: how to help improve or maintain performance while also keeping the person safe from injury.

When working with athletes the goal may be to help the athlete running faster, lift heavier weights, or improve their ability to strike a ball with better accuracy and consistency while working to keep them healthy enough to train and compete at very high levels of performance. For those rehabbing from an injury, how quickly and effectively can the rehab proceed without resulting in further injury or other performance setbacks? It is a never-ending balancing act to push the boundaries of human performance while attempting to keep the person from being injured.

Equipment advances in speed skiing provide a real-world example of how working to improve performance can also increase the likelihood of severe injury for participants if something should go wrong.

One or more interactive elements has been excluded from this version of the text. You can view them online here: https://pb.cognella.com/83647-1b/?p=25#oembed-4

Please refer to the interactive ebook in Cognella Active Learning for interactive/media content.

The extremely aerodynamically efficient skin suits worn by speed skiers help them to reach speeds of greater than 245 km/hr as they rocket down the slope. Any mistake at that speed can result in severe injury. They are moving so fast that if they fall the heat generated from friction as they slide down the mountain trying to slow down in their very slippery suits often results in second- and third-degree burns, not to mention the bumps, bruises, and possible broken bones they are likely to suffer from a crash at such speeds.

Where Does Biomechanics Fit in the Area of Movement Sciences?

Under the umbrella term of kinesiology there are many subspecialties that merit study for students working toward degrees in human movement–related fields. Where does biomechanics fit in, and how is it related to areas such as exercise physiology and motor behavior? In many cases biomechanics acts as a bridge between the more biological-focused courses and those that are more related to the mechanics of movement. Figure 1.1 illustrates the bridge biomechanics provides that links many of the subspecialties of kinesiology and shows its important role in tying them together.

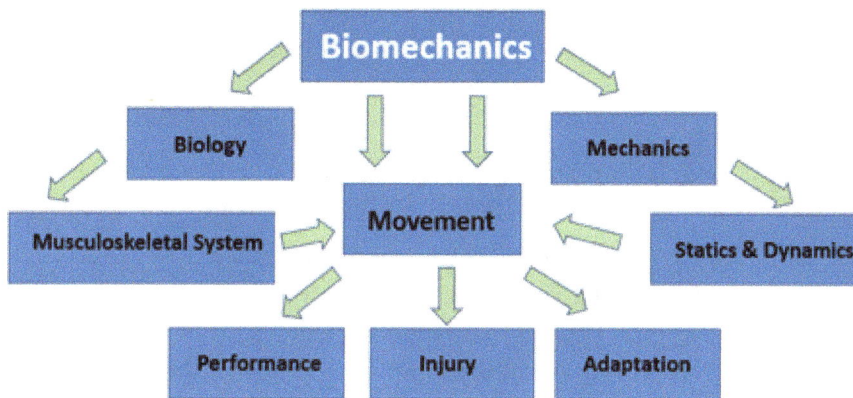

Biomechanics relationship to movement

Figure 1.1   Biomechanics relationship to movement.

Where Did Biomechanics Come From?

From our earliest known human records, such as cave paintings dating back over 40,000 years, to the ancient records of virtually every civilization around the world, art and literature are full of images of human, animal, and cosmic motion. Motion is one of the basic tenants of life as we know it. It allows us to explore our environment and provides us with the means to survive. It is so basic that it is one of the very first indicators of life, a baby kicking within its mother's womb, as well as a measure used to determine the death of an individual, when they can no longer breath.

Have you ever watched someone walk? Not just seen them stroll past, but actually taken the time to focus on how they perform one of the most basic types of human movement? If you have, you likely noticed that each person has a unique movement style. That movement style is more specific to that person than their fingerprints. It is so individually specific that it can be used to uniquely identify them from any other person on earth. How a person walks is an outward expression of all of the physical and emotional experiences they have experienced during their lives. It's their movement signature that cannot be faked or reproduced by anyone else. Biomechanical analysis of gait confirms the unique aspects of this and a wide variety of human and animal movement patterns. Yes, there are similarities between how individuals perform different movement tasks, and we are all governed by the same physical laws of movement, but we each place our own special stamp on the types of movement we use to navigate our world. Biomechanics can help us identify the similarities and differences that makes each one of us special from a movement standpoint.

All of us have experienced and observed motion throughout our lives, but few have truly understood what motion is. How does motion start, what causes it to change, and what are the ranges of motion for humans, animals, and other objects that we encounter every day? To begin to answer those questions we will apply the science of biomechanics. This text is designed to provide a brief glimpse into the biomechanics of motion and help you to better understand you, those around you, and the world in which we live!

The "Fathers" of Biomechanics

It wasn't until the late 1960s and early 1970s that the term biomechanics began to be widely used to describe this area of motion science that views all bodies in motion as mechanical systems governed by the principles of mechanical physics. Prior to that time descriptors such as movement studies, exercise science, kinesiology, and others served as umbrella terms under which the mechanics of motion was housed. As more students studying movement sciences gained access to computers it became possible for a much larger group to learn and conduct research related to movement based on the mechanical properties of a body. It was the right time for this area of study to establish its own academic identity, and after much discussion the term *biomechanics* (*bio* for living or once living and *mechanics* for the branch of physics related to mechanical motion) emerged as the term to be applied to this unique area of motion study. Today's students of biomechanics have at their fingertips technology and resources that the early biomechanists (the correct term for someone who practices biomechanics) couldn't even dream of. The hand and manual calculator-based results of the analysis of human gait reported in the seminal work by Braune and Fischer took over a decade to complete and required the invention of a suite of specialized equipment to biomechanically analyze the walking patterns of a handful of study participants. Now the calculations and the special tools needed to perform that level of gait analysis are available to almost every student who takes a biomechanics class.

There were three men who standout in the history of biomechanics for their contributions to the three main areas of biomechanics (anatomy, physics, and instrumentation) that deserve a little special attention. The men are Giovanni Borelli, Sir Isaac Newton, and Eadweard Muybridge. Of the three, only Sir Isaac Newton is widely recognized for his genius, but the other two hold special places of honor in the field of biomechanics. Each is considered a "father" of modern biomechanics for their significant contributions to this field of science.

Ironically, it is almost a certainty that none of the fathers of biomechanics ever heard the word *biomechanics* spoken or saw it in written in text, nor could they have realized that their life's work would significantly contribute to the eventual creation of the field of biomechanics, yet they will be forever tied to its inception.

Anatomy

Giovanni Alphonso Borelli (1608–1679)
Giovanni Borelli was born in Naples, Italy, and lived his whole life in the that Mediterranean country. He is remembered as a Renaissance Italian physiologist, physicist, and mathematician (https:\\en.wikipedia.org/

wiki/ Giovanni_Alfonso_Borelli). But in the field of biomechanics we remember him as a "bone collector" whose posthumous text *de Motu Animalium* or *On the Movement of Animals* marked the first widely referenced text on the anatomical/mechanical characteristics of the human body.

Borelli conducted his research into the mechanical properties of the human body during a time when such study was strictly prohibited by the Catholic Church. If found guilty of performing such work a person could be excommunicated from the Church, resulting in a loss of any hope of attaining heaven during the afterlife. That threat was more than enough to keep most from exploring how the interval functions of the body worked. But not Borelli. He secretly acquired human specimens that he dissected and carefully documented the musculoskeletal structure and function of their bodies. His work led to a couple of chapters inserted toward the end of the *de Motu Animalium* that were followed by multiple chapters dealing with anatomical information on other forms of animals. The book itself was published after his death by his son so that Giovanni wouldn't be in peril of being found out by the Church and denied his chance for eternal bliss. Whether he truly believed the Church teachings or was concerned with its possible punishments, he took no chance.

To ensure his contributions to biomechanics are not forgotten, the highest individual award in the area of biomechanics presented by the American Society of Biomechanics is the "Borelli award."

Physics

Sir Isaac Newton

Sir Isaac Newton was born in England and gained worldwide prominence in a variety of scientific disciplines, including mathematics (inventor of calculus), physics (laws of motion and gravity), and astronomy (reflecting telescope). Because during his life two calendars were widely in use in Europe, his birthday is reported to be either on Christmas Day 1642 (Julian calendar) or January 4' 1643 (Gregorian Calendar), and death on March 20' 1726 (Julian calendar) or March 31' 1727 (Gregorian calendar). And no, that is not a typo in the year of his death; look it up if you don't believe me!

Newton was credited with developing calculus during a forced break from his studies at Cambridge University due to a plague outbreak in England at the time. It was his study of the physical world and attempts to match his observations with the mathematics of his day that led him to develop a form of mathematics that helps us understand functions related to situations of continual change over time, such as most forms of human motion.

It was Newton's ability to grasp the "big picture" and summarize it into understandable mathematical equations that lead to his laws of motion and gravity, which enable us to better understand motion in our world. His influence in the application of classic mechanical physics led to the term *Newtonian physics*—a way to express through formulas the thought processes used to study, understand, and predict the outcomes of most forms of mechanical systems in motion.

Instrumentation

Eadweard Muybridge (1830–1904)

Eadweard Muybridge was born in England but immigrated to the United States at the age of 20. At 30 he suffered a severe head injury and returned to England to recuperate. It was during that time he found his professional calling as a photographer. He returned to the United States and moved to San Francisco, where he set up shop as a photographer of natural wild landscapes.

Photographic technology at the time made it almost impossible to capture a clear, nonblurred image of any object that was moving. Always interested in advancing the art of photography and using it to enrich himself, he set about a series of experiments attempting to modify his cameras to capture short duration snapshots. By inventing a high-speed mechanical shutter mechanism that could be attached to the lens of his cameras he discovered a way to clearly capture images of animals during motion. He didn't know it at the time, but that technical breakthrough might have saved his life!

It was around the time he invented the high-speed shutter mechanism that a personal issue looked to put an end to his work permanently. Having shot and killed his wife's lover, Muybridge was put on trial for murder. A murder conviction would have likely resulted in him being hung. Lucky for him, he had made some rich and powerful friends as a photographer and inventor.

One such powerful friend was Leland Stanford (former governor of California and founder of Stanford University). Stanford was a regular client of Muybridge, having purchased many of Muybridge's photographs. At the time, all artistic representations of a horse galloping showed at least one hoof in contact with the ground. It's said that Stanford didn't believe that to be the case but had no way to prove his suspicions. Legend has i, that Stanford made an open wager of $25,000 payable to any person who could prove that a horse when if full gallop would at some point have all of its hooves off the ground. Muybridge, being in desperate need of money to hire the right lawyers to have him acquitted of the murder charge, sought out Stanford and told him he had the technology to win his bet if Stanford could provide him with access to a horse and racetrack. Fortunately for Muybridge, Stanford agreed.

Muybridge was given access to one of Stanford's racehorses and use of his race track in Palo Alto, California, starting in 1873. By carefully setting up 24 individual cameras, each spaced 1 foot apart with trip wires used to snap successive pictures as a horse raced by, Muybridge was able to successfully capture the silhouette of the horse and rider galloping down the track. Those images showed that a horse is completely airborne at some point during a full gallop (see Figure 1.2), providing the proof Stanford was looking for (Ball, 2013).

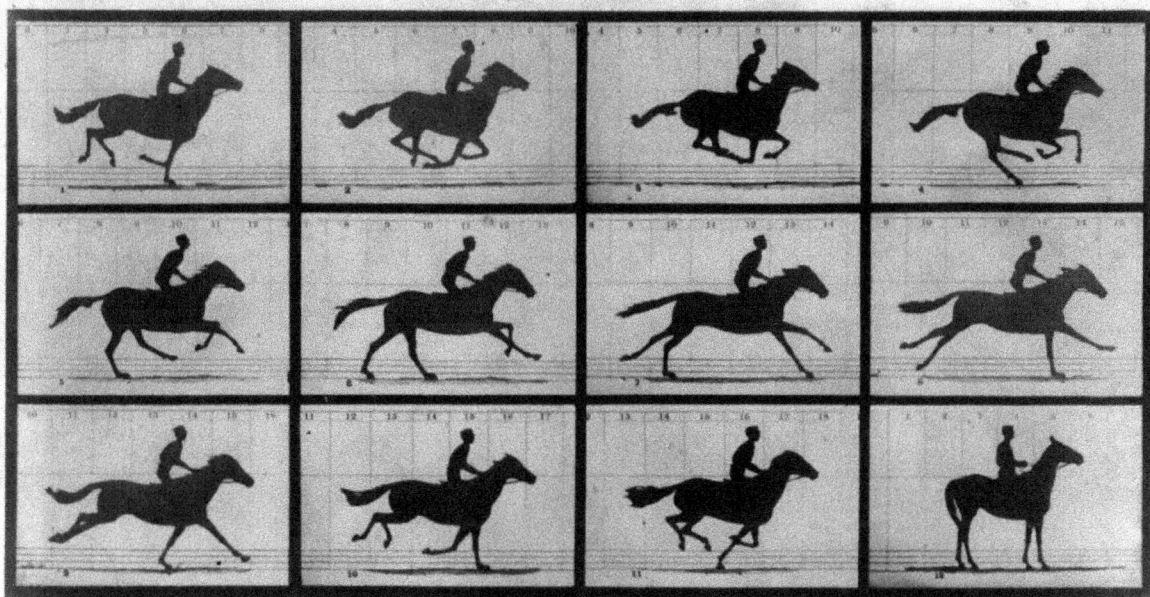

THE HORSE IN MOTION.

Illustrated by
MUYBRIDGE.

"SALLIE GARDNER," owned by LELAND STANFORD; running at a 1.40 gait over the Palo Alto track, 19th June, 1878.

Figure 1.2   Horse galloping.

Regardless of whether there was a bet, Muybridge had earned enough money through his dealings with the rich and famous to afford the best legal defense in his murder trial. He was acquitted of murder and returned to his tinkering with cameras. Eventually he invented a way of sequentially projecting the snapshot images of moving objects at a high rate of speed. This resulted in the viewer believing that they were seeing actual motion and not a series of still images. He named his invention the zoopraxiscope (Figure 1.3).

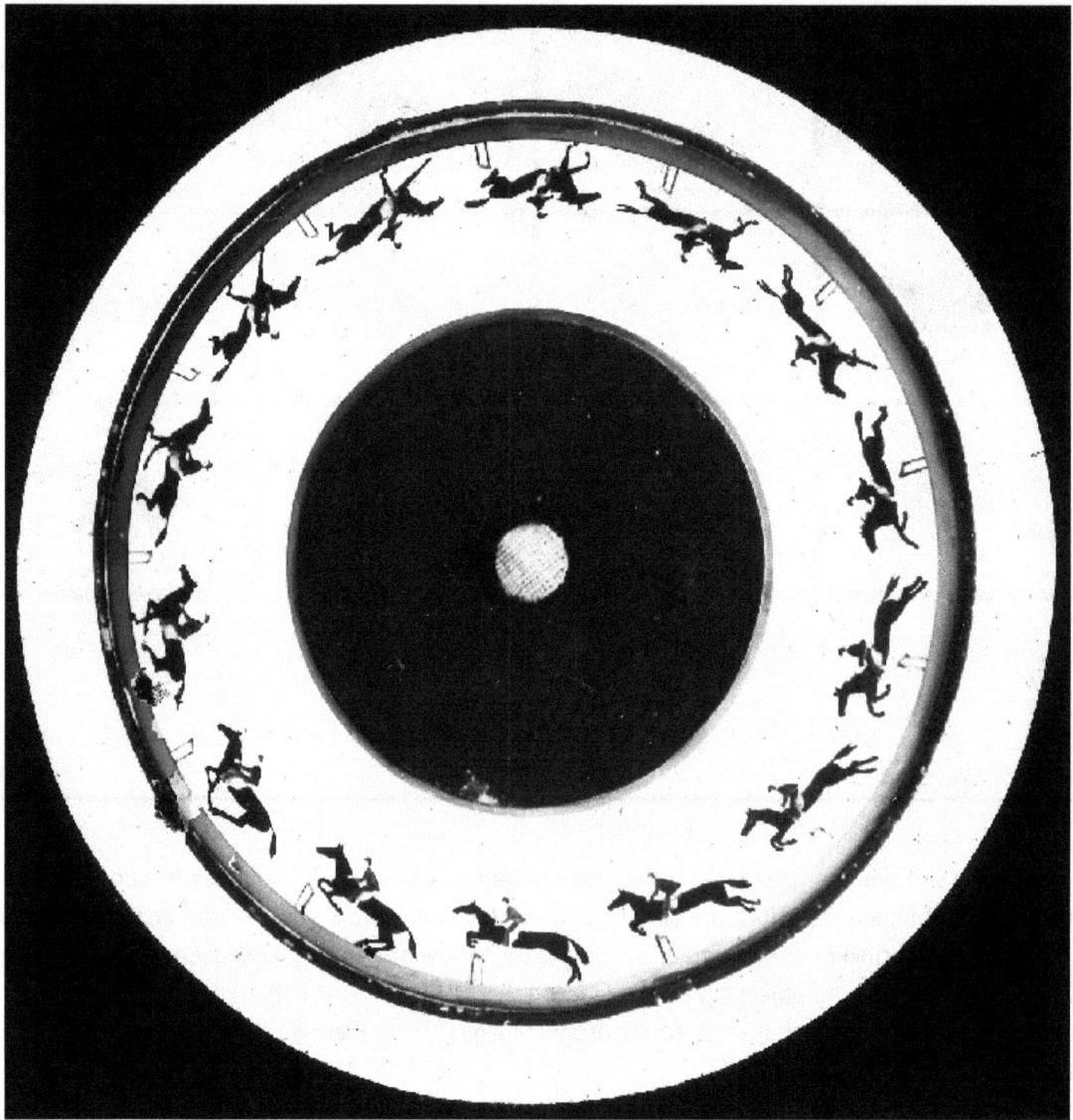

Figure 1.3   Zoopraxiscope record of horse movement.

The zoopraxiscope was the first motion picture projector and the predecessor of cinematography and the various forms videography used today.

More on the life and times of Eadweard Muybridge can be found in this video:

One or more interactive elements has been excluded from this version of the text. You can view them online here:
https://pb.cognella.com/83647-1b/?p=25#oembed-5

To ensure his contributions to biomechanics are not forgotten, the highest individual award in the area of biomechanics presented annually by the International Society of Biomechanics is called the "Muybridge award."

Penn State Water Tower

Biomechanics was a relatively new label used in the area of human movement science when Dr. Richard Nelson founded the biomechanics laboratory in the Water Tower on the Penn State University campus in State College, Pennsylvania, in 1967. Nelson realized that a revolution in technology was starting that would allow for the human machine to be studied in ways never before possible. He, along with Drs. Dewey Morehouse and Peter Cavanaugh, created one of the most important early centers for the training of future biomechanists. Between the students who studied under the trio and the many visiting scholars that spent time in the tower over the years, a legacy was created that links many biomechanists across the world to this humble structure that is still producing outstanding contributors to the area of biomechanics.

Women in Biomechanics: Shaping the Future of Movement Analysis

Biomechanics is a newly recognized field of science, first defined in the English language during the mid to late 1800s. It is a hybrid term formed from the ancient Greek words *bios* (life) and *mechanika* (mechanics) to describe the study of living or once living creatures, their movement patterns/possibilities, and their underlying structural makeup. It wasn't until the 1960s that the term began to be considered a subspecialty of kinesiology, similar to exercise physiology or motor development.

Women have played an increasingly important role in the areas of biomechanical research and education, with many contributing greatly to the biomechanical knowledge base of today. Two of the more widely recognized women in biomechanics are Drs. Jaquelin Perry and Jill McNitt-Gray.

In 1992 Perry published *Gait Analysis: Normal and Pathological Function*, a seminal work that was updated in 2010 and continues to be a widely used by those who study/treat lower extremity function. Perry was widely acknowledged as one of the leading researchers, scholars, and clinicians in the area of polio. She continued to be an active clinician almost until the day she died at the age of 94 in March of 2013.

McNitt-Gray is a professor at the University of Southern California, where she studies the mechanisms organisms use to control and distribute mechanical load during goal-directed multijoint movements involving external loading. A product of the Penn State Biomechanics program, she has been an extremely active researcher, educator, and scholar for more than 3 decades (USC Dornsife, n.d.).

Who Are Biomechanists Today and in the Future? (or, You Might Be a Biomechanist If . . .)

Some people have spent a lifetime of work and study to better understand how humans and animals move, are injured, and successfully return to activity. But you don't have to go to school and earn degrees that say biomechanics to become a biomechanist. Anyone who is curious about and wonders at how they or other things move is a biomechanist.

An infant, amazed and fascinated by the sights and sounds of the environment in which they find themselves uses their senses to make sense of the world around them. They are a biomechanist. Eventually they will learn to move themselves, first by crawling, then, after many failed attempts, walking. Through trial and error, they learn to apply their understanding of motion to achieve their ultimate goal of controlled movement in the form of human locomotion. That is biomechanics. The junior high student trying to figure out how to gain control over their bodies again following a growth spurt is functioning as a biomechanist. The "invincible" young adult trying all kinds of different, and often dangerous, combinations of human and machine pairing, from bike riding to snowboarding, is a biomechanist. Older adults attempting to stay active and healthy while juggling careers and family demands are biomechanists. The elderly adapting to the reality of declining health and vitality by using canes and walkers to assist them as they move are continuing their lifelong application of the principles of biomechanics. Regardless if your career path leads to sports, health care, teaching, coaching, private industry, or almost any area involving performance or understanding human and/or animal movement, biomechanics will have value for you.

Summary

Biomechanics is a field of science that attempts to better understand the movement possibilities of living or once living organisms through the application of knowledge in the areas of anatomy, physics, and instrumentation. The application of biomechanics across a wide range of needs, from athletics to combatting neurodegenerative diseases, have helped individuals improve/maintain their movement ability while decreasing and/or reducing the severity of injuries sustained while attempting to reach their movement goals. We are all biomechanists!

Takeaways

- Biomechanics is a hybrid science that uses the knowledge of biology and musculoskeletal anatomy to predict the movement and injury potential of living or once living organisms.
- The main areas of biomechanical research are sports, daily life, and medicine.
- The goals of biomechanics are improving/maintaining function while limiting injury and improving recovery outcomes when injuries do occur.
- The "fathers of biomechanics" and their main area of expertise are Giovanni Borelli (anatomy), Sir Isaac Newton (physics), and Eadweard Muybridge (instrumentation).

- We are all biomechanists with our own movement goals and aspirations.
  -

References

Ball, E. (2013). *The inventor and the tycoon*. Doubleday.

Braune, W., & Fishcher, O. (2011). *The Human Gait*. Springer Berlin, Heidelberg.

Perry, J. & Burnfield, J. M. (2010.) *Gait analysis: normal and pathological function (2nd edition)*. Thorofare: SLACK Incorporated, 576.

USC Dorsnife. (n.d.). Jill McNitt-Gray. https://dornsife.usc.edu/labs/biomech/mcnitt-gray

Image Credits

Fig. 1.2: Source: https://commons.wikimedia.org/wiki/File:The_Horse_in_Motion.jpg.

Fig. 1.3: Source: https://artsandculture.google.com/asset/zoopraxiscope-disc-eadweard-muybridge/QgFEWJoEKUWqAQ.

Chapter 2

Areas of Biomechanical Research

Preparing to Learn: *Watch*

In sports the proper application of force and body orientation during complex movements allow athletes to accomplish extraordinary feats. As you watch the following videos focus on the many different aspects of the motion that must be performed in exactly the right sequence with exactly the right amount of effort to assure success.

Every day we waste much of the energy we put into movement. What if we could harness that lost kinetic energy and convert it into electricity that we could use in other ways?

(Only watch from 0:00 to 3:55)

One or more interactive elements has been excluded from this version of the text. You can view them online here: https://pb.cognella.com/83647-1b/?p=26#oembed-1

Please refer to the interactive ebook in Cognella Active Learning for interactive/media content.

Advances in patient assessment and rehab can be furthered through the correct use of instrumentation and applied biomechanical knowledge.

One or more interactive elements has been excluded from this version of the text. You can view them online here: https://pb.cognella.com/83647-1b/?p=26#oembed-2

Please refer to the interactive ebook in Cognella Active Learning for interactive/media content.

Preparing to Learn: *Respond*

Directions: Based on what you saw in the videos, respond to the following questions:

1. Why is it important to note that the high jumper generated a maximum foot strike force of over eight times his body weight during less than 2 tenths of a second?
2. If we can't light whole cities with human power, is it worth it to retrofit gyms and pedestrian walkways with kinetic energy–capture systems?
3. How does having specialized equipment designed to measure information about gait, balance, and strength benefit those working with people who have Parkinson's disease?

Introduction to the Chapter

Biomechanics shows up in many forms of basic and applied research. This chapter will highlight the three primary areas of biomechanical research and present some examples of how biomechanists have and are changing the world of movement for the better.

Learning Objectives

After completing this chapter, students should be able to do the following:

- List the three main areas of biomechanical research
- Provide examples of each of the three main areas of biomechanical research
- Explain how the Fosbury flop used knowledge of the center of mass to change the sport of high jumping
- Explain the dangers of the "diabetic foot triad" to a diabetic patient
- List some of the instruments used to capture/analyze data by biomechanists for medical research
- Be able to identify biomechanical applications/innovations and match them to specific areas of biomechanical research

In this chapter we will explore how biomechanics has been applied in three areas of human movement: sport, daily life, and medicine. The goals of biomechanics are to improve and/or maintain performance while attempting to reduce the likelihood injury. Those goals are found across the three major areas of biomechanical research and application.

Advances in technology during the past half century have spurred the development of specialized instrumentation that makes it easier than ever before to gather and analyze an ever-growing number of movement-related parameters. This ability to record unbiased data has spread across all areas of biomechanical research and applications, bringing biomechanics out of the laboratory and into the lives of more people every day.

Sports

Are we as athletes getting bigger, stronger, and faster, or has human movement potential stayed relatively unchanged over centuries? Could it be those innovations in sports equipment, training, nutrition, and rehab practices account for much if not all of the noted improvement in human athletic performance? Is it possible that the application of sport sciences like biomechanics is responsible for the improvements seen in sport?

One or more interactive elements has been excluded from this version of the text. You can view them online here:
https://pb.cognella.com/83647-1b/?p=26#oembed-3

Please refer to the interactive ebook in Cognella Active Learning for interactive/media content.

Probably the most recognizable area of biomechanics for the general public is related to the design of athletic footwear. Go to any sports store anywhere in the world or look online for athletic apparel and you will find a wide variety of different shoes in different colors and shapes created by a host of manufacturers. The majority of those shoes have something in common: They are built to meet the goals of biomechanics. Almost all athletic footwear is designed to improve/maintain performance while attempting to reduce injury in the wearer.

Maybe the best-known maker of athletic footwear is the company Nike. Nike was founded by Phil Knight and his track coach Bill Bowerman in 1964. They met when Phil was member of the University of Oregon track team that Bowerman coached.

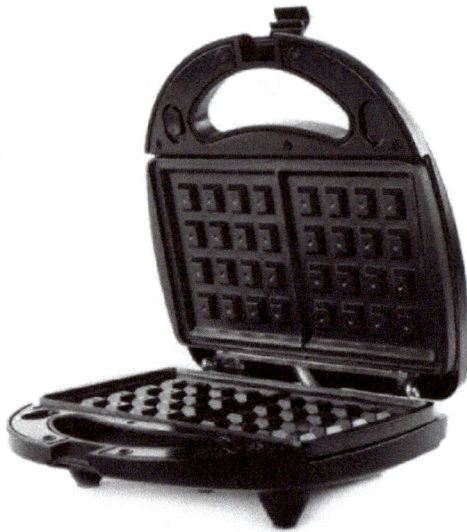

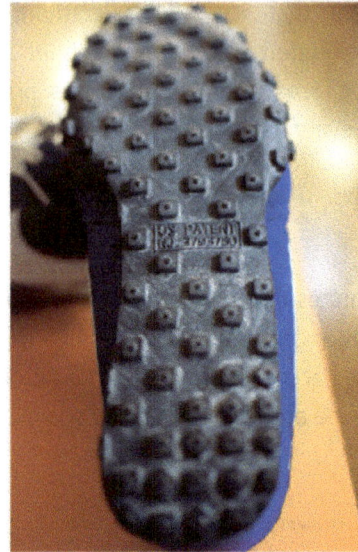

Figure 2.1   Nike formula: athlete + waffle iron = waffle training flat.

There is some question as to who created the first Nike waffle trainer, Knight or Bowerman, but there is no doubt that the advent of today's multibillion-dollar athletic shoe market is linked to the invention of this unique training shoe with the waffle-like sole design.

Their intent was to create a new-generation running shoe that would provide both stability and additional traction. The shape that would change athletic shoes forever was found at the breakfast table (Figure 2.1). They called their invention the waffle trainer because of the shape of the sole of the shoe, which resembled a waffle and is not that surprising when you realize that the actual sole of the first prototype shoes was created with the use of Mrs. Bowerman's waffle maker! (National Museum of American History, n.d.; Enterprises Explained, 2021).

After a series of improvements from their original design, Knight and Bowerman decided to start selling the waffle trainer to other aspiring athletes. That was the start of Nike.

Their plan was simple in hindsight: Develop shoes based on the biomechanical understanding of human needs relative to athletics, and once they had perfected their design, market them to the athletic public. Today there are many manufacturers around the world that create biomechanically correct athletic shoes designed to meet the needs of virtually every known form of athletic pursuit.

Good Shoes, Bad Shoes

However, not everyone believes that athletic shoes are necessarily a good idea for the athlete; in fact, there have been a number of studies that have shown that wearing athletic shoes can increase joint stress forces and may possibly result in higher injury rates for those who wear athletic shoes during training or participation in sport as compared to those who go unshod or barefoot (Jenkins & Cauthon, 2011; Kerrigan et al., 2009).

Shoes were originally designed to provide protection to a wearer's feet. They were not created in an attempt to provide an advantage from a movement standpoint but primarily to reduce the injuries sustained by individuals walking over uneven, rocky ground. Wearing shoes does provide a certain level of protection for the feet, but over time wearing shoes for most of the day results in modifications in our basic movement patterns. Walking, running, and jumping all are learned skills (Figure 2.2), and for those of us who have grown up wearing shoes, often from a very early age, we unconsciously adapted our biomechanics to adapt to wearing shoes during activities.

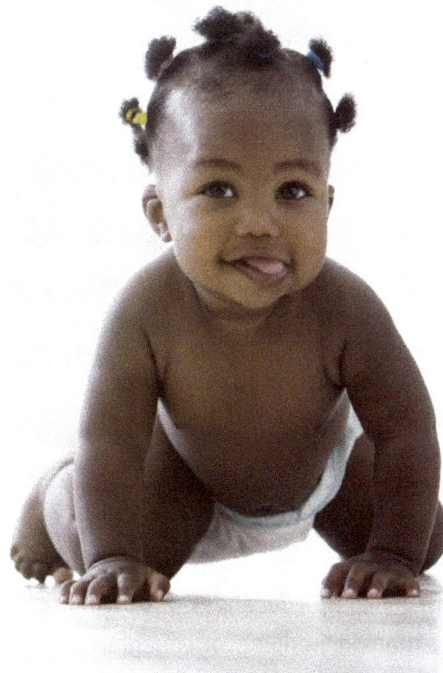

Figure 2.2   Baby learning to crawl.

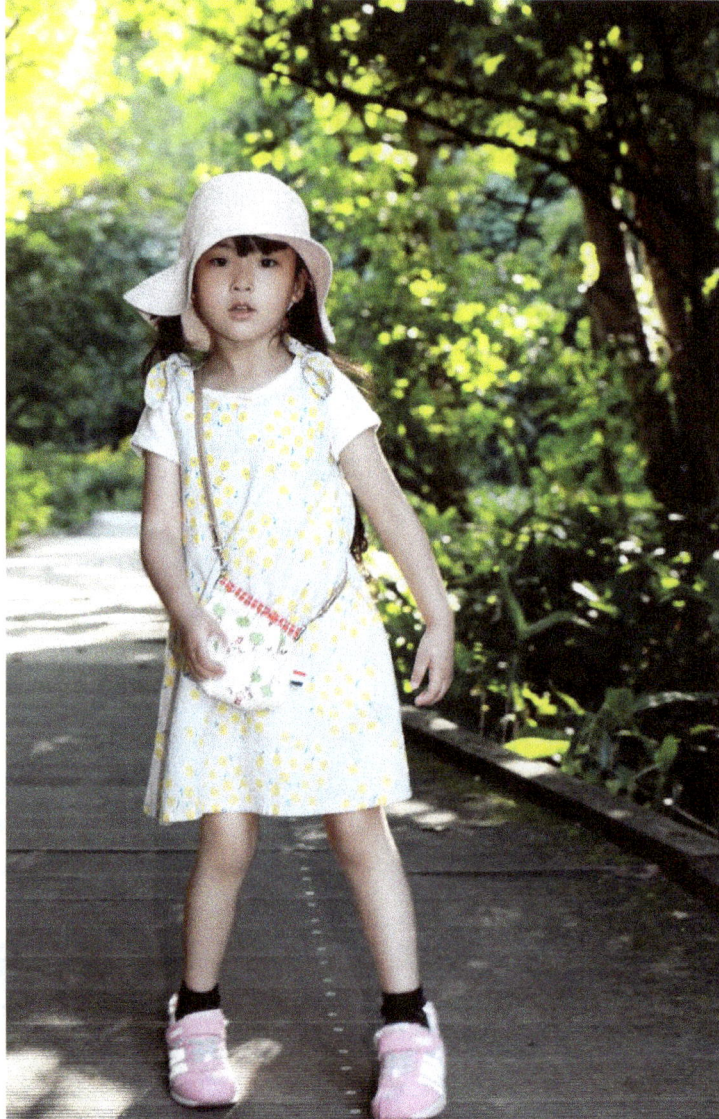

Figure 2.3   Toddler standing in bare feet.

For us to revert to a natural state of unshod movement could result in injuries. So, if you are considering giving up your shoes or starting to wear any of the minimalist athletic shoes on the market to wear while running, jumping, or engaging in any other form of athletic activity, be aware that you've spent your life wearing shoes and adapting to them to be who you are. To begin walking or running without shoes is inviting injury without a solid plan to relearn those skills without the use of shoes (Figure 2.3).

If you don't believe that you have adapted to wearing shoes, try this little experiment. First, determine what type of foot striker you are when you run. If you strike heel first on each step, you are a rear foot striker; land on the middle or arch, and you are a mid-foot striker; others are fore-foot or toe strikers. Now try running without shoes on a hard surface like a paved road. For those of you who are rear foot or toe strikers, how long did it take for you to modify your running style to become a mid-foot striker? Put your running shoes back on and try it again. Chances are you revert to your "normal" foot strike pattern. It's the shoes!

No one knows exactly how athletic shoes will change in the future. One thing we do know is that every time humans wearing athletic shoes perform a feat that appears superhuman people will obsess over and analyze it, and at some point they will question what those shoes did or did not do for the athlete.

A good example of this phenomenon of not accepting an exceptional performance as an unaided athletic achievement is the controversy surrounding the Nike Vaporfly high-performance running shoe. There have been many articles written about how the Nike Vaporfly provides a mechanical advantage to the wearer and that it somehow generates a running economy superior to other athletic footwear. Some feel it provides an unfair advantage and should be banned from competition. And that may be. Advances in shoe design, making them lighter and stronger while at the same time extremely flexible, allows athletes to return to the before-shoes form of running biomechanics. It will take us a while to adjust to this new technology, but continued advancements in shoe technology should allow athletes of the future to perform better than ever before Healey & Hoogkamer, 2022, Castellanos-Salamanca et al. 2023, Patoz et al. 2022, Rodrigo-Carranza et al. 2021.

Something that will not happen any time soon, if ever, is the invention of an athletic shoe that provides such a large mechanical advantage to the wearer that it truly can make a good runner into an elite runner. One of the more outrageous conspiracy-type theories about the Nike Vaporfly claims the shoes somehow create energy with use, then somehow transfer that energy to the runner, giving them an unfair advantage. The first law of thermodynamics proves that is impossible: You cannot create energy in a closed system, and no human movement is capable of creating more energy on its own than the cost of that movement Goldstein, 2023, Nigg & Sasa 2020.

So as long as we live in the real world governed by the laws of motion and not in an imaginary world of science fiction, people can improve their performance while reducing injuries by choosing the most biomechanically efficient footwear. But you can rest assured that footwear is not going to somehow aid performance by breaking the laws of physics. Elite athletes generate their "superhuman" feats, not by wearing some magical shoes, but by matching their unique athletic abilities with the best equipment technology currently available.

Praying Mantis

As long as people participate in sports, they will look to others, elite performers, in their particular activities as role models to mimic. This happens at the junior high level to the super elite level. There are scores of examples of different athletes we believe surely must know themselves and their sport better than any anyone else, and yet when they come against an opponent who is superior, they look to that person, trying to dissect and understand how they managed to achieve their level of excellence. Like everyone, all athletes have their blind spots. And that goes for even the best in the world. An example is something that happened years ago in elite cycling. One of the top cyclists at the time was an American cyclist named Floyd Landis, who had recently won the Tour de France and was considered the best cyclist in the world. Floyd had a unique riding style that other cyclists noticed and tried to copy. Always looking to improve themselves or those they trained, those in and around the sport watched closely as Floyd rose to the top of his sport.

One of the things that they noticed was a unique hand/arm configuration that Floyd adopted during his time trial races. A time trial is a shorter distance race in which cyclists are sent out individually at specified intervals and attempt to complete the race in the shortest time. Floyd's riding style was different from any of the other top competitors, and those observing the sport felt that his time trial superiority might be tied to his unique positioning on the bike during those events.

Other cyclists tried to copy his riding style but never attained his level of success. It was only later that we found out the reason that Floyd had adopted this unique riding position, and it wasn't because he had somehow stumbled onto a new magical position that allowed him to go faster than his competitors. It was an adaptation necessitated by a health issue he was dealing with and a way for him to reduce his pain while riding. Floyd had a degenerative hip problem that would not allow him to sit on a bike in what would be considered a normal conventional riding position without being in great pain. That led he and his coach to experiment with different ways for him to sit on and ride his bike, particularly during the time trial phases of the long tours. What they came up with was called the "praying mantis" style of bike riding (see Figure 2.4). It was called that because of the similarities between the posture of a praying mantis and how Floyd looked when wearing his signature yellow and green biking apparel as he rocketed along the time trial courses.

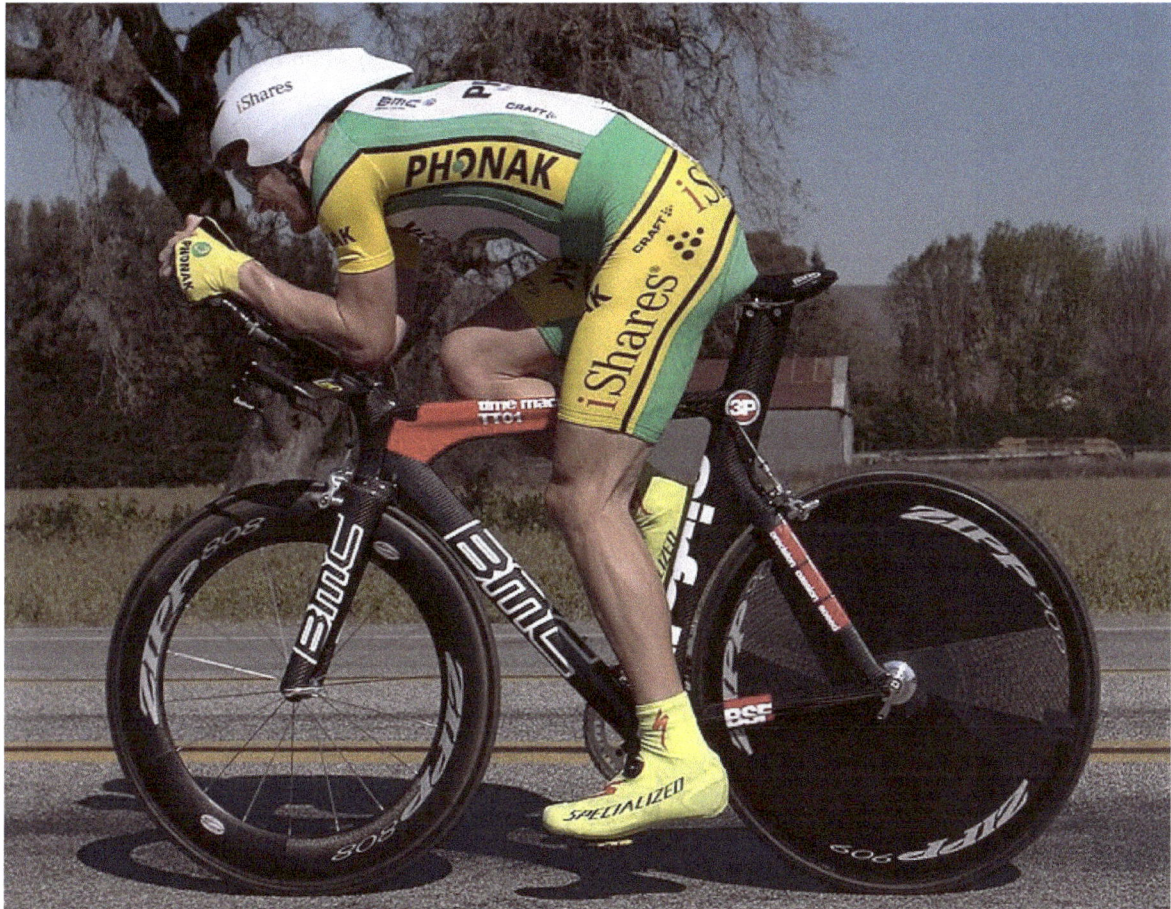

Figure 2.4   Floyd Landis, "praying mantis."

Even at the very highest level of athletic performance, sometimes people miss the reason for the improvement and/or modification of an athlete's performance as opposed to what they believe is the cause of that athletic success.

Fosbury Flop

Occasionally there is a significant breakthrough in a sport technique championed by a lone individual that is eventually adopted by everyone participating in the sport. The Fosbury flop in high jumping is one such example. The lone athlete was a man named Dick Fosbury, who decided to use his understanding of human movement potential, applied physics, and the use of a unique sport technique to succeed in his sport. Fosbury understood that the goal of his sport was to have the human body pass over a suspended bar at a height higher than anyone else during competition. This seems like a very simple and straightforward way of determining who is the best high jumper. To win, jump over a bar without knocking it off its standards, at a height higher than anyone else in the competition. Due to a combination of equipment limitations, two different techniques for jumping had developed before Fosbury's innovation. Prior to Fosbury all athletes used either the "scissors kick" (Figure 2.5) or the "western roll" (Figure 2.6) when high jumping.

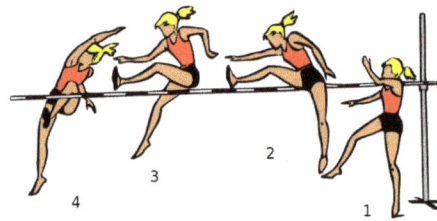

Figure 2.5   Scissor kick jumping style.

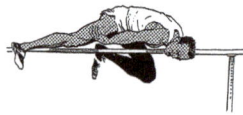

Figure 2.6   Western role jumping style.

Then along came Fosbury, and the way athletes hurled their bodies over the bar changed forever. He looked at the requirements of his sport through the lens of a biomechanist and realized that athletes were trying to do things the hard way. The rules stated that the athlete had to clear the bar without knocking the bar off the standards to record a successful jump. However, there was nothing in the rules that said the person had to have their center of mass (COM) go over the bar. That realization was Fosbury's moment of genius. He understood that an object's COM is acted upon by gravity, accelerating it down toward the center of the earth. Gravity is what limits how high a person can jump. You must "beat" gravity for a period of time to become and stay airborne. Because people can contort their bodies into many different orientations (Figure 2.7), including ones in which their COM falls outside the physical confines of the body (see Chapter 8), Fosbury realized that there might be a way to have the human body clear the bar but have the COM pass through or even under the bar, essentially allowing a person to successfully clear a height even through their COM doesn't!

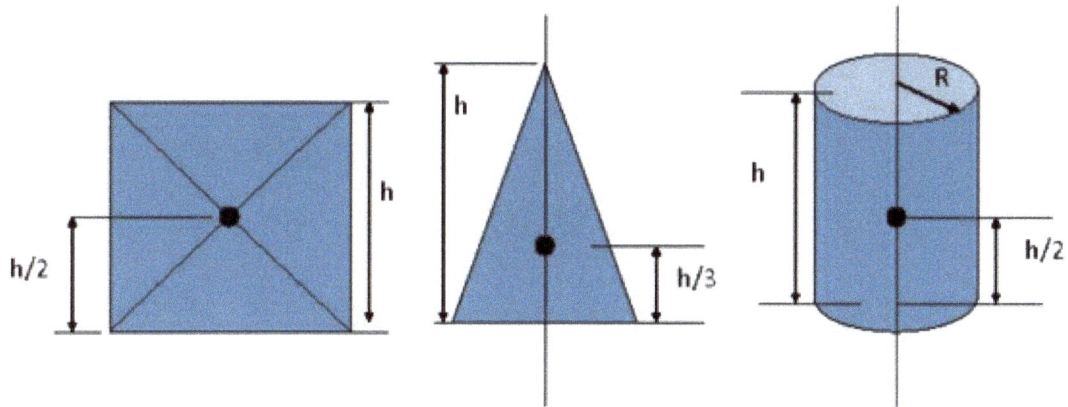

Figure 2.7   COM locations.

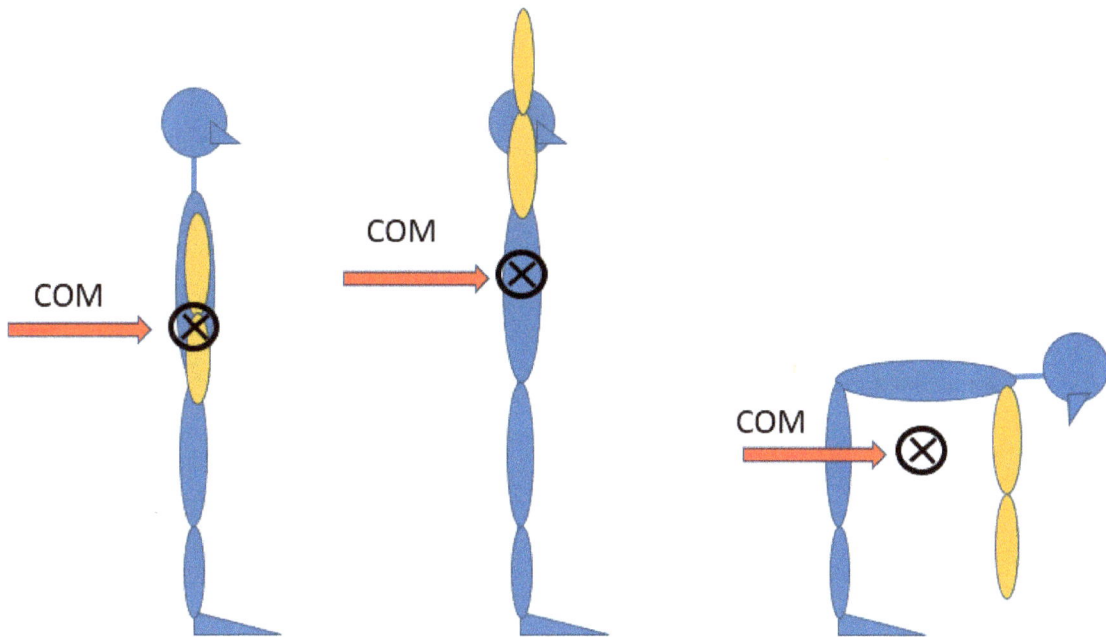

Figure 2.8   COM location in various poses.

After some experimentation, he came upon a jumping technique that did just that, allowing his body to clear the bar with his COM going under the bar (Figure 2.8). The limiting factor for how high he could jump was based on how high he could project his COM upward against the force of gravity. This new technique didn't require him to push his COM higher, but it did allow his body to clear a bar at a higher height with the same effort! Perfecting his technique of twisting, arching his back, and clearing the bar head first on his back resulted in the high jump technique now known as the Fosbury flop. The technique (depicted in Figure 2.9) proved so successful that he won a Gold medal in the 1968 Olympics in the high jump, and his style of jumping has been universally adopted by high jumpers around the world.

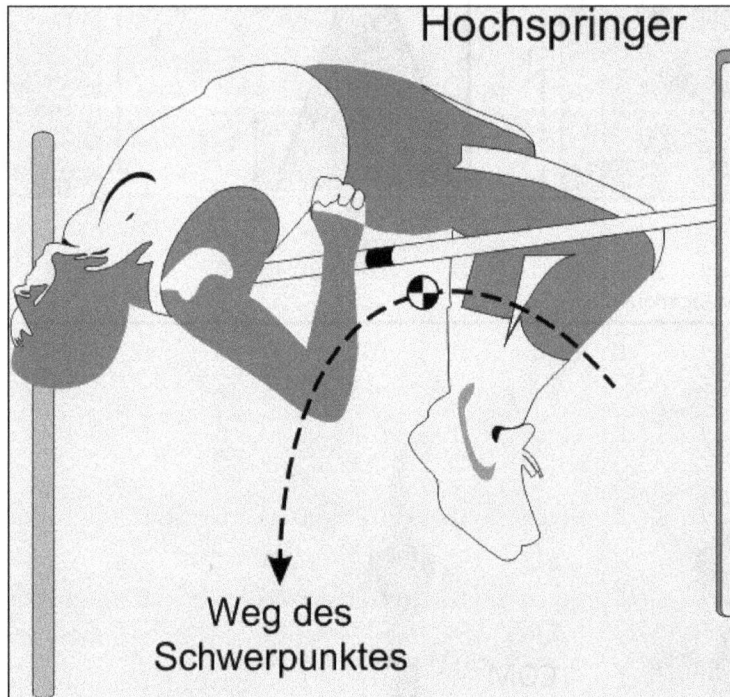

Figure 2.9   Fosbury flop diagram.

It was an example of a movement problem solved through the application of biomechanics!

Trap or Hex Bar

Biomechanical research has improved a wide variety of sport performance. One such improvement found in the area of weightlifting is the creation of something called a trap or hex bar. The trap bar is the outcome of biomechanists understanding the mechanical and anatomical requirements of individuals lifting weights to strengthen the muscles of their lower body.

Traditionally, the method used to strengthen the body from the hips down in weightlifting is to perform a lift called a high bar back squat (HBBS), which starts with the weight bar balanced across the shoulders behind the neck, often with additional weight plates added to the far ends of the bar. The lifter, while balancing the weight bar across their shoulders, squats down to a point where their thighs are roughly parallel to the ground, then returns to their starting position. In doing so this motion strengthens the muscles surrounding the major joints of the lower body from the hips to knees to ankles. The HBBS can be a dangerous lift for athletes if done incorrectly since the weight of the bar is located high above the body's COM and requires the lifter to always use stabilizing trunk muscles throughout the lift to balance the weight. Any uncontrolled shifting of the weight forward, backward, or side to side could lead to injury.

One or more interactive elements has been excluded from this version of the text. You can view them online here: https://pb.cognella.com/83647-1b/?p=26#oembed-4

Please refer to the interactive ebook in Cognella Active Learning for interactive/media content.

One or more interactive elements has been excluded from this version of the text. You can view them online here: https://pb.cognella.com/83647-1b/?p=26#oembed-5

Please refer to the interactive ebook in Cognella Active Learning for interactive/media content.

The HBBS works the major muscle groups of the lower body, the quadriceps, hamstrings, gastrocnemius, and soleus muscles. When done correctly, the exercise, targets and strengthens the entire lower body. However, the use of poor technique or attempting to lift too heavy a load can result in injury.

People who lift weights with the goal of competing in Olympic lifts, such as the snatch or clean and jerk, should train using the HBBS as part of their practices. But other athletes, such as basketball, football, soccer, tennis, or volleyball players, who spend time in the weight room, do so to strengthen their bodies to better perform their chosen sport, not to compete in Olympic lifting competitions. For those athletes, finding a safer, less technical lift alternative to the HBBS should be strongly considered.

Using a trap bar provides the same lower body strengthening as the HBBS but with much less risk of injury. The trap bar is a biomechanical innovation that allows the same motion and the same strength-related benefits as performing a HBBS exercise but is much safer. Using a trap bar requires a person to step into the center of the bar, grasping the bar with both hands and standing up and squatting down, all the while keeping the load of the bar below the person's COM. Using a trap bar might reduce the maximum weight a person can lift during a single attempt, but overall lifting volume can be maintained or increased by increasing the number of reps during training. Being smart and staying healthy in the weight room is a good way to improve at your sport!

Daily Life

You don't need to be an athlete to benefit from a knowledge and application of Biomechanics. Every day, we move, we sit, we stand, we lift things to accomplish what is necessary to live our lives. Those movements may not garner as much attention as hitting a homerun in the World Series, but for most of us to be able to accomplish those simple everyday actions is much more important to our daily lives, than that homerun.

Human to Electrical Power

Understanding what it takes to create and maintain motion allows the biomechanist to see the world of possibilities motion provides for people. One of the things that has been noticed is how inefficient certain types of motion are, but those inefficiencies can sometimes lead to interesting innovations. An example of this is related to mechanical energy loss when a person uses a stationary bike to exercise. As the person repeatedly activates muscles to push pedals and rotate weighted flywheels (Figure 2.10), much of the energy they put into the system is lost. Yes, the person is exercising, improving strength, flexibility, and cardiac capacity, but the mechanical outcome leaves a lot of unused energy on the table.

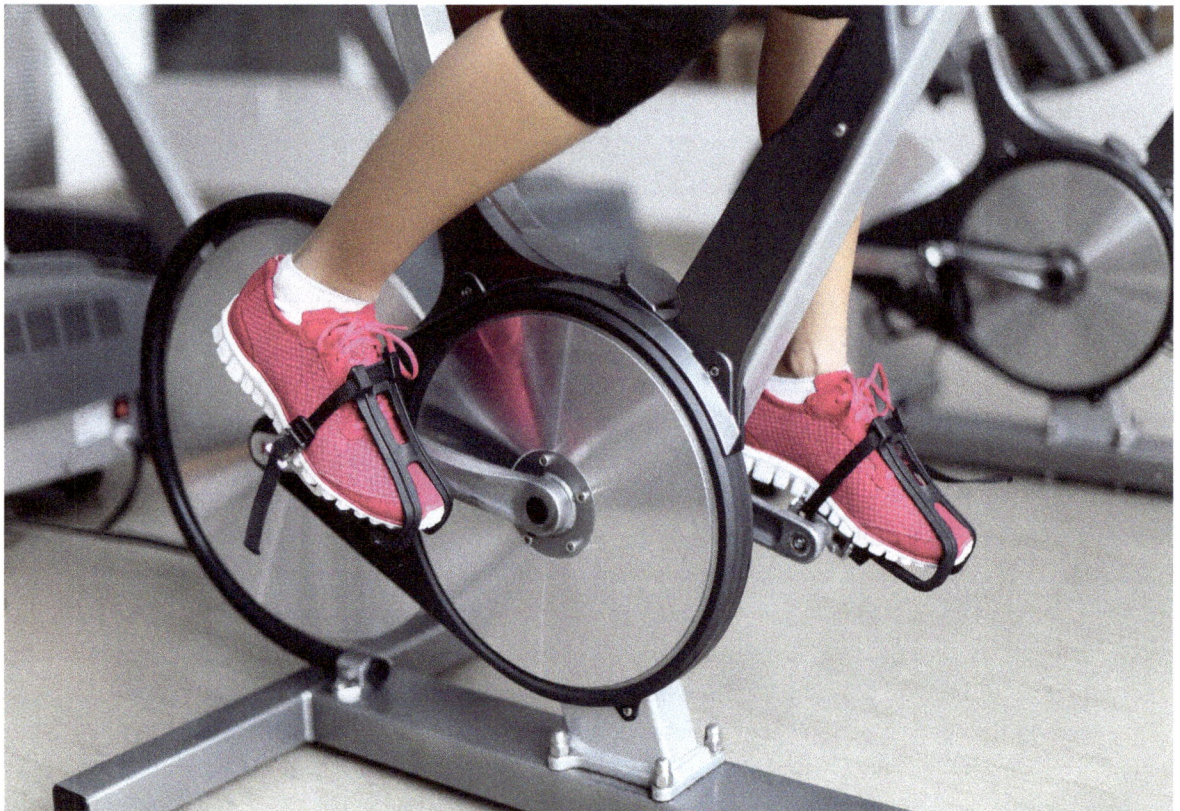

Figure 2.10   Rotating flywheel.

What if some of the wasted mechanical and kinetic energy could be converted into electrical energy? That idea has been around for a long time. Ever since the invention of electric dynamo by Michael Faraday in 1831 ("Michael Faraday," n.d.) people have been attempting to turn pedal power into electric power. Now with advances in electronics, and the improvements in exercise cycles, it may be time to revisit this thought. What a great way to put exercise science into practice by applying the science of biomechanics to improving people's lives through the generation of clean energy as a byproduct of exercise.

That is what companies like SportArt (Silver, 2016) are doing with a line of exercise equipment, including cycles, treadmills, and elliptical machines that generate electricity as a person exercises. If that electricity can be returned to the grid or stored for future onsite use in the homes and facilities where a person exercises, they can benefit from free electricity. With wider range goals, it has been suggested that some or all of the generated energy could be given back to the local community to help reduce the economic burden of individuals least able to afford their electricity costs. It's a win-win-win situation: You exercise and get healthier, you light the lights in your home, and you help those in need in your community!

EMG and Recording Templates of Motion

Electromyography (EMG) is a technique utilized by biomechanists and others to record the electrical signals generated by muscle when actively attempting to generate force. This technique uses either surface (adhered to the outside of the skin over a muscle belly) or indwelling fine wire (inserted into the muscle) electrodes.

When a person does any of the many complicated movement activities they engage in during a typical day, from standing to walking, sitting, jumping, turning, lifting, and so on, they do so by accurately following a learned set of motor instructions. That "recipe" for motion requires muscles to be activated in a very specific sequence, for a given period of time, and at the appropriate force levels to accomplish the intended movements. Think about it: To do something like standing up from a seated position takes the properly coordinated muscle actions of over 30 major muscles!

Most of us learned how to perform a wide array of complex everyday movements when we were very young. Once we mastered them, we have continued to be able to perform those movements with little effort or thought. But what happens if the pathway from the brain to our muscles is somehow damaged through injury or disease and we can no longer control our muscles we wish? What if there was a "recipe" book of common daily movements that with the aid of advances in biomedical technology could help us regain our movement independence? While that may sound like science fiction, it is becoming science fact as biomechanists continue to map complex human movements using EMG technology. It's hoped that in the near future these efforts will leave the laboratory and make significant improvements in the lives of people who need of help (Weintraub, 2023).

Car Safety

Today's cars, trucks, and SUVs are more comfortable and safer than ever. This is not a car commercial but a statement of fact based on the significant changes made to protect the human occupants of motor vehicles. An applied understanding of the physics of motion and how changes in motion affect people has led to major safety improvements such as air bags, crumple zones, multipoint safety belts, and more. All such changes are based on the physics of motion and the best way to dissipate and/or redirect the damaging forces produced in crashes by shunting them from passengers. That means that people with the skill set of biomechanists (understanding human anatomy, physics, and technology) have been involved in making cars safer and more comfortable.

One or more interactive elements has been excluded from this version of the text. You can view them online here: https://pb.cognella.com/83647-1b/?p=26#oembed-6

Please refer to the interactive ebook in Cognella Active Learning for interactive/media content.

Air bags do not prevent crashes or reduce the impact force of the crash. They do, however, take advantage of two well-understood concepts of force application: pressure and impulse. Pressure is the outcome of force applied over a given area. Think about what happens when you stand on your bare feet on a flat, solid surface. Not much, right? That is because the area of the plantar surface of your feet is large enough that when the weight of your body (force) creates pressure (force/area) it is low enough to not cause any harm or discomfort. What happens if instead of a flat solid surface you step onto a sharp rock? You have the same body weight (force), but the sharp point of the rock (small area) creates a high, localized pressure, resulting in pain and possible injury.

How does that relate to airbags? Air bags produce a large area for your upper body to impact with as the car violently stops. Without the air bag you would strike smaller structures such as the steering wheel or dashboard, which have a smaller contact area than the airbag. Those structures represent the sharp rock; the deployed airbag represents the soles of your feet. In one situation the impact force is applied over a small area (interior vehicle structures), resulting in a high, damaging pressure. With the airbags inflated (large surface air of the bag), the same impact force results in a much lower pressure, making it less likely you will be injured.

Okay, but what about car crumple zones? How do they help? They don't reduce force or change impact area. That's correct, but what crumple zones do is increase the time it takes to slow and stop the car. That increase in time reduces the accelerations (changes in velocity) that can injure a person by changing the impulse of the crash. Impulse is the product of force (impact force) times the time of force application (crumple zones' increase time). This may seem a little counter intuitive since you might think that a smaller impulse would be less damaging. However, you need to understand how an impulse was generated to understand its relationship to injury.

If you wore a hat for 10 hours, the impulse exerted by the hat on your head could be calculated by multiplying the hat weight times the number of seconds you wore it. For example, the result might be impulse = 1.5 N * 36,000 s $\Rightarrow$ 54,000 Ns. That appears to be a very large number, and it is, but the effect of that specific impulse on a person when it is created that way is negligible unless you are concerned about "hat head."

The same impulse generated during a 1-second car crash would mean that the person in the car would experience an average of 54,000 N, about 12,140 pounds or over 6 tons of force during the crash! If that force was applied over a 4 cm^2 area, the pressure experienced would be 13,500 N/cm^2 or about 2,700 times the normal pressure measured under the forefoot while standing.

By extending the time to 3 seconds because of crumple zone engineering and having an airbag deploy (increasing the contact area by a factor of 10), the force you experience is reduced by about 67%, resulting in an impact pressure of ~222 N/cm^2, providing you a much better chance of surviving the crash! It's all biomechanics, and it is being used to make you safer.

One or more interactive elements has been excluded from this version of the text. You can view them online here:
https://pb.cognella.com/83647-1b/?p=26#oembed-7

Please refer to the interactive ebook in Cognella Active Learning for interactive/media content.

Forensics (Subspecialty of Daily Life)

Biomechanical forensics focuses on the ability of a biomechanist to provide insight in legal cases that often revolve around injury or death and the related liability of parties involved in a lawsuit. Again, the biomechanist finds themselves in a unique position to tell the whole story in a way that can make sense to a judge, jury, or parties in dispute. While the medical experts may speak regarding issues of anatomy and an engineer can rightly discuss the mechanics, the biomechanist routinely works with both anatomy and mechanics related to human movement and injury.

An example of forensic biomechanics might be explaining what happened just prior to, during, and following a residential pool diving accident. Even assuming there was no video record of the diving accident, a biomechanist can tell the whole story of what happened and why.

What can be determined related to an accident that left a young male paralyzed with multiple broken cervical vertebrae? After collecting pertinent information about the pool environment at the time of the accident (pool geometry, water depth, poolside run-up, etc.); physical characteristics of the injured person (height, weight, age, athletic ability, etc.); depositions of any eyewitnesses, including the injured person; medical records; an accident report; and other data, it is possible to simulate, with a high degree of certainty, how the failed dive was performed.

Statistics from previously published documented injuries provide boundaries for the biomechanist to compare their results with the actual medical report of injury. For example, it is known that the cervical vertebrae of a healthy young adult male will fail under a load of 900 pounds when the load is applied through compression from the top of the head over a time less than 20 milliseconds. It is also known that the skull will fracture under the same conditions with a load in excess of 1,700 pounds. Therefore, if the model created results in loads in between 900 and 1,700 pounds it is reasonable to assume that cervical vertebrae would fracture while the skull would remain intact. This would provide support for the story that the biomechanist could then present in court regarding how the dive was actually performed. That information would indicate if the young man performed an "unsafe" dive. However, if he did perform a "safe" dive, yet was still injured, that part of the dispute can be removed, and other areas should be reviewed to determine liability (Gabrielsen, et. al., 2001).

Through the application of biomechanical principles, it is often possible to go back in time, or forward into the future, to explain the outcome of a given set of actions. In this way, the biomechanist becomes a teller of truth in areas in which the outcome is in dispute.

Medicine

Maybe the most important area of biomechanical research and application is in the area of medicine and health care. It is here that advances in maintaining or improving performance while reducing injury have the potential to directly affect a huge segment of the population. Following are several examples of areas medicine and biomechanics meet.

Balance and Gait

Two of the most important motor functions that humans perform throughout most of their lives are standing/balancing on two feet and walking upright on two legs. Balance and gait are central motor skills for most people to live an independent and active life. Aging reduces overall physical ability, including our capacity to balance and walk. Too often compromised balance and gait function result in significant life-altering changes, especially as a person becomes more susceptible to falls as they age.

What can be done to minimize the likelihood of falls and improve or maintain gait function for the elderly? Understanding what is required for balance is a good start. Balance can be improved by lowering a body's COM and increasing its base of support. Think about Figures 2.11a and b.

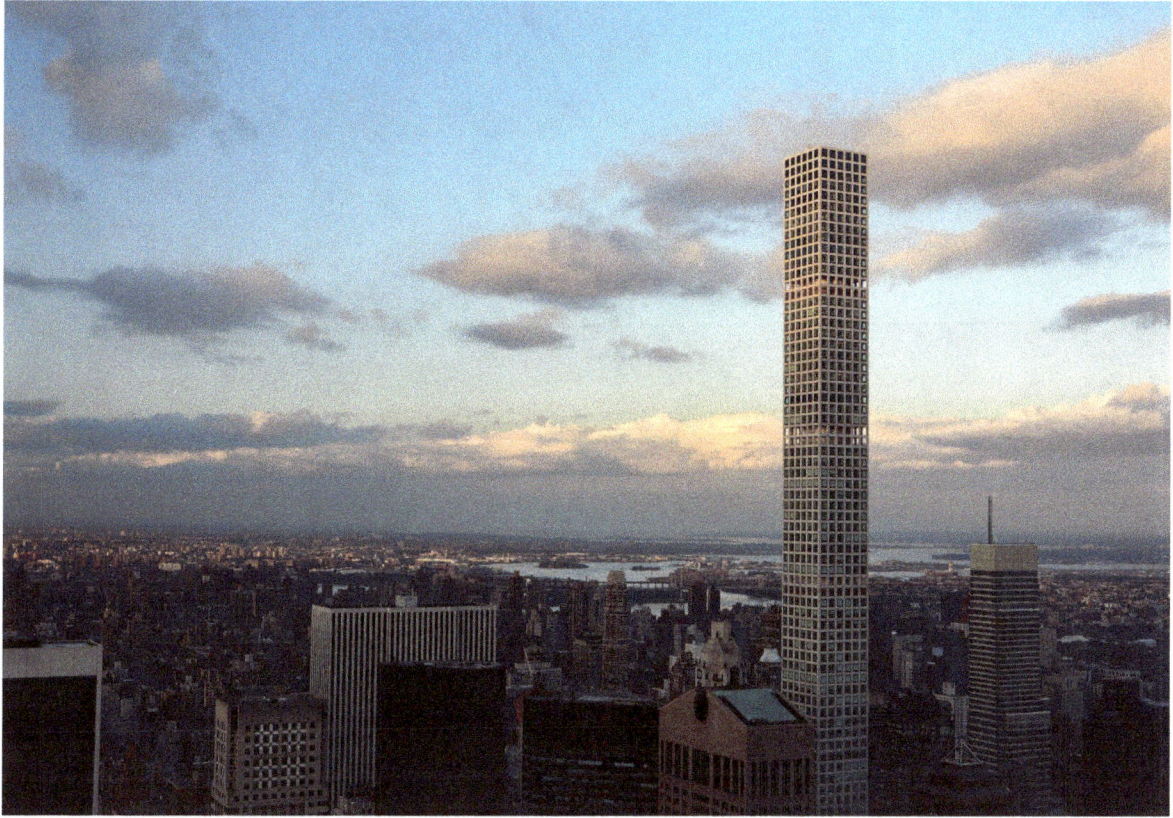

Figure 2.11a   Tall building.

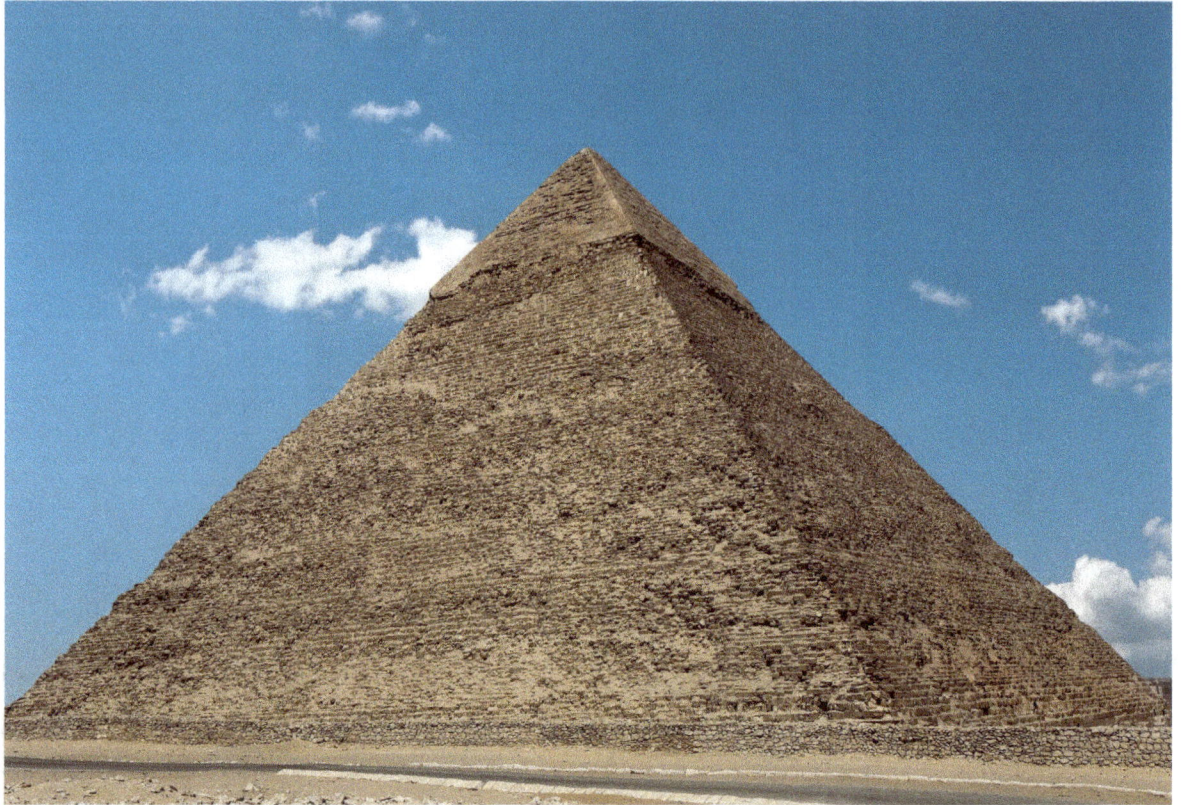

Figure 2.11b   Pyramid.

Which image is more likely to be balanced and stay stable? A pyramid is designed with a large base of support and has a low center of mass, which makes the solution easy if we want to recommend a strategy that will reduce falls: Sit down and keep your feet on the floor (Figure 2.12).

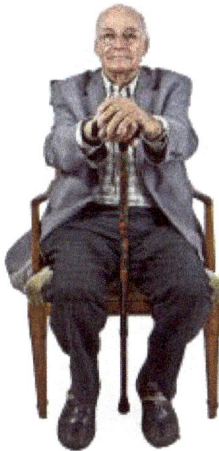

Figure 2.12   Older person sitting down.

Unfortunately, such a position is terrible for self-propelled motion such as walking. Walking is essentially an act of repeated falling, catching yourself, balancing, then falling again.

How to improve balance and gait? One possible solution is to increase the points of contact with the ground. Walking or balance for humans usually involves at most two points of contact with the ground while standing or walking. Through the use of a cane (Figure 2.13) or walker (Figure 2.14), a person can add more points of contact to improve balance/stability, but in the case of using a walker, they may sacrifice freedom of movement and reduce their gait speed. To solve that problem biomechanists are working to create "smart walkers" that will monitor the needs of the user and modify the movement options provided by the walker to help maintain a safe and independent option of gait for the elderly (Technical Research Centre of Finland, 2015).

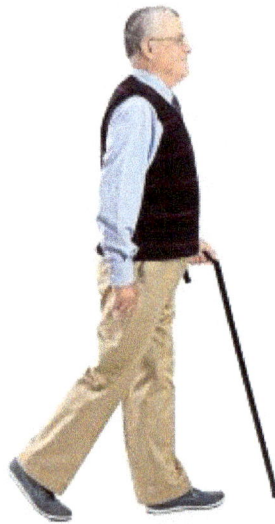

Figure 2.13   Walking with a cane.

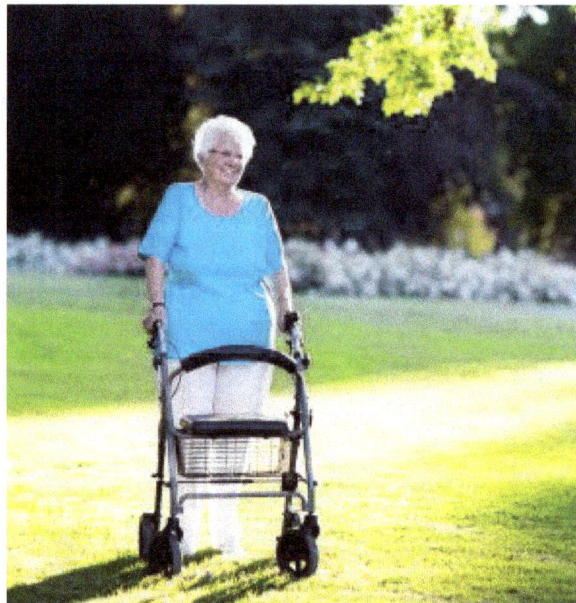

Figure 2.14   Walking with a walker.

Diabetic Foot Neuropathy

Diabetes is a chronic condition related to the body's ability to regulate sugar usage. The outcome of the disease often leads to the damage of capillary beds in the extremities, which result in a loss of blood flow (ischemia) in those areas. Ischemia may cause tissue and nerve damage (neuropathy). This leaves the person with cold hands and feet, and a loss of feeling in those regions. Neuropathy in turn increases the person's susceptibility to very poor outcomes when some kind of trauma or damage happens in the areas without feeling.

The diabetic foot triad (Figure 2.15) is well documented in the medical world and describes how the ischemia leads to neuropathy, then ulcers in the areas that sustain some form of injury (Figure 2.16).

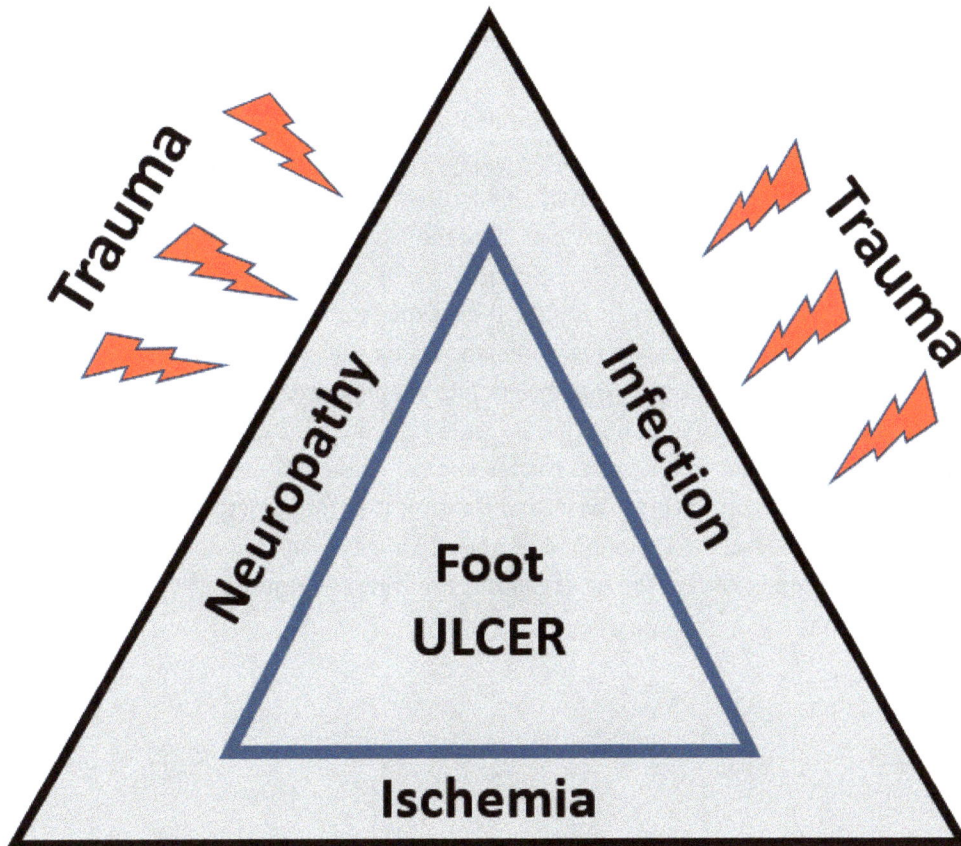

Diabetic Foot Triad

Figure 2.15   Diabetic foot triad diagram.

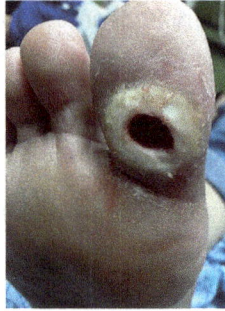

Figure 2.16   Diabetic foot neuropathy outcome.

These ulcers can usually be treated if identified before they progress to the point that significant damage has been done. However, ulcers may grow unchecked when a person has little or no feeling in that area of the body. If that is the case, the condition can go unnoticed until it may be too late to treat the affected area. Radical surgery and loss of some or all of the foot/ankle/lower leg is often the only option at that point.

While biomechanists cannot cure diabetes, their expertise in force measurement technology has allowed them to develop insole pressure measurement systems like the one shown in Figure 2.17, which can provide the patient and their doctors with insight into the high-pressure zones of the foot that are most likely to develop ulcers. By modifying the clinical insole measurement technology used in the lab, it has been possible to create versions that patients can take home. These daily wear insole pressure shoe inserts can now record information on a regular basis and transmit it to their doctor's office between visits. This daily monitoring greatly reduces the likelihood of a severe ulcer forming undetected. If identified early, it is often possible to successfully treat the ulcer without resorting to surgery and/or amputation.

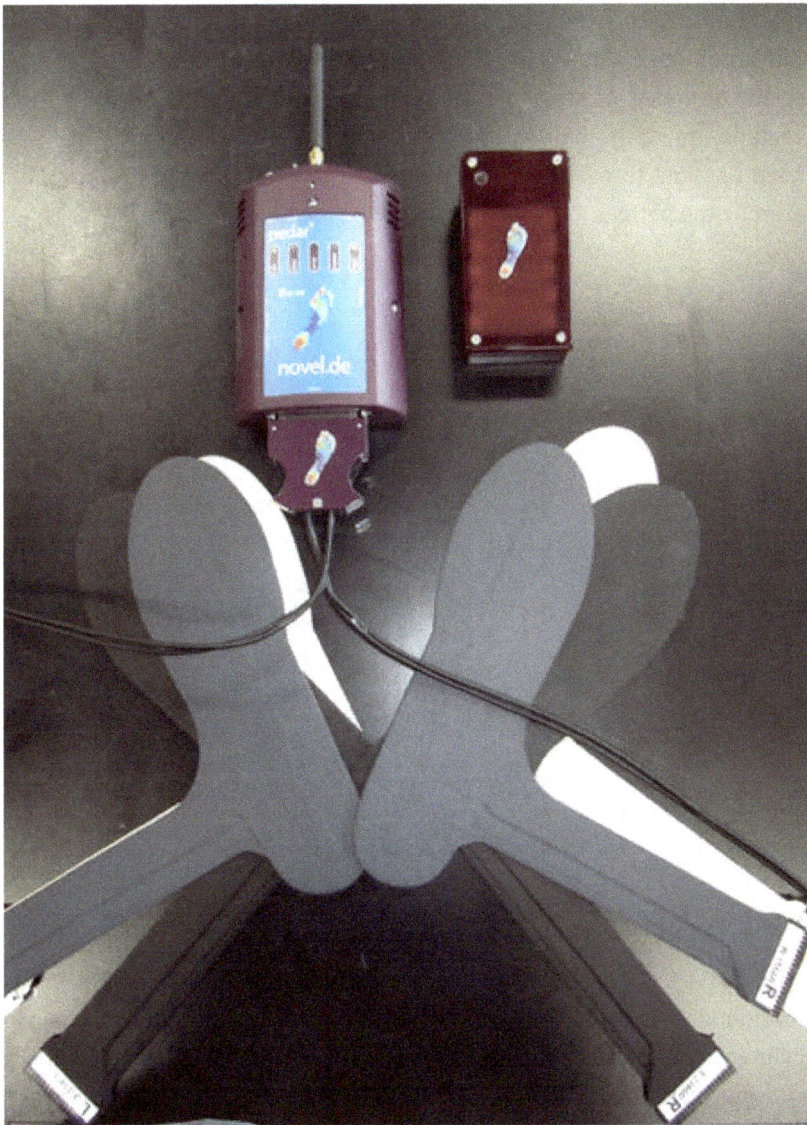

Figure 2.17   Insole pressure measurements.

Parkinson's Disease

Parkinson's disease (PD) is a chronic neurodegenerative disease that presents with, among other things, upper body tremor, increased likelihood of falls, shuffling, and freezing of gait. The underlying cause of those symptoms is the body's inability to adequately synthesize and utilize the neurotransmitter dopamine.

Biomechanists who work with Parkinson's patients are reevaluating the standard practice of care related to recommendations of what and how PD patients deal with the symptoms of the disease.

Biomechanists are not going to cure the disease, but they can improve and prolong the movement function and balance capabilities of those with PD.

By using specially designed wireless sensors such as that produced by ADPM Wearable Technologies (Figure 2.18), the balance and gait abilities of PD patients can be determined. Once a baseline has been established, it is then possible to evaluate the possible benefits of various exercise and/or drug therapy strategies undertaken by the patient.

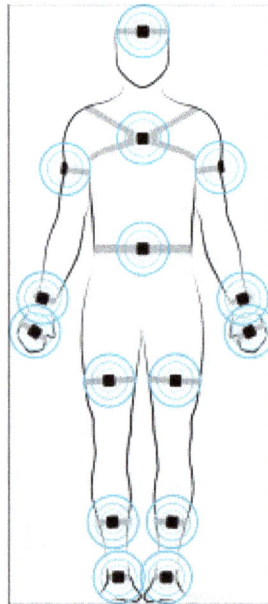

Figure 2.18   Sensor locations.

This kind of evaluation has led to the revelation that Parkinson's patients may gain significant benefit from modified high intensity interval training (HIIT) that had previously been deemed too strenuous or even potentially dangerous for that group. Finding a safe and effective type of HIIT training for a population that is mostly older and physically challenged has proven difficult, but it appears that using a machine called a reACT eccentric trainer may provide the answer.

Recent studies have shown that a little more than 5 minutes of exercise per week on the reACT trainer has resulted in measurable improvement in gait and balance for Parkinson's patients.

Summary

Biomechanics plays an increasingly important role in allowing individuals across the spectrum of human movement, from birth to death, to live active and healthy lives. Innovations related to movement come from a variety of sources, from athletes to sport scientists to health care professionals. By utilizing a basic knowledge of musculoskeletal anatomy, applied mechanical physics, and advances in technology, biomechanists continue to aspire to improve or maintain movement performance while minimizing injury for us all.

List of Key Takeaways

- There are three main areas of biomechanical research: sports, daily life, and medicine.
- Regardless of the area of research, the goals of biomechanics, to improve/maintain performance while working to prevent the severity and frequency of injury, continue to be applied.
- In any form of biomechanical research, the anatomical structures impacted by the work, the physics of the movements being studied, and the proper use of instrumentation remain central to the efforts of the biomechanists involved.
- Specialized equipment can provide information about movement far beyond what our senses can reveal.

References

Castellanos-Salamanca, M, Rodrigo-Carranza, V, Rodríguez-Barbero, S, González-Ravé, J, Santos-Concejero, J, González-Mohíno, F. (2023). Effects of the Nike ZoomX Vaporfly Next% 2 shoe on long-interval training performance, kinematics, neuromuscular parameters, running power and fatigue: Effects of the Nike ZoomX Vaporlfy Next% 2 on interval training performance. European journal of sport science, p.1-14

Enterprises Explained. (2021, September 11). How a waffle iron changed the shoe industry [Video]. https://www.youtube.com/watch?v=TvIHQwOj1R4

"Michael Faraday." Wikipedia, Wikimedia Foundation, 5 June 2023, https://en.wikipedia.org/wiki/Michael_Faraday

Gabrielsen, A., M., McElhaney, J., and O'Brien, R. (2001). *Diving Injuries: Research Findings and Recommendations for Reducing Catastrophic Injuries*. CRC Press ISBN 0-8493-2370-3.

Goldstein, A. (2023, January 23). Do super shoes work for regular marathoners? Runner's World. https://www.runnersworld.com/gear/a42723316/super-shoes-performance-effect/

Healey, L. A. & Hoogkamer, W. (2022). Longitudinal bending stiffness does not affect running economy in Nike Vaporfly Shoes. Journal of sport and health science, Vol.11 (3), p.285-29

Jenkins, D. W., & Cauthon, D. J. (2011). Barefoot running claims and controversies. Journal of the American Podiatric Medical Association, 101(3). https://doi.org/10.7547/1010231

Kerrigan, D. C., Franz, J. R., Keenan, G. S., Dicharry, J., Croce, U. D., & Wilder, R. P. (2009). The effect of running shoes on lower extremity joint torques. PM&R, 1(12), 1058–1063. https://doi.org/10.1016/j.pmrj.2009.09.011

National Museum of American History. (n.d.). Nike LDV with "waffle" sole. https://americanhistory.si.edu/collections/search/object/nmah_1413776#:~:text=In%201972%2C%20Bill%20Bowerman%20applied,which%20Bill%20subsequently%20ruined%20while

Nigg, B.M. & Sasa, C. (2020). Effects of running shoe construction on performance in long distance running. Human Performance Laboratory, Faculty of Kinesiology, University of Calgary, Calgary, Canada https://orcid.org/0000-0003-0794-834X Pages 133-138 | Published online: 17 Jun 2020

Patoz, A, Lussiana, T, Breine, B, Gindre, C. (2022). The Nike Vaporfly 4%: a game changer to improve performance without biomechanical explanation yet. Footwear science, Vol.14 (3), p.147-150.

Rodrigo-Carranza, V, González-Mohíno, F, Santos-Concejero, J, González-Ravé, J. (2021). Comment on "A Pragmatic Approach to Resolving Technological Unfairness: The Case of Nike's Vaporfly and Alphafly Running Footwear"Sports Medicine - Open, Vol.7 (1).

Silver, A. (2016, December 22). Are stationary bikes that generate electricity making a comeback? IEEE Spectrum. https://spectrum.ieee.org/bikes-that-generate-electricity-are-making-a-comeback

Technical Research Centre of Finland. (2015, October 1). Smart walkers for elderly with new technology. Science Daily. https://www.sciencedaily.com/releases/2015/10/151001095419.htm

Weintraub, K. (2023, February 20) "New frontier" in therapy helps 2 stroke patients move again – and gives hope to many more. USA Today. https://www.usatoday.com/story/news/health/2023/02/20/stroke-patients-stimulator-implant-trial/11272868002/

Image Credits

Fig. 2.1a: Copyright © 2020 Depositphotos/NewAfrica.
Fig. 2.1b: Copyright © by Kazuhiro Keino (CC BY 2.0) at https://commons.wikimedia.org/wiki/
File:Nike_Waffle_Racer_Vintage_(11023100684).jpg.
Fig. 2.2: Copyright © 2011 Depositphotos/monkeybusiness.
Fig. 2.3: Copyright © by MIKI Yoshihito (CC BY 2.0) at https://commons.wikimedia.org/wiki/
File:A_toddler_explores_the_wetlands,_Japan;_August_2020_(02).jpg.
Fig. 2.4: Copyright © by Michael David Murphy (CC BY-SA 2.0) at https://commons.wikimedia.org/wiki/File:Floyd-landis-toctt.jpg.
Fig. 2.5: Source: https://commons.wikimedia.org/wiki/File:High_jump_cissors.svg.
Fig. 2.6: Source: https://commons.wikimedia.org/wiki/File:High_Jump_(PSF).png.
Fig. 2.9: Copyright © by Ralf Pfeifer (CC BY-SA 3.0) at https://commons.wikimedia.org/wiki/File:Fosbury.gif.
Fig. 2.10: Copyright © 2014 Depositphotos/Maridav.
Fig. 2.11a: Copyright © by Epistola8 (CC BY-SA 4.0) at https://commons.wikimedia.org/wiki/File:432_Park_Avenue,_NY.jpg.
Fig. 2.11b: Copyright © 2012 Depositphotos/papik1.
Fig. 2.12: Copyright © 2011 Depositphotos/Hackman.
Fig. 2.13: Copyright © 2014 Depositphotos/ljsphotography.
Fig. 2.14: Copyright © 2016 Depositphotos/FamVeldman.
Fig. 2.16: Copyright © by Mark A. Dreyer (CC BY 4.0) at https://commons.wikimedia.org/wiki/File:Diabetic_Foot_Ulcer.jpg.
Fig. 2.17: Copyright © by P0todd0p (CC BY-SA 3.0) at https://commons.wikimedia.org/wiki/File:Example_insole_pressure_device.jpg.
Fig. 2.18: Copyright © by APDM Wearable Technologies, a Clario Company. Reprinted with permission.

Chapter 3

Equipment

Tools of the Trade

Preparing to Learn: *Watch*

What do you see when you watch a fast movement, and what are you missing? By using high-speed videography, fast-action complex movement can be seen and appreciated in a whole new way.

See Video: Golf Ball Golf Ball 70,000fps 150mph at: https://www.youtube.com/watch?v=AkB81u5IM3I

Forces literally make the world go around. But forces are almost impossible to accurately measure without the use of specialized instrumentation. Dynamography refers to a wide range of force and pressure measuring systems.

One or more interactive elements has been excluded from this version of the text. You can view them online here: https://pb.cognella.com/83647-1b/?p=47#oembed-2

Please refer to the interactive ebook in Cognella Active Learning for interactive/media content.

Preparing to Learn: *Respond*

Directions: Based on what you saw in the videos, respond to the following questions:

1. Were you surprised by how much a golf ball deforms during impact? Could you see such a change with just your eyes? What other sport impact would you like to see in high speed, and do you think the results would be similar to what you saw with the golf ball?

2. How could the use of force sensor systems as shown in video 3.2 be of use across the three main areas of biomechanical research? Explain.

Introduction to the Chapter

At its core, biomechanics is a problem-solving science. How much? How fast? What is the best way to jump high? Why were they injured? How can I measure that?—these are the types of questions confronting biomechanists every day. To help answer those questions, biomechanists have developed an ever-expanding "tool kit" of techniques, formulas, procedures, sensors, software, and experience that are applied when a question arises. In this chapter, you will be introduced into the world of solving problems, biomechanics style!

How can you describe a complex human movement sequence to someone? Do you have the vocabulary to adequately explain the movement to someone who didn't see it or is completely unfamiliar with the activity? Would a picture or video help? How about trying to demonstrate the movement yourself? It can be difficult if not impossible at times to describe or explain human movement without personal training in or experience with the movement, knowledge of a specialized vocabulary, and/or a visual record of the event that can be played back so the person can see the movement as you try to explain its intricacies. If you don't believe me, try explaining American baseball to someone who has never seen or played the sport. Or, to give you a different perspective, have someone explain the sport of cricket to you if you have never watched or played the game, and see how that goes!

It's hard enough trying to describe a motion from a time and position change standpoint, but how do you explain the internal and external effects of forces on a person? Again, your current vocabulary is probably lacking, and certainly having some measurements to provide the sizes of the forces involved would be helpful.

In this chapter the biomechanical areas that provide the terms and tools to describe and measure motion and forces will be presented: kinematics, kinetics, and instruments designed to measure a variety of movement-related values.

Learning Objectives

After completing this chapter, students should be able to do the following:

- Define qualitative or quantitative
- Explain the differences among accuracy, repeatability, and precision
- Define kinematics and kinetics
- Give examples of kinematic and kinetic measurement devices
- Be able to suggest what instruments would best meet the needs of a biomechanist studying a variety of human movements

Qualitative and Quantitative Research and Problem Solving

Problems fall into two broad categories: those with numbers and those without numbers.

Qualitative

Qualitative refers to evaluating some event, object, or condition without the use or need of numbers. It allows the observer to use various terms or expressions that convey information about the characteristics of the situation without the need to measure, calculate, or count as part of the evaluation process. Many adjectives, such as good, bad, fast, slow, large, and heavy, are often used when assessing and sharing the outcome of a qualitative analysis. For example, a doctor describing an aging patient's general health as "good" may be all that is needed to set the patient at ease related to some new aches and pains. A coach telling an athlete that she is disappointed in her athlete's performance conveys that the athlete did not meet expectations and must work harder. A young person describing the number of stars in the sky on a cloudless night as "Wow!" is enough to relay their appreciation for what they observe when gazing upward. All are examples of qualitative analysis of a situation and word choices used to share that assessment with someone.

Qualitative analysis can be very general or extremely specific in nature, depending on the analyst and the audience receiving the results of the analysis. We all perform qualitative analysis of our world all the time. The basis for our ability to qualitatively evaluate situations is based on the information we gather and process through our senses, primarily vision, sound, and touch, along with our experiences/history related to similar situations from our past. Depending on our training, it is possible to be extremely accurate with our understanding and evaluation of even very chaotic and fast-moving changes in our environment. An example is an American football official who almost always is correct with interpreting and making the correct decisions about whether a play was executed with or without penalties, even as 22 large men rush around and collide with one another on every single play.

See Video: : Santonio Holmes Incredible Game-Winning TD in Super Bowl XLIII at:
https://www.youtube.com/watch?v=oEoTvQJKhpE

While qualitative analyses are based on individual experience and the information gathered by our senses, it is possible to generate both very accurate and highly repeatable outcomes when solving qualitative problems. Qualitative analysis ***does not*** equal an inferior analysis!

Quantitative

Quantitative pertains to the use of numbers when analyzing an event or solving a problem. While qualitative analysis relies heavily on the experience or skill of the analyst and what they gather with their senses, qualitative analysis utilizes specially designed measurement systems and mathematical formulas to arrive at a number that "quantifies" or describes something with a number, uniquely defining its value on a number line.

The numbers associated with a quantitative problem can come from (a) recorded observations of the event being studied,(b) sensors designed to record and output quantities related to the event, (c) software created to tabulate and/or illustrate the values associated with the event, or (d) related formulas that when solved generate numbers representing the event.

Possible examples demonstrating how to record someone's pulse immediately following a bout of strenuous exercise include the following:

- Counting the number of heart beats by taking someone's pulse manually
- Using a smartwatch to record and display a person's heart rate
- Software created to tabulate and/or illustrate a person's pulse
- Formulas to predict a person's pulse

Numbers are numbers. They are not, unto themselves, good or bad; however, when numbers are paired with a qualitative assessment of their values related to the experience of the observer, they may be classified as good or bad, or any of a host of other quality-related meanings. The same ordinal value, or number, can have widely different qualitative descriptors depending on the circumstances and what the number represents.

For example, if you were a Major League Baseball player and were successful at getting a hit half of the times you went to bat, 50%, you would be a superstar and paid millions of dollars a year to play your sport. If the same value, 50%, represented how many valves in your heart were working properly, you would be in grave danger and would require immediate heart surgery to prevent you from dying! It is important to understand terms related to the "goodness" of measurement values.

Measurement Devices

Measurement devices are pieces of scientific equipment or formulas that provide the user with values that can be used to better understand the circumstances being studied. There are several terms associated with measurements that are often used interchangeably, when in fact they are quite different in their meanings. Terms such as accuracy, repeatability, and precision are often used to indicate that the numbers generated through measurement or calculation are correct according to widely accepted standards. If a number or outcome is **accurate** it must match a preestablished value that has been accepted as the correct value for that situation. An example is an accurate reading of 1 kilogram from a scale when a standard 1-kilogram object (according to the International System of Units [SI]) was placed on the scale. **Repeatability** is a condition in which the same outcome value is reported each time a measurement is taken given the same measurement circumstances. *Measurement repeatability does not ensure that the measurement is accurate.* It simply means that if the same object were placed on the same scale 100 times, the reading would be the same for each of the 100 measurements. If the scale reports accurate values, then the outcome is 100 correct and accurate values. If the scale produced repeatable measurements but was not accurate, the same value would appear 100 times, but it would be wrong each time. **Precision** indicates how similar one measurement is to another of the same item or condition. If that standard 1-kilogram mass was placed on a scale and the value reported was 1.0001 kg, that would indicate a measurement precision of 1/10,000 of a kilogram from measurement to measurement. Precision does not assume that the values are accurate, just that the measurement device has the ability to report and detect very small differences between measurements.

Kinematics and Kinetics

Kinematics is a branch of mechanics that describes motion related to time and space. Kinematics ignores the forces that cause or change motion. Motion requires an object to change its position from one observation time to another. Terms such as distance, displacement, speed, velocity, acceleration, and jerk all describe motion as an object changes its position over time. Kinematics will be covered in much greater detail in Chapters 5 and 6. For now, understanding that kinematics is a description of motion related to time and space is enough for us to explore how certain techniques, technologies, and formulas can assist us in capturing and analyzing kinematic variables.

Kinematic Tools

Any tool, device, or process that provides information about the time it takes and the space through which an object moves can be classified as a kinematic tool. Some devices that measure time, such as chronographs or timing mats, can provide very accurate measures of the time of movement. Other tools, such as tape measures, laser tracking devices, or trundle wheels, are useful in recording position change information. All fit into the kinematic measuring tool kit. Some devices or sensors are especially suited for capturing both time and space information simultaneously, such as radar, lidar, or GPS trackers.

There are a myriad of kinematic sensors, tools, and systems, and more are created each day. In this section we will focus on the kinematic tool that is by far the most used by researchers and the general public to capture, analyze, and share kinematic data: video.

The most universally used type of kinematic measurement device was developed in the 1960s around the use of a charged couple device (CCD) light-capturing sensor. That sensor, the CCD, is at the heart of the technology that we call videography. It was modeled on the structures in the human eye (rods and cones) found in the retina that sense and respond to light. The CCD uses a grid of light-sensitive diodes to gather information about the intensity of photons striking the sensor over a given time period, then reports a value indicating how much light struck each area of the sensor. That information is then translated into a map of pixels (picture elements) that when viewed appear to be a picture to the human observer. The advent of the CCD-based video camcorder allowed instantaneous image capture and storage without the need for conventional film, which needed to be chemically processed after capture and before images were visible.) To find more information about digital image sensors watch this video: https://www.youtube.com/watch?v=_djfA0ermCM.)

Since most people are visual learners and we rely on our eyes to provide us with visual information of our world, it is no surprise that the image technology that we use is modeled on the structure and function of the human eye (Figure 3.1a). Today's video cameras, like the human eye, have a way of completely stopping light from entering the sensor (eye: eye lid, camera: lens cap) a protective outer shield (eye: cornea

, camera: filter), a structure for limiting light entering the eye (eye: iris, camera: aperture), a structure to focus light onto the sensor (eye: lens, camera: lens), light-capturing sensor (eye: retina, camera: CCD), a structure to transport information for the sensor to storage (eye: optic nerve, camera: data bus), and storage for the image data (eye: brain, camera: secondary memory) (Figure 3.1b).

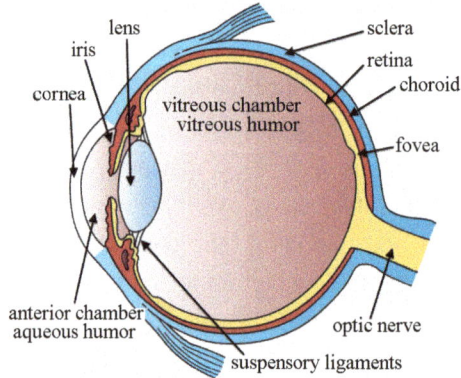

Figure 3.1a   Human eye.

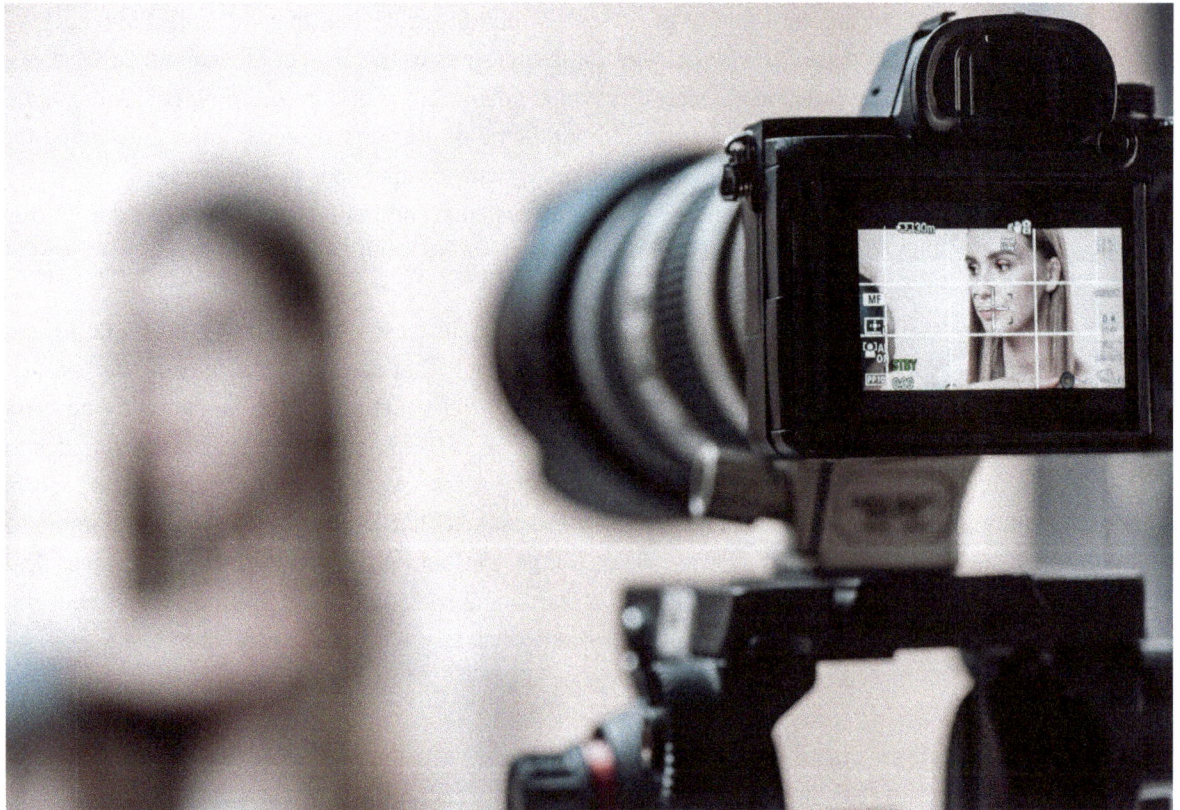

Figure 3.1b   Video camcorder.

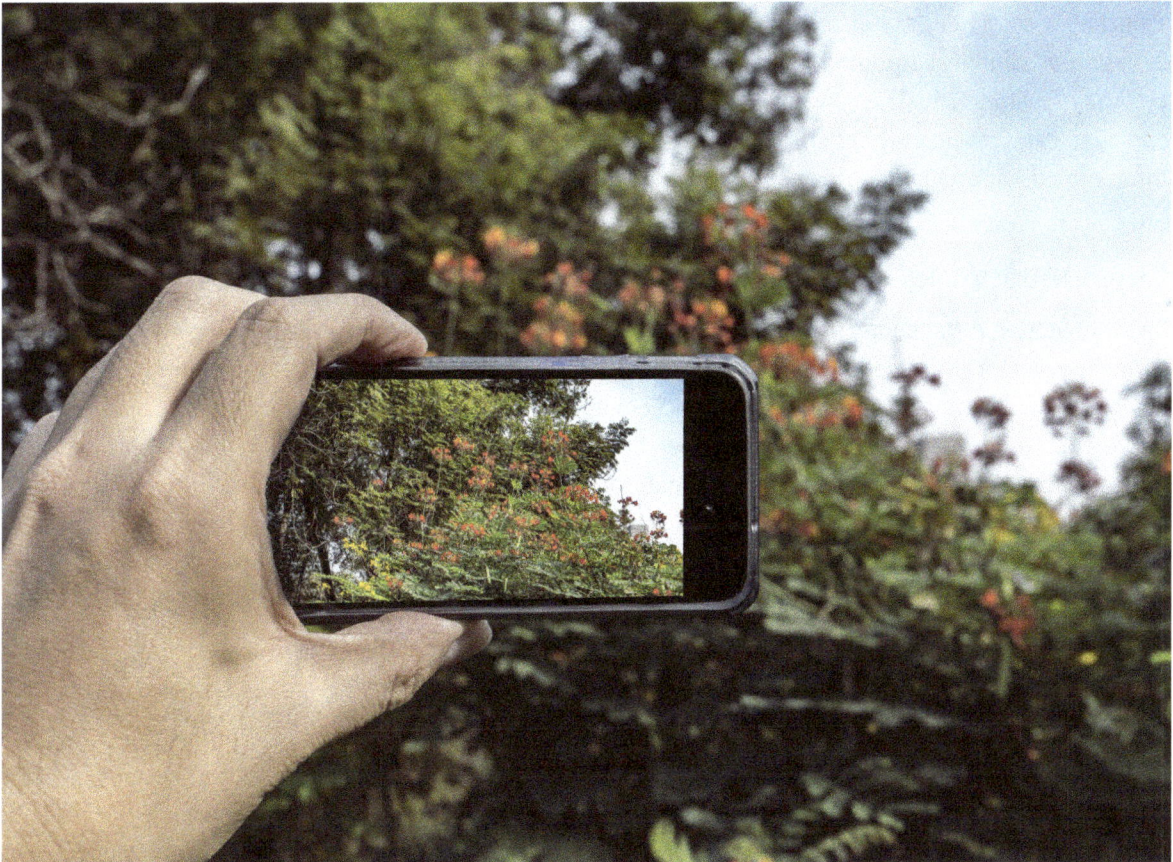

Figure 3.1c   Smartphone.

Improvements surpassing the human eye with today's video technology center around the ability to accurately share perfect reproductions of the captured images and play them back for viewing as often as needed by one or more people (Figure 3.1c). Video images can also be played back and analyzed at speeds faster or slower than real time, and since the images are digital in nature, they are perfectly suited for analysis using computers.

Videography is the most widely used qualitative and quantitative technology currently available for capturing kinematic information. It provides both a precise time code of events, due to the fixed interval of image capture, and the visual record that it creates allows any observed position change of objects to be easily tracked and measured.

The human eye captures and processes new visual images at a rate of 15–20 images per second, or 15–20 Hz. That means that still image information flashed before the human eye at greater than that rate cannot be preserved as still images to the observer. The person is tricked into believing that what they are seeing is not still images but a stream of continual image information. This is especially true when the majority of the information in each image remains the same, as would be the case when an object moves across the field of view of a recording video camera. When such images are played back and viewed by a person at a rate of greater than 20 images or pictures per second, the human mind interprets what it is seeing as continual smooth motion, just as we would experience viewing some type of motion in our everyday environment. This is what Eadweard Muybridge (Chapter 1) realized when he became the first person to capture and play back high-quality still images of objects in motion, which led to his invention of the zoopraxiscope and later others' inventions of motion pictures and eventually the video we have today.

Kinematic Variable Measurement Technology

Instrumentation is frequently used to augment our human senses to record, analyze, and share information about movement. New sensor technology is constantly being created, and more traditional forms of kinematic data capture are being enhanced. Common to all of this instrumentation is the fact that the information it allows us to gather and analyze helps us to understand the complex relationship between time and space as we study how people, animals, or objects move.

The following is not intended to be a comprehensive list of kinematic sensors or motion-capture systems used in biomechanics but rather an attempt to demonstrate the breadth and variety of tools used. The reader will find more information related to the individual technologies listed by following the links found with each listed item.

Optical Measurement Systems

Devices that capture, store, and replay images fall into the broad category of optical systems. A basic component of all optical systems is light. Most but not all optical systems used by biomechanists work with light from the visible portion of the electromagnetic spectrum; however, some systems work with thermal imaging devices that record data from the infrared portion of the spectrum. The systems use lenses to focus incoming light onto light-sensitive sensors that report the amount of photon-based energy striking the sensor and convert it into chemical or electrical signals that can be processed and stored. They can record single or multiple images over a given time period. Their output is stored and can then be retrieved for review later or compared to previous recordings of similar movements.

Examples of image based kinematic measurement systems include the following:

- **Videography**: An electronic optical system that records visible light-based images at a fixed collection frequency onto varying forms of magnetic storage media. The stored images can be shared, replayed, compared to previous recordings, and manipulated with specialized video editing software.
- **Photography**: The process of recording the image generated by light striking a light-sensitive material. The word itself comes from the Greek *photos* (light) and *graphein* (to draw) and has been in use since the 1830s (Rosenblum et al., n.d.).
- **Computer vision**: The process of utilizing specialized software and hardware to scan, evaluate, and provide responses to digital imagery.
- **Magnetic Resonance Imager (MRI)**: A device that applies color to a digital image frame based on the time required for water molecules in the body to return to their normal orientation after

being subjected to a powerful magnetic pulse. This technology, mainly used in medical applications, provides a way to generate noninvasive images of tissue under the surface of human skin.

Motion-Tracking Systems

Systems that use markers or sensors or regional image contrast changes to track motion are generally classified as motion-tracking systems. Here are some examples of motion tracking technology:

- **Passive optical markers system**: Motion-capture systems that rely on unpowered markers to identify points of interest on the human or animal body. The marker locations often identify joint centers or other important structural locations of body segments. The marker locations are joined to create stick or solid-body representations of the organism being studied.
- **Active optical markers system**: Similar to passive marker systems in all respects, except these markers generate a constant or intermittent signal uniquely identifying the marker location in 2- or 3D space that is recorded by the motion-capture system.
- **Goniometers- and electogoniometers-based system**: Instruments used to determine the angle between two segments of the body. Goniometers provide an angular value for nonmoving body segments, whereas electrogoniometers can record constant angular measurements for segments in motion.
- **Exoskeletons**: Structures worn over the body that by design helps support the body while augmenting the body's natural physical abilities to help overcome injury or increase the strength and stamina of the wearer.
- **Inertial tracking system**: A way of tracking the movement of body segments through the use of inertial sensors such as gyroscopes to report information on movement and orientation.

Temporal Measurement Technology

Temporal measurement technology includes devices and mechanisms designed to record or use changes in time for determination of kinematic variables. Some of the more familiar devices used to measure time are listed:

- **Chronographs**: A device specifically built to record and report time with great precision and accuracy.
- **Switch mat**: An electromechanical device that starts and stops a timer when a load threshold is surpassed or removed from the sensor.
- **Radar**: A measurement device that determines the velocity of an object moving toward or away from the device by determining the time it takes for an electromagnetic wave pulse to travel to and be reflected back from an object. That time difference, along with the known speed of the wave pulse, allows for the calculation of the velocity of the object relative to the radar transmitter.

- **Lidar**: A device similar to radar, but instead of electromagnetic wave pulses, it uses a laser pulse to determine time differences and the velocity of a moving object.
- **Photocells**: A type of resistor that creates a voltage when struck with light. When coupled with a timer, they can function as an on/off switch since when light strikes the photocell there is a voltage (on) and when the stream of light is interrupted or extinguished (off) no voltage comes from the photocell.

Kinetic Tools and Instrumentation

Kinetics is the study of forces and how they are related to motion. Forces are the pushes or pulls that cause or change the motion states of objects. Forces are measured and reported in units of Newtons in the SI system or pounds in the English system of weights and measures. They are vectors that have magnitude and direction and must have a point of application to accelerate or attempt to accelerate a mass. Forces can be internal or external. Forces can be detected through our senses, but it is very difficult for humans to accurately report precise values of force without the use of measurement instrumentation.

The study of force measurement and recording is called **dynamography**. It encompasses a wide range of sensor technology and instrumentation specifically designed to report on the effects of forces. The sophistication of dynamographic devices range from the simple balance scale to extremely complex touch screen force transducers found in smartphones. Whether simple or complex, all dynamometers measure force.

Some dynamometers are considered transducers. A **transducer** is a type of sensor that reports an electrical signal proportional to the amount of force acting on the sensor. The ability of a touchscreen to register a force that is converted into an electrical impulse that results in some change on the screen when you touch the icon for an app indicates that the touchscreen is a force transducer.

Regardless of whether they are mechanical, as with the balance scale, or electrical, as with the touchscreen, dynamometers measure force. For the biomechanist, a must-have type of force dynamometer is the force plate. Industrial or research-quality force plates are very accurate and precise devices. They allow the user to collect force data at varying collection rates, often surpassing 1,000 samples per second and having a measurement precision of a fraction of a Newton.

Focus on Force Plates

A **force plate** can be thought of as an exceptionally accurate bathroom scale that can sample and report on forces acting on its surface. The actual sensors in the force plate fall into two broad categories of mechanical (strain gauge, beam load cells) or electrical (piezoelectric, capacitance, piezo resistance). Most high-quality force plates allow for the simultaneous collection of six channels of force-related data (Figure3.2). Those six channels represent force in the x, y, z directions and the associated moments or torque values in the same x, y, z values.

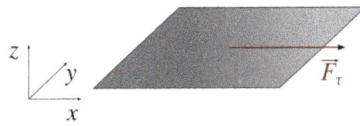

Figure 3.2   Six-channel force plate.

A force plate system refers to a force plate connected to a computer that records, processes, displays, and stores the force and moment data reported by the force plate. A properly calibrated force plate will report zero force and zero moments when nothing contacts the surface of the plate. As long as a person or object is in contact with the plate, a steady stream of data will be reported. Figure 3.3 is an example of vertical (z) force data recorded from a force plate as a person executed a countermovement vertical jump.

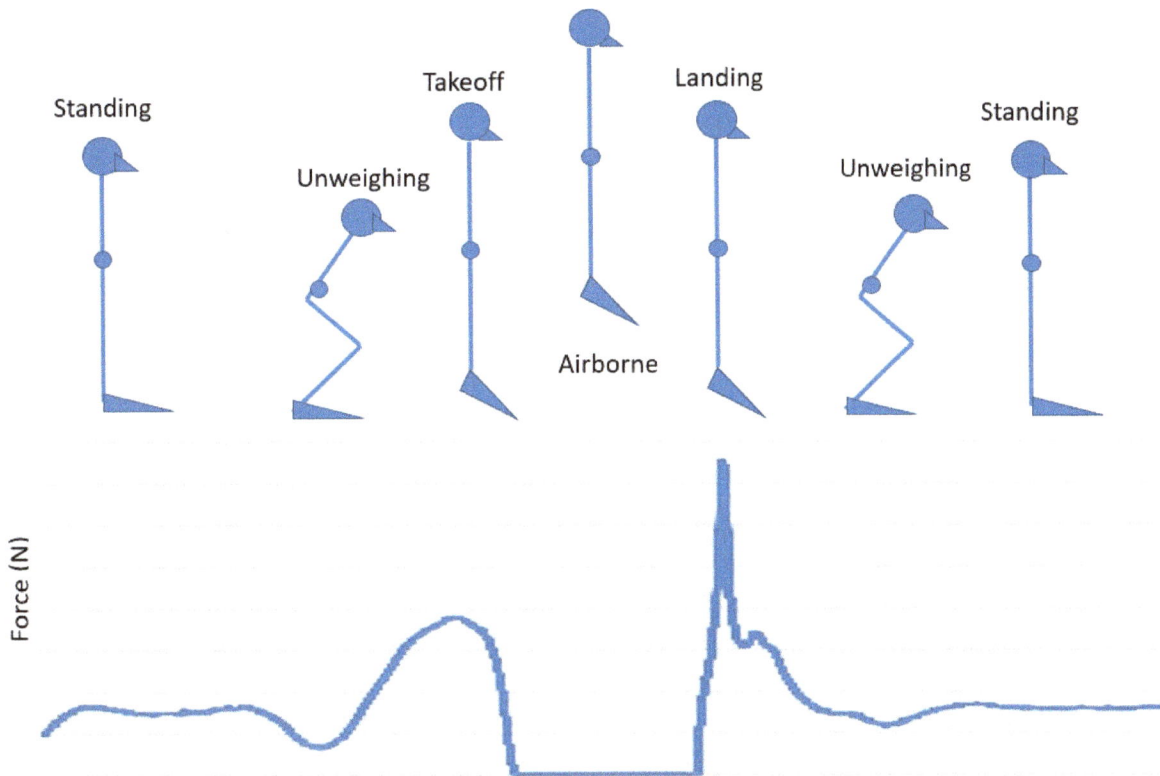

Figure 3.3   Counter-movement jump ground reaction force curve.

Force plates are often used to measure ground reaction forces (GRF) to better understand the dynamics of gait.

Pedography

Force and pressure (force/area) measurements at the plantar surface of the foot provide a wealth of information related to gait, balance, and the general health status of individuals. Due to the importance of understanding how forces are generated and transmitted through the foot/ankle complex, a host of dynamographic devices have been created specifically for reporting force and pressure data from that region of the body. Whether to identify pressure "hot spots" on the foot of a diabetic patient or evaluate the changes in force application when an athlete changes models of athletic footwear, being able to map how force acts at the sole of the foot is important.

Force plates can and do provide useful information regarding GRFs, but they have the limitation of only reporting information of single-aggregated force value during foot contact with the plate and do not provide a data map of force across the entire sole of the foot.

Pressure Measurement

Pressure mats and**insole pressure measurement systems** provide pressure data at discrete locations across the entire plantar surface of the foot. This allows for a much greater ability to identify exactly where and how much pressure is acting on the various regions of the foot during all conditions of foot contact. As shown in Figure 3.4, pressure mats are instrumented walkways that utilize thousands of individual sensors embedded in the mat to capture foot pressure data for multiple foot strikes as a person walks. Insole pressure measurement systems use instrumented insoles worn inside the shoe to report in-shoe pressure values as a person performs a wide variety of gait-related activities (Paromed, emed, ProtoKinetics, etc.).

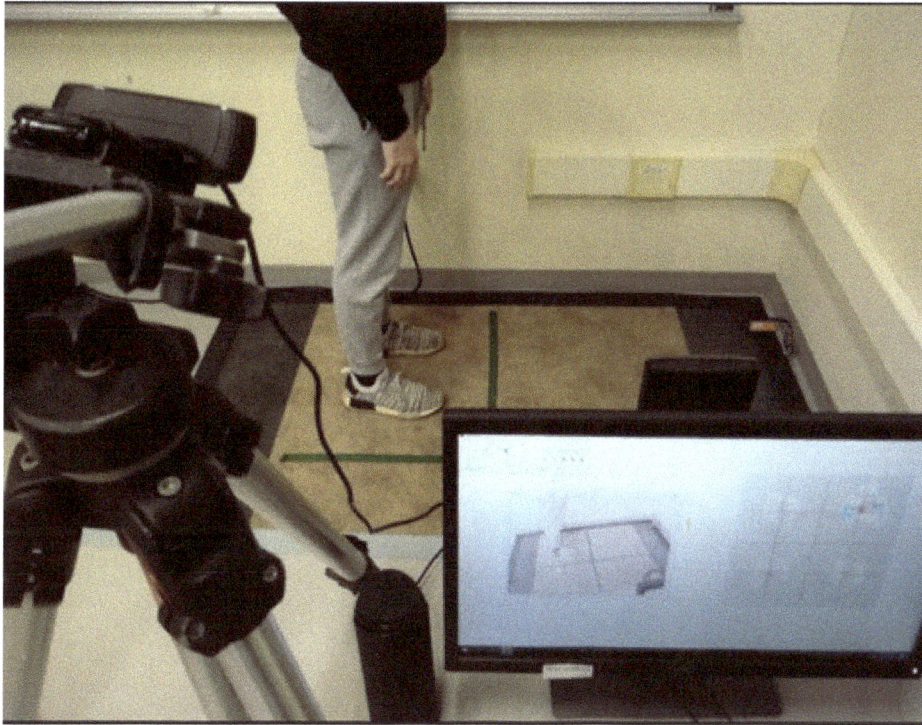

Figure 3.4   Using a pressure mat.

Dynamometers

Hand or **grip strength dynamometers** are devices that measure the amount of hand muscle force a person can generate. A handheld dynamometer (Figure3.5) falls into the category of isometric dynamometers, which provide a method of measuring maximum static concentric and eccentric muscle force at major joints of the body. To record force production during movement, an isokinetic dynamometer (Figure 3.6), a device that measures dynamic concentric and eccentric muscle force across major joints, should be used.

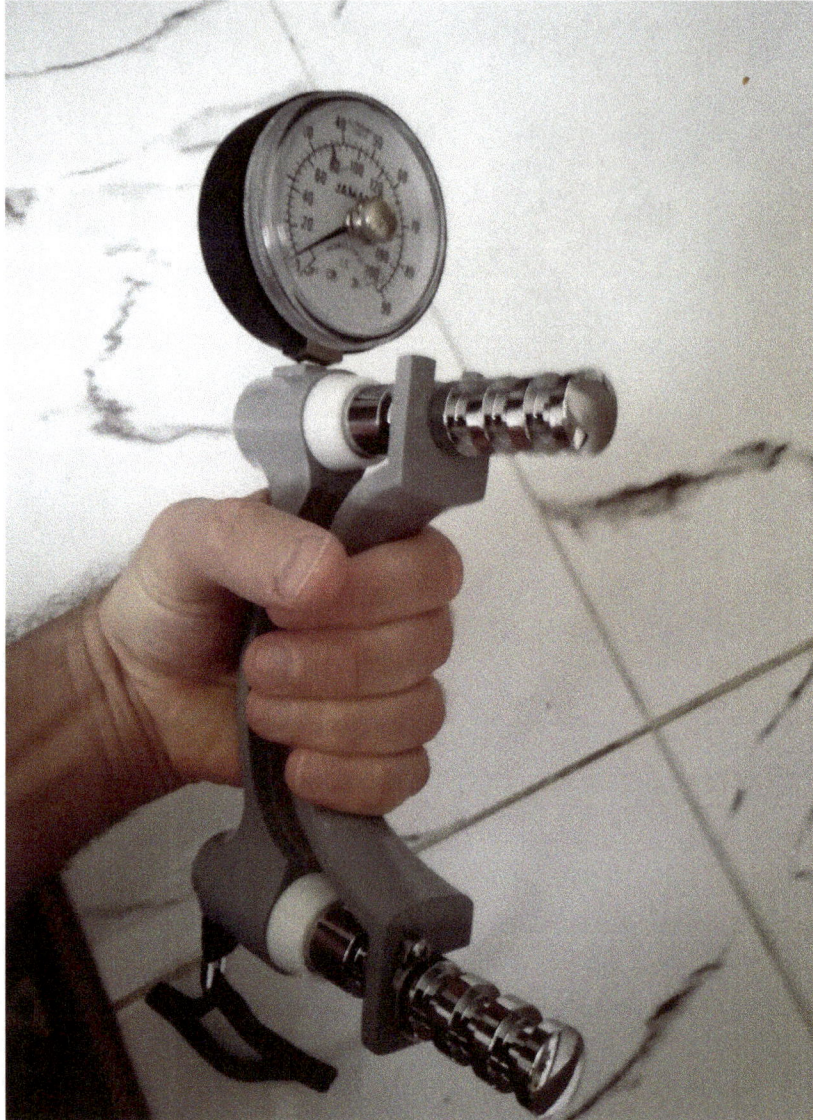

Figure 3.5   Hand grip dynamometer.

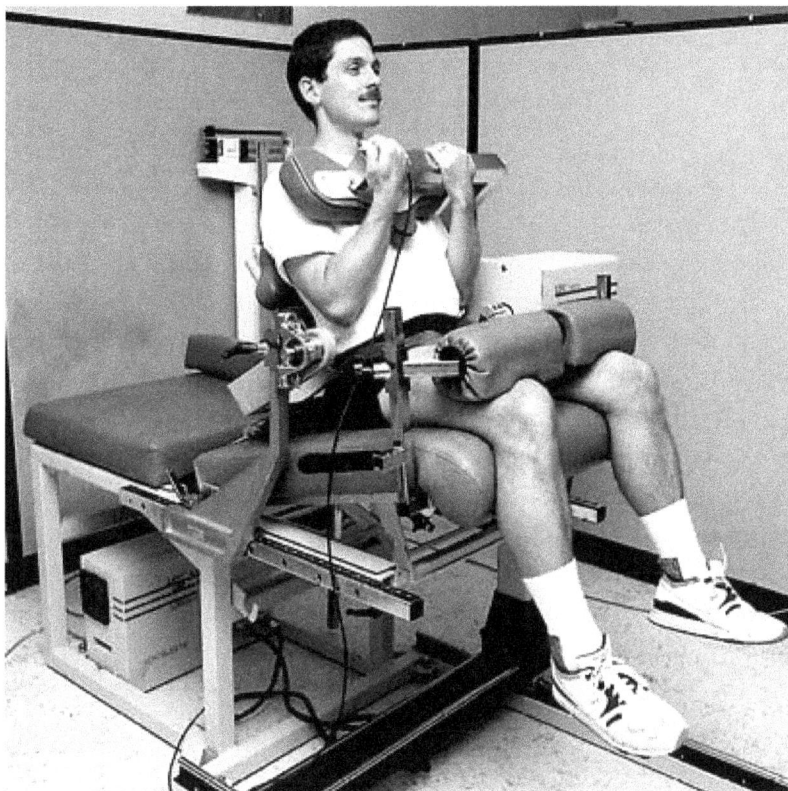

Figure 3.6   Using an isokinetic dynamometer.

How to Measure Forces While Moving Through a Fluid

Wind tunnels are specially constructed enclosures that allow for the testing of the aerodynamic characteristics of various objects, including people. Such a facility allows the operators to control the wind speed inside the tunnel and make measurements related to the effects of air movement around objects. One or more fans generate wind speeds ranging from a few meters per second when measuring aerodynamic drag on sporting equipment, like bicycles, up to over 1800 m/s when evaluating supersonic aircraft. The airflow has to be smoothed so that it doesn't generate turbulence before it passes over the object. That smooth, or laminar, airflow is created by passing the turbulent air generated by the fan blades through a series of fins or blades, which results in air traveling parallel to the interior walls of the tunnel. The tunnel itself is built with no hard edges and with extremely smooth surfaces to reduce turbulence. By using such a device, it is possible to determine the aerodynamic properties of any object that fits in the tunnel.

One or more interactive elements has been excluded from this version of the text. You can view them online here: https://pb.cognella.com/83647-1b/?p=47#oembed-3

Please refer to the interactive ebook in Cognella Active Learning for interactive/media content.

Such analysis is critical to determine the best configurations for people and objects to minimize wind resistance or drag. Reducing drag can significantly improve performance in areas such as cycling where it is estimated that up to 90% of the energy that must be generated by a cyclist is used to overcome air resistance (Debraux et. al. 2011). (You can see how air resistance factors into energy costs in cycling yourself here: https://www.tribology-abc.com/calculators/cycling.htm.)

Air is not the only fluid that people move through during sport or daily activity settings. Water is a fluid that is much more viscous than air and can greatly inhibit movement. To study the effects of motion through liquid, a device similar to a wind tunnel has been created. This device is called a **swimming flume**.

A swimming flume uses a configuration similar to a wind tunnel, a long smooth space through which low turbulence water flow passes around an object being studied. Propellers are used to create a constant stream of water through the swimming flume. If a person is being studied in the flume the water speed will be set to match the swimming velocity of the swimmer. That way the swimmer will remain in the same location in the flume while water rushes around them. Changes in water speed can be made, and the effects of those changes can be determined. That way, swimming stroke mechanics can be optimized and the effects of modifications in swimwear, and the use of goggles, caps, and flippers, can be understood.

Computer Simulations

Computers allow researchers and clinicians to model a wide variety of human, animal, and object movement. Computer modeling and simulations provide the ability to quickly and safely run "what if" scenarios related to motion. They provide the person running the simulation the ability to evaluate the outcome of computer programs designed to model the physics of movement for any object. Once a movement simulation program is written and verified against known values, it is possible to change starting parameters and let the computer solve for the movement outcome. It is possible for the simulation to be run as many times as necessary to determine the most optimal outcome. This provides a way of testing all of the possible combinations of starting conditions to generate a highly accurate prediction of the movement outcome.

The following is a projectile motion simulator by Walter Fendt: https://www.walter-fendt.de/html5/phen/projectile_en.htm.

Movement Vocabulary

Watch the following video clip.

One or more interactive elements has been excluded from this version of the text. You can view them online here: *https://pb.cognella.com/83647-1b/?p=47#oembed-4*

Please refer to the interactive ebook in Cognella Active Learning for interactive/media content.

Now think of how you would describe to someone what you saw with enough detail that the person could duplicate exactly the movement sequence shown in the video. You aren't allowed to demonstrate or show them what the motion looked like. You can only talk to them about the movement so that they replicate it themselves. What are the chances that they would perform the movement correctly? Probably zero! It's not your fault; it's a difficult task because most of us don't have a sufficient vocabulary to provide the precise instructions necessary to describe even a very simple three-dimensional movement accurately.

We live in a three-dimensional world (height, width, depth), and qualitative terms such as up, down, right, and left often ignore the possibility of forward or backward, or may be too general to guarantee a proper outcome or understanding when using only words. In biomechanics we need to establish at least a minimum set of vocabulary that will allow us to describe location, orientation, and basic movements of the segments of the human body.

Cardinal Planes

To facilitate our ability to accurately describe body orientation and movement, three cardinal planes have been identified that align with the three dimensions in which we exist. Up and down can be identified relative to the **transverse plane**, right and left by the **sagittal plane**, and forward and backward by the **frontal or coronal plane** (Figure 3.7). In the anatomical starting position (standing upright with arms extended and palms forward) the cardinal planes bisect the body into equal halves of equal mass. The intersection of the three cardinal planes is the center of mass of the whole body.

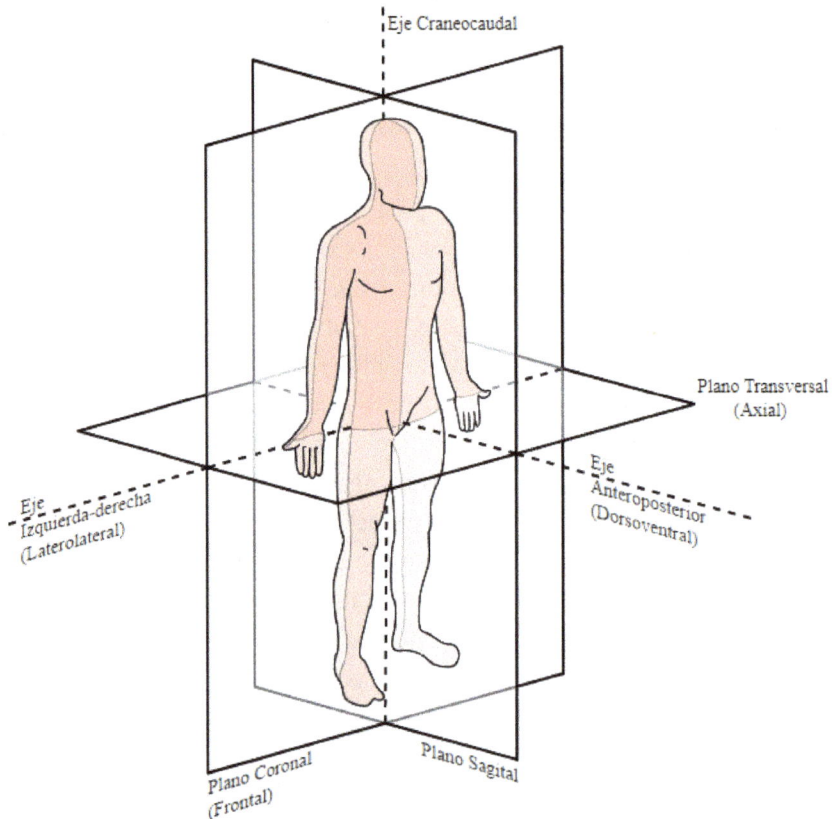

Figure 3.7   Anatomical planes.

Each of the cardinal planes has a corresponding axis of rotation around which body segments may rotate, sliding the segment along the plane. The plane and axis pairs are **transverse–longitudinal**, **frontal–anteroposterior**, and **sagittal–mediolateral**. Each axis is oriented perpendicular to the plane. Movement terms are often paired with a term associated with a movement in the opposite direction and are usually associated with a specific plane.

One or more interactive elements has been excluded from this version of the text. You can view them online here:
https://pb.cognella.com/83647-1b/?p=47#oembed-1
Please refer to the interactive ebook in Cognella Active Learning for interactive/media content.

When determining the primary plane of motion, it is best to think of how the planes are oriented related to the body. The transverse plane bisects the body up and down, the frontal front to back, and the sagittal side to side. A motion like walking would be considered a movement primarily in the sagittal plane because the segments in motion (legs and arms) could be considered to slide along the sagittal plane during the activity. A movement such as a jumping jack would have the arms and legs sliding along the frontal plane and thus would be considered a frontal plane movement.

Location and Directional Terms

It is also helpful to have directional terms available to describe a location or travel orientation in a specific direction related to the parts of the body. Location or movement toward the head is considered **superior** while location or direction leading to the feet is considered **inferior**. Location or direction toward the center of the body is considered **proximal**, and location or direction away from the center of the body is **distal**. Finally, location or direction away from the midline, or sagittal plane of the body, is considered **lateral**, while location or direction toward the midline is **medial**. The midline is equivalent to the cardinal plane from your viewpoint when describing an orientation or movement.

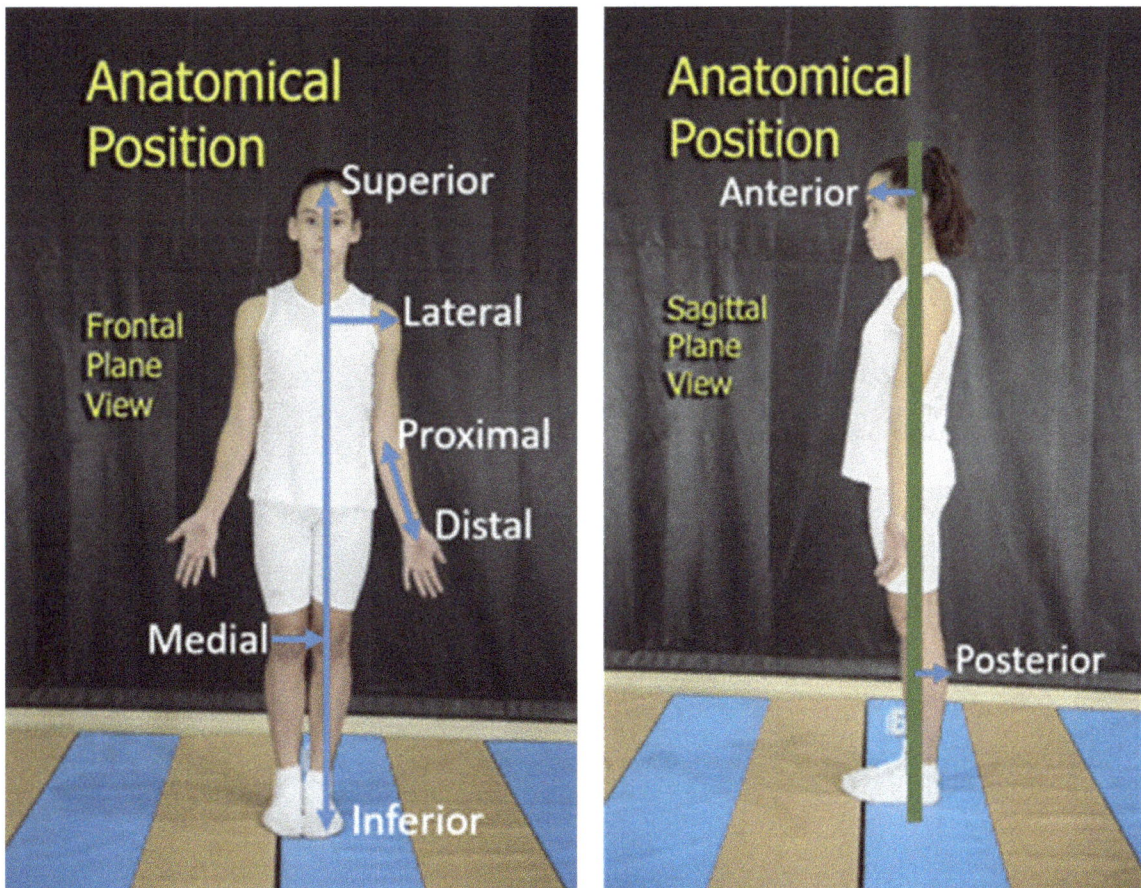

Figure 3.8   Images illustrating directional terms related to frontal and sagittal plane.

A general rule related to the severity of injury is that injuries that are **superior**, **medial**, and **proximal** are more severe and life-threatening (head injury) than those that are inferior, lateral, and distal (stubbing your little toe).

Table 3.1 Anatomical and Common Terms and Descriptors

Plane	Axis	Bisects the Body (Common Descriptors)	Bisects the Body (Anatomical Descriptors)
Sagittal	Mediolateral	Right and left	Medial and lateral
Frontal	Anteroposterior	Front and back	Anterior and posterior
Transverse	Longitudinal	Up and down	Superior and inferior

There are many different terms used to describe everyday orientations and movements of the body. In the Table 3.2 some of the most common terms are presented.

Table 3.2 Common Planer Motions

Plane	Motion Pair	Motion Outcome	Joints	Examples
Sagittal	Flexion and extension	Flexion decreases angle distance between segments Extension increases angular distance between segments	Wrist, elbow, shoulder, spine, hips, knees	Biceps curl or knee motion during a squatting movement
	Dorsiflexion and plantarflexion	Dorsiflexion: pulling the dorsal (top) of the foot toward the lower leg Plantarflexion: pushing the sole of the foot downward	Ankle	Keeping your heel on the ground while lifting your toes up or rising on your toes
Frontal plane	Flexion and extension	Body segments move right or left away from the midline in flexion and back with extension	Spine	Head or trunk, right or left flexion and extension
	Abduction and adduction	Body segments rotate away (abduction) or toward (adduction) of the midline	Shoulders, hips	Swinging upper arm from side to parallel to the ground
	Deviation (radial and ulnar)	The hand rotates toward the ulna or radius bone of the forearm	Wrist	Rotating wrist to move thumb away (radial) or toward (ulnar) the midline
	Inversion and eversion	Turns the plantar side of the foot toward or away from the midline	Ankle	Rolling the foot so only the lateral side or the medial side sole is touching the ground

Table 3.2 Common Planer Motions

Transverse plane	Right and left spinal rotation	Rotate a body segment around the longitudinal axis	Spine	Rotating your head to look over your right or left shoulder
	Internal or external flexion	Rotate the arm toward the anterior or posterior of the body	Shoulder	With forearm parallel to the ground, rotating the shoulder to bring the hand in front or to the side of the body
	Radioulnar supination and pronation	With forearms parallel to the floor, rotate the palm of the hand upward (supination) or downward (pronation)	Forearm	With your forearm parallel to the ground, rotating your hand so the palm is pointed toward the floor
	Internal or external flexion	Rotate the leg in a medial (internal flexion) or lateral (external flexion)	Hip	Standing straight up, lifting a leg and rotating it at the hip to point your foot to the right or left

Summary

Qualitative and quantitative movement problems can be solved using a variety of instrumentation, mathematical formulas, and movement-based specific vocabulary. Both kinematic and kinetic problems may be qualitative and quantitative in nature, and may require a combination of tools to solve. While the instruments and equipment used by biomechanists come in many forms, they are all designed to provide accurate, precise, and repeatable results. In addition to being able to work with a variety of equipment, a biomechanist must have a strong vocabulary and understanding of directional, location, and movement terms to successfully share their knowledge with others.

List of Key Takeaways

- Kinetics is the study of force and how it effects motion. Force is a special type of vector that, in addition to having a magnitude and direction, must also have a point of application to be relevant. To gauge how a force may affect the motion state of an object, the mass of the object must be known.
- Forces occur in many forms, but all must have time to act. The combination of force times time provides a value called impulse that is directly related to the momentum of an object. The relationship between changes in momentum allows for the calculation of force, if certain kinematic values and the mass of the object are known.
- Dynamography describes the instruments and processes of force and pressure measurement.
- Many of the mechanical tools used by a biomechanist to capture and analyze motion are based on human or animal sensory organs such as the eyes or ears.

- Knowledge of the cardinal planes and axes of motion allow for very specific descriptions of the location and directional movement of segments of the human body.

References

Debraux, P., Grappe, F., Manolova, A. V., Bertucci, W. (2011) Aerodynamic drag in cycling: methods of assessment. Sports Biomechanics. 10(3), 197-218.

Rosenblum, M., Gernsheim, H. E. R., Newhall, B., & Grundberg, A. (n.d.). History of photography. Britannica. https://www.britannica.com/technology/photography

Image Credits

Fig. 3.1a: Copyright © by Holly Fischer (CC BY 3.0) at https://commons.wikimedia.org/wiki/File:Three_Main_Layers_of_the_Eye.png.

Fig. 3.1b: Copyright © 2019 Depositphotos/DmittriyAnaniev.

Fig. 3.1c: Copyright © 2016 Depositphotos/somdul.

Fig. 3.2: Source: https://commons.wikimedia.org/wiki/File:Shear_force_on_a_plate.svg.

Fig. 3.5: Source: https://commons.wikimedia.org/wiki/File:Hand_dynamometer.jpg.

Fig. 3.6: Source: https://lsda.jsc.nasa.gov/Hardware/hardw/309.

Fig. 3.7: Copyright © by Edoarado (CC BY-SA 3.0) at https://commons.wikimedia.org/wiki/File:Planos_anat%C3%B3micos.svg.

Chapter 4

More Tools

Math

Preparing to Learn: *Watch*

Being able to run fast is the result of being able to control a host of factors that both help you get from point A to point B and those that try to stop you, or at least slow you down during the activity.

🖥 *One or more interactive elements has been excluded from this version of the text. You can view them online here: https://pb.cognella.com/83647-1b/?p=50#oembed-1*
Please refer to the interactive ebook in Cognella Active Learning for interactive/media content.

I'm sure many of you play video games. Did you ever wonder how information about direction of the characters in the game is automatically understood and factored into their movements within the gaming space? Well, it's all done with vectors.

Note that some of the terms or expressions used by the creator of this video do not exactly match how vectors are described later in this chapter; however, both are correct.

One or more interactive elements has been excluded from this version of the text. You can view them online here: https://pb.cognella.com/83647-1b/?p=50#oembed-2

Please refer to the interactive ebook in Cognella Active Learning for interactive/media content.

Preparing to Learn: *Respond*

Directions: Based on what you saw in the videos, respond to the following questions:

1. What symbol was used to represent forces during running? What forces play a key role in the success or failure of runners attempting to run fast?
2. Explain why video game developers need to understand human motion and the mathematics associated with position change to create realistic game situations for players?

Introduction to the Chapter

Mathematics provides the biomechanist with a universally accepted set of tools that can be used to understand movement in an unbiased and objective fashion. The properties of geometric shapes and relationships that can easily be applied to the kinematics and kinetics of motion make a working knowledge of some basic mathematic principles critical to the problem solving that needs to be done in biomechanics.

In this chapter we will see how being able to visually represent bodies using stick figures, accurately draw spatial diagrams illustrating the locations of multiple bodies interacting, and using vector algebra to link similar kinematic and kinetic variables together to understand the past or predict the future are valuable skills to the biomechanist.

A review of basic trigonometry and vector algebra will be provided in this chapter. Vectors are ideal mathematical constructs used to represent any variable that contains both magnitude and direction. Common examples of vector quantities are force, velocity, and momentum. They, along with, many other kinematic and kinetic values, are commonly used by biomechanists to understand and solve problems related to complex motion. Conventions associated with how to report and use vectors in 2D space will be presented in this chapter along with "recipes" for solving vector-related problems.

Learning Objectives

After completing this chapter, students should be able to do the following:

- Define scalar and vectors

- List examples of both kinematic and kinetic variables that are scalars and vectors
- Demonstrate how to draw accurate stick figures and use the tip-to-tale method of vector addition to solve vector problems
- Solve for the horizontal and vertical components of any vector
- Determine the resultant of two or more vectors
- Use trig functions to determine the direction angle of any resultant vector

The Human Machine

The human machine can be modeled and understood using a series of equations and formulas to accurately describe the human musculoskeletal system and the movements it can perform. However, that system is made up of over 200 bones, 600 muscles, 900 ligaments, and 4,000 tendons! It's complicated! In an attempt to simplify solving problems related to such a complicated machine, biomechanists often make assumptions that reduce the complexity of the problem but do not invalidate their results.

Some of assumptions and simplifications that biomechanists often make include the following

- Thinking of the body as being made up of smaller motion units called motion segments. Motion segments are usually two body segments connected at a joint center. This simplification allows for the evaluation of a specific motion segment in isolation from the rest of the body.
- Thinking of muscles as small force generators that pull on their points of insertion, which eliminates dealing the complex physiology associated with skeletal muscle.
- Assuming the mass of each body segment is located at a single point, which makes calculations of torque or moment of inertia much easier to understand.
- Considering our bodies a series of simple machines such as levers and pulleys all powered by our muscles. Those machines have specific properties that are well documented in the area of physics called mechanics.

The assumptions used in this text are similar to those frequently used by biomechanists every day in laboratory, classroom, and real-world settings. It is accepted and understood that the solutions found using such assumptions are "good enough" to accurately predict real-world outcomes but may not match exactly measured responses of human performance.

This text is not calculus based, as it is designed for the general undergraduate biomechanics class; however, some basic concepts, such as functions that change over time (differentiation ⇒ ex. displacement to velocity to acceleration) and the concern for determining the area under a curve (integration ⇒ acceleration to velocity to displacement), will be discussed (Figure 4.1). In general, a working knowledge of algebra and trigonometry will provide all of the math background needed to understand and appreciate the information presented here.

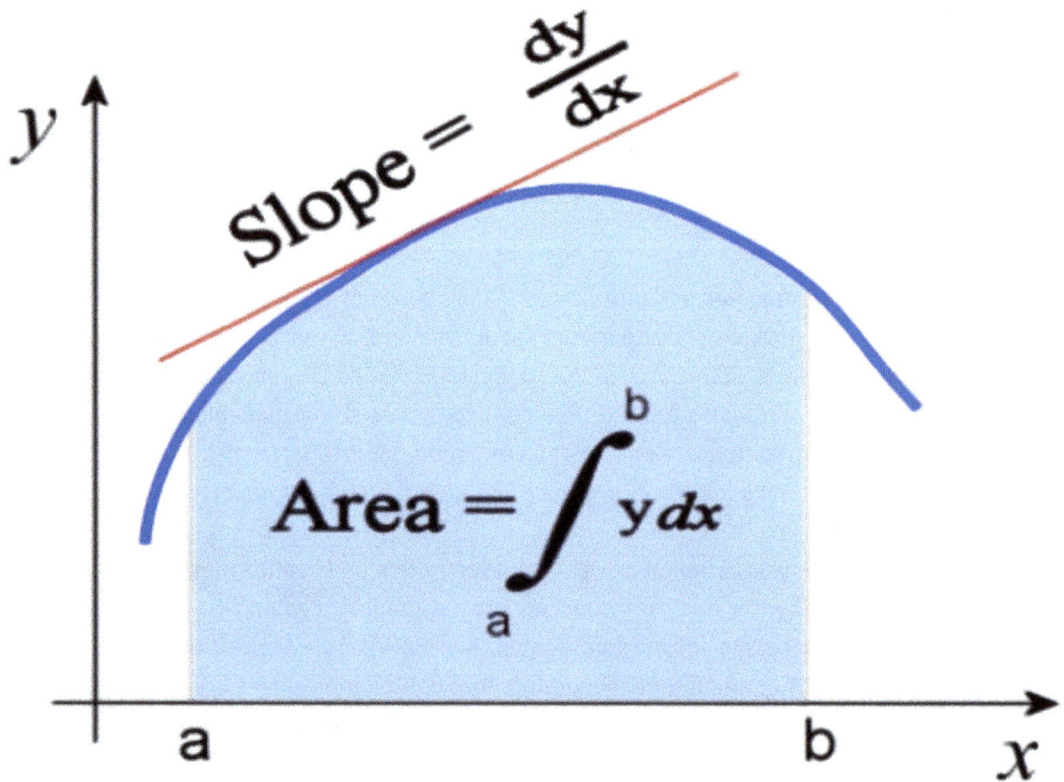

$$\text{Slope} = \frac{dy}{dx}$$

$$\text{Area} = \int_a^b y\, dx$$

Figure 4.1   Slope and area.

Stick Figures

Before we get to a review of the math you will need, we must reinvent our way of looking at the human body. Biomechanists view the human body as a series of motion or movement segments that are comprised of two individual body segments connected at a joint. For example, the forearm is connected to the upper arm at the elbow. That movement segment (bone - joint - bone), can be depicted as Figure 4.2.

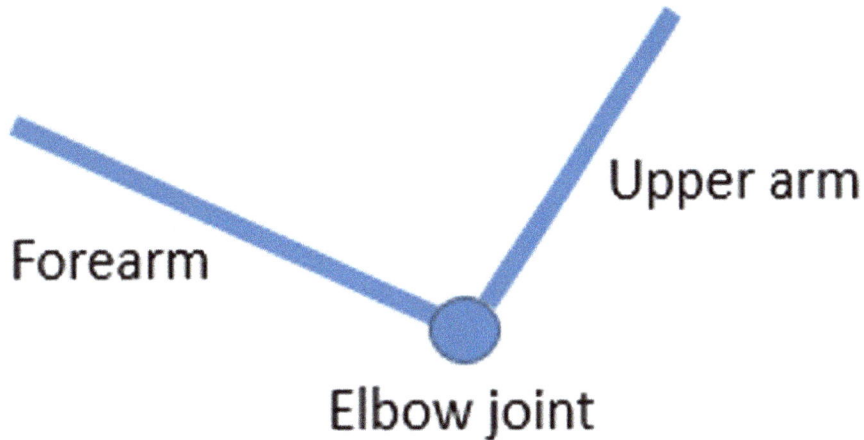

Figure 4.2   Elbow joint.

Notice that the actual names of the bones in the forearm or upper arm are not stated. This "stick figure" representation uses lines to identify segments of the body, not individual bones or structures such as tendons, ligaments, and muscles that are found in the segments. The same is true for the joints. They are simply a point that connects segments. Following that method of representing body segments and joints, the entire right side of the body can be drawn as Figure 4.3.

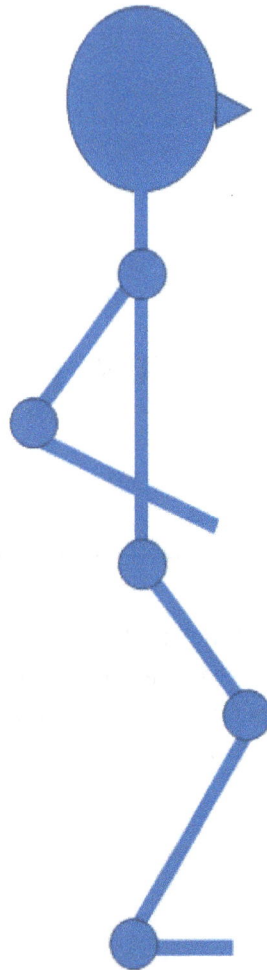

Figure 4.3   Stick figure.

Stick figures provide a starting point for the discussion and analysis of the movement potential of the human body. In this way, it is possible for body orientation to be easily illustrated and the movement segments to be isolated for analysis. They allow us to view some or all of the body as a "kinetic chain" that links the body segments together, which allows us to explain and understand the effects of loads (forces) applied anywhere on the body. The concept of a kinetic chain also makes it possible to track events through the kinetic chain such as determining the outcome of a load held in the hand and why that may require the movement of the center of pressure location under the feet to maintain balance. It's all connected!

Trigonometry and Human Body

Why do you need to know how to apply basic trigonometry if you are in a class focused on studying the biomechanics of motion? Trigonometry provides us with a mathematical tool to better understand and predict how the kinetic chain will change its orientation when forces are applied to it.

Trigonometry is the mathematics of triangles, the length of their sides and the angles that are found within them. Because biomechanists use stick figures to represent the human body and the orientation of any movement segment can be described knowing its relative angle (angle between two adjacent body segments), trigonometry is the perfect tool to provide answers related to segment length and the joint angles of the body at any time.

Though a movement segment is not a complete triangle, it can easily be converted into one by connecting the segment ends not joined at the joint. See the examples in Figures 4.4 and 4.5.

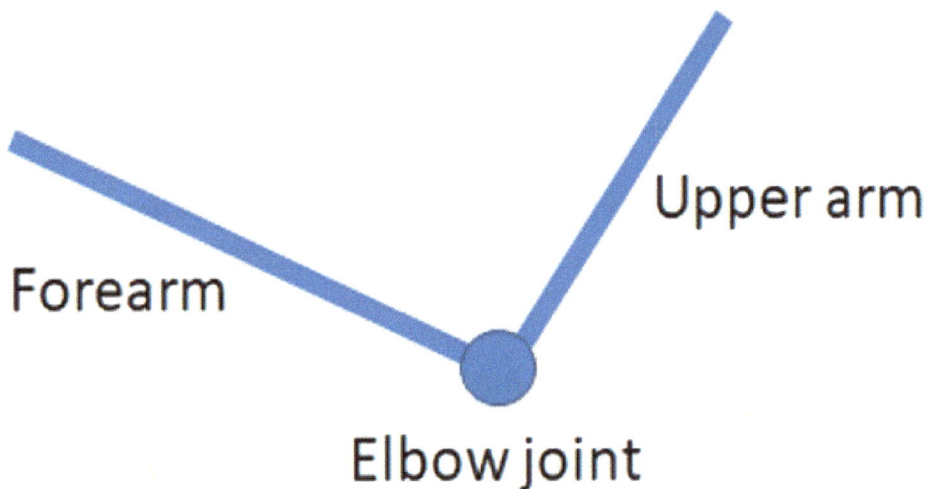

Figure 4.4   Elbow joint.

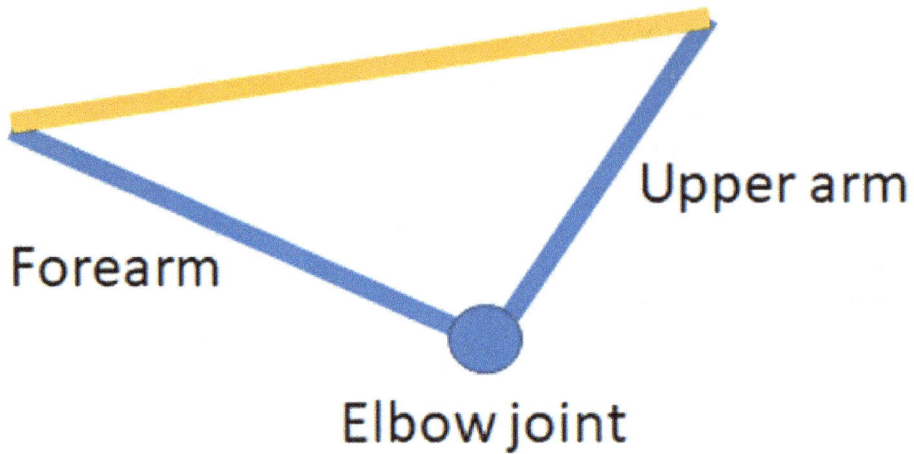

Figure 4.5   Upper body triangle.

If we strip the segment and joint names we are left with Figure 4.6, a triangle.

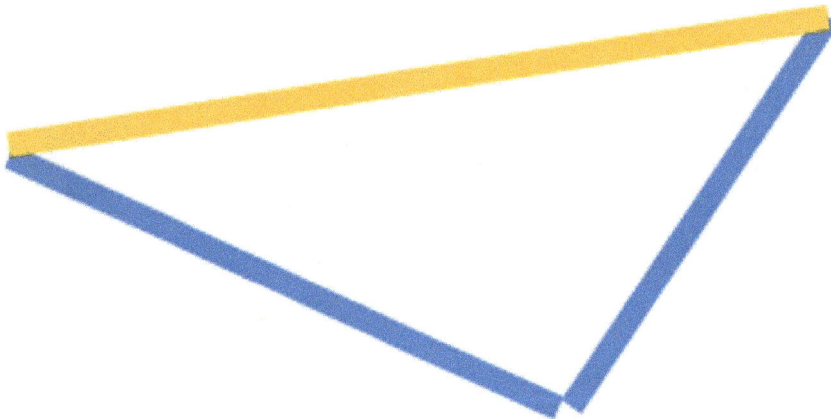

Figure 4.6   Triangle.

Trig Functions

Triangles come in two forms: right triangles as shown in Figure 4.7 (triangles with one internal angle of 90 degrees) and non−right triangles, Figure 4.8, (triangles with no internal angle of 90 degrees).

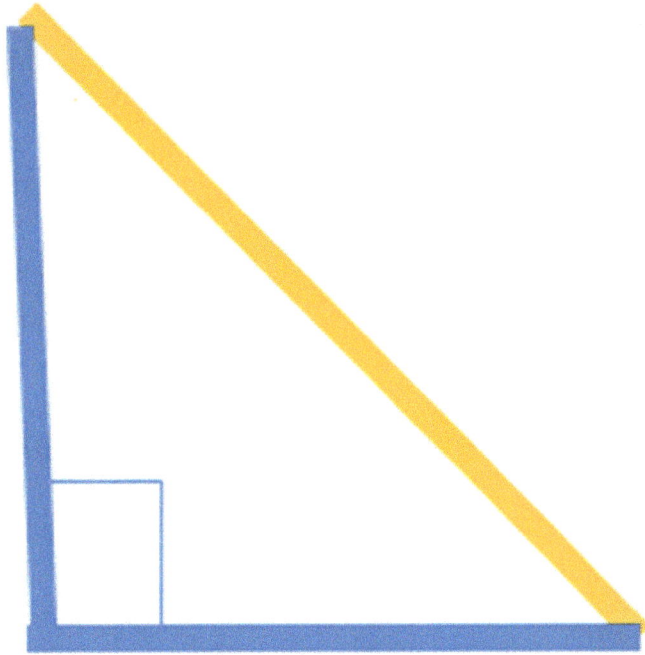

Figure 4.7   **Right triangle.**

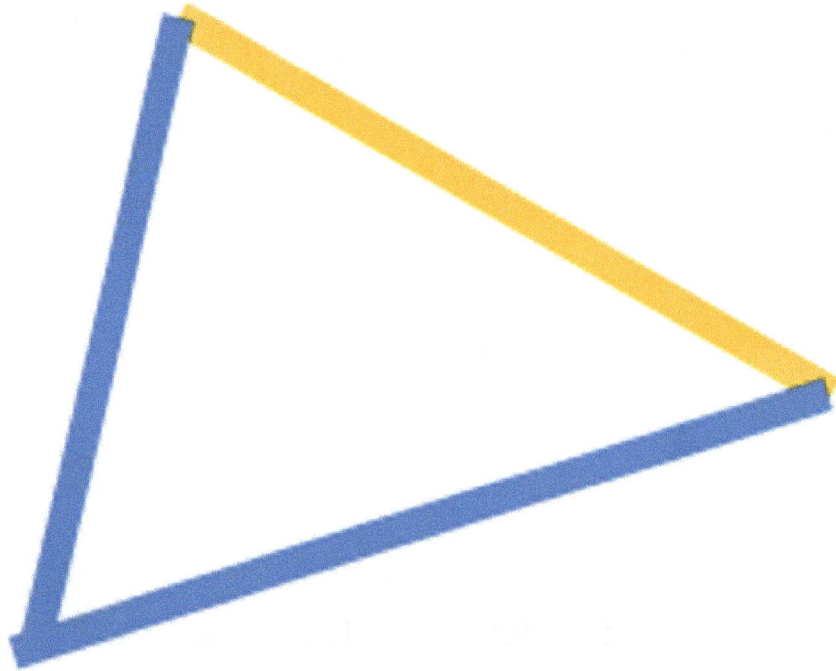

Figure 4.8   Non–right triangle.

All triangles have three sides, and all triangles have for the sum of their three internal angles a value of 180 degrees.

For the sake of consistency, we will refer to the shortest side of our triangles as side A, the middle-sized side as B, and the longest (hypotenuse) as side C (Figures 4.9 and 4.10). We will also name all angles with Greek symbols and relate them to the sides of our triangles:

α (alpha) = the smallest internal angle of the triangle located across from side A

β (beta) = the middle-sized internal angle of the triangle located across from side B

γ (gamma) = the largest internal angle of the triangle located across from side C

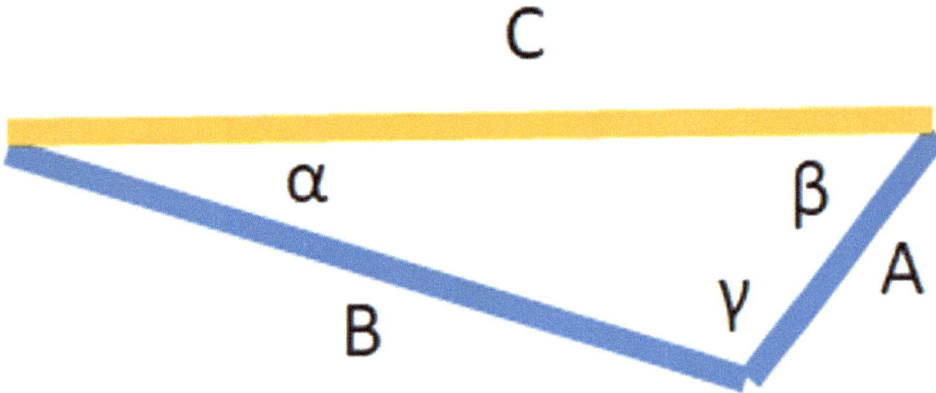

Figure 4.9   Labeled triangle.

There are several trigonometry functions specifically related to determining the sizes of the sides of right triangles. You are probably familiar with the **Pythagorean theorem** that states that the square of the length of the longest side (hypotenuse) in a right triangle is equal to the sum of the squares of the lengths of the other two sides: $C^2 = A^2 + B^2$ or that $C = \sqrt{A^2 + B^2}$.

In addition, there are three functions that describe the ratio of the sizes of the sides of right triangles to the non–ninety degree angles found in the triangles: sine, cosine, and tangent. The form of each function is as follows:

sin(angle) = opposite side from angle / hypotenuse

cos(angle) = adjacent side from angle / hypotenuse

tan(angle) = opposite side from angle / adjacent side from angle

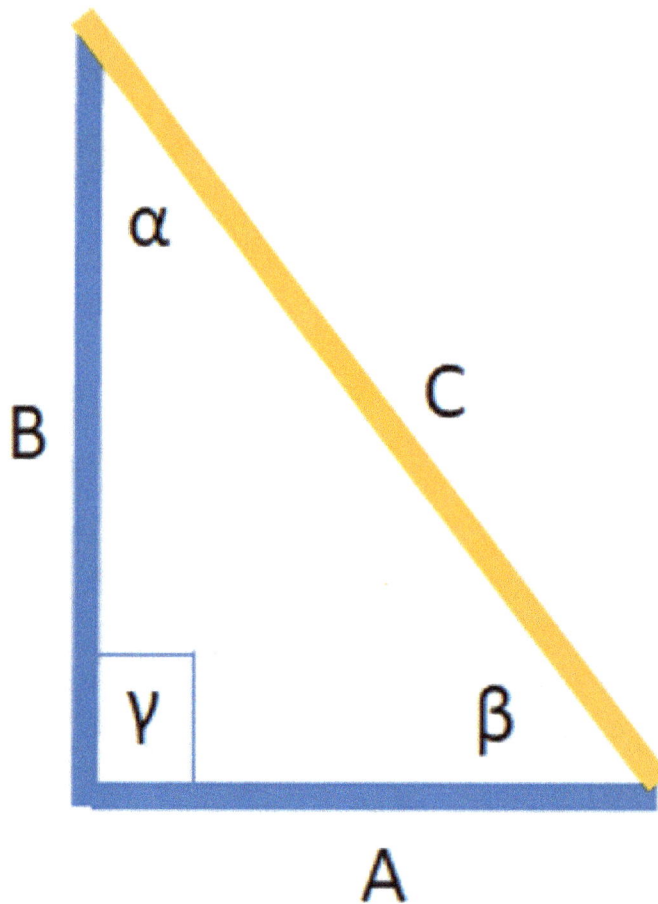

Figure 4.10   Labeled right triangle.

| sin (α) = A/C | cos (α) = B/C | tan (α) = A/B |
| sin (β) = B/C | cos (β) = A/C | tan (β) = B/A |

All those forms of the basic trig functions provide the user with information regarding the ratio of one side to another side in a right triangle. There are no units associated with sine, cosine, or tangent since both the numerator and denominator of the ratios have the same units of length. With the same units in the numerator and denominator, the units of length will cancel out and result in a ratio value with no associated units.

For example, the sine of angle alpha (α) a triangle with sides of 3 cm, 4 cm, and 5 cm, Figure 4.11, would be sin(α) = 3 cm / 5 cm ⇒ 0.6. That result, 0.6, means that the smallest side (A) of that particular triangle is 60% as large as the largest side (C).

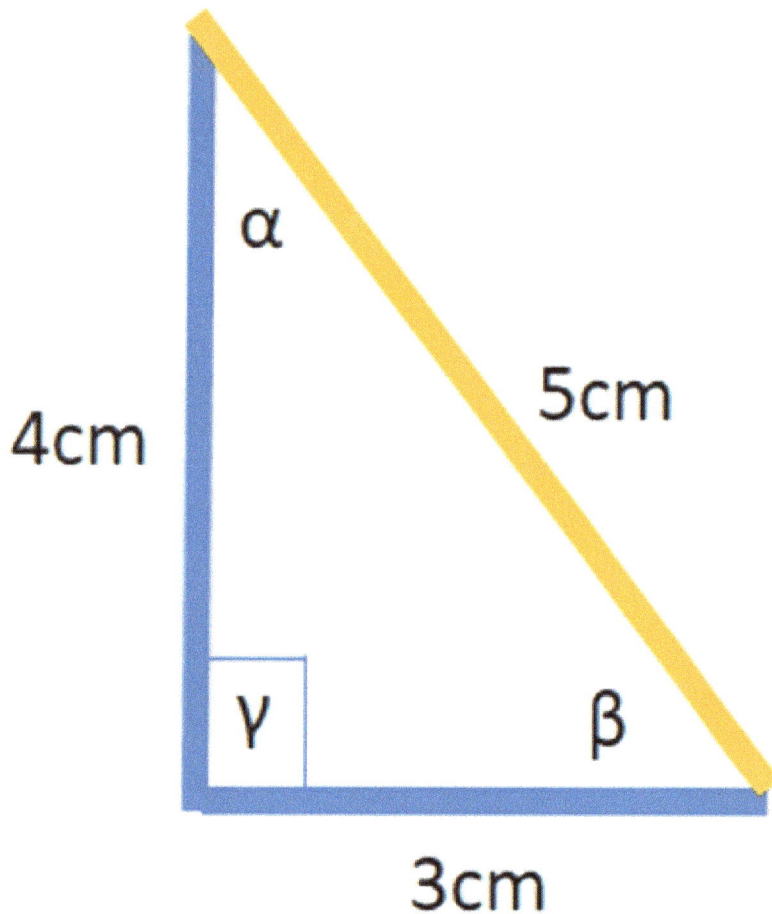

Figure 4.11   3-4-5 right triangle.

It is possible to find the size of the angles α and β using the functions sine, cosine, or tangent, but the base equations must be slightly modified through the use of algebra:

$$\sin(\alpha) = A/C \Rightarrow \qquad \alpha = (A/C)/\sin \Rightarrow \qquad \alpha = \sin^{-1}(A/C)$$
$$\cos(\alpha) = B/C \Rightarrow \qquad \alpha = (B/C)/\cos \Rightarrow \qquad \alpha = \cos^{-1}(B/C)$$
$$\tan(\alpha) = A/B \Rightarrow \qquad \alpha = (A/B)/\tan \Rightarrow \qquad \alpha = \tan^{-1}(A/B)$$
$$\sin(\beta) = B/C \Rightarrow \qquad \beta = (B/C)/\sin \Rightarrow \qquad \beta = \sin^{-1}(B/C)$$
$$\cos(\beta) = A/C \Rightarrow \qquad \beta = (A/C)/\cos \Rightarrow \qquad \beta = \cos^{-1}(A/C)$$
$$\tan(\beta) = B/A \Rightarrow \qquad \beta = (B/A)/\tan \Rightarrow \qquad \beta = \tan^{-1}(B/A)$$

To find the angular value for α using sine for the same 3 cm, 4 cm, 5 cm triangle, you would use the equation $\alpha = \sin^{-1}(A/C)$, which is $\alpha = \sin^{-1}(3 \text{ cm} / 5 \text{ cm}) \Rightarrow 36.9$ deg. β can be found with sine using the same procedure: $\beta = \sin^{-1}(B/C)$, which is $\beta = \sin^{-1}(4 \text{ cm} / 5 \text{ cm}) \Rightarrow 53.1$ deg. You can check those values by remembering that the sum of the interior angles for any triangle equals 180 degrees. Therefore, $\alpha + \beta + \gamma$ = 180 degrees $\Rightarrow$ 36.1 deg + 53.1 deg + 90 deg = 180 deg ✔.

How does that work related to the human movement segment of the upper and lower arm? With that knowledge you can determine the angles formed when an upper arm of 30 cm is oriented at 90 degrees to a forearm of 27 cm, as well as the distance between the shoulder and wrist when the arm is in that orientation (Figure 4.12).

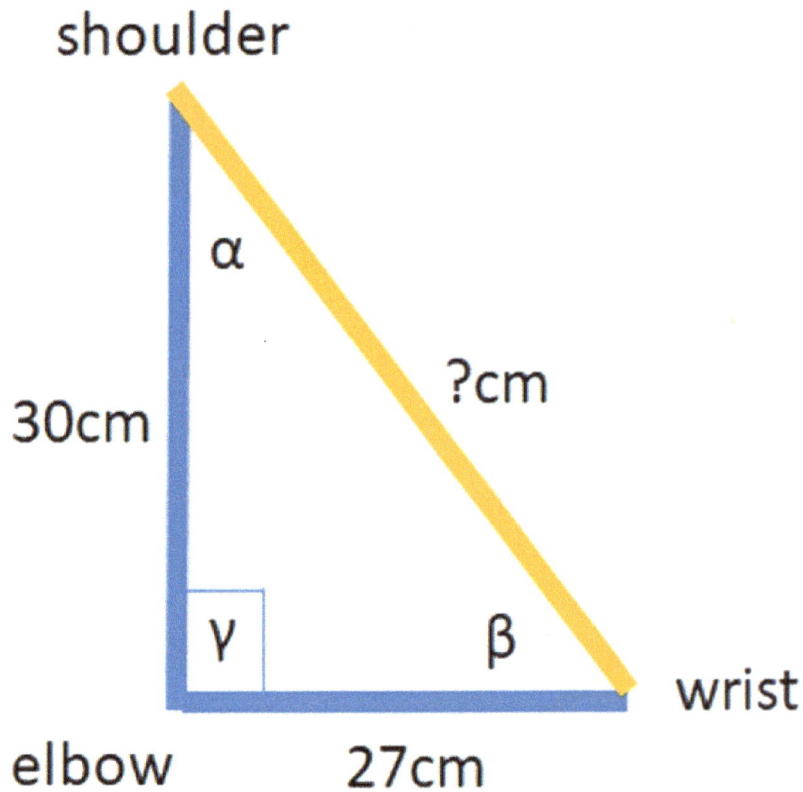

shoulder

α

?cm

30cm

γ

β

wrist

elbow   27cm

Figure 4.12   Upper body—labeled right triangle.

We can use tangent to find α as tan (α) = A/B ⇒ α = tan^{-1} (A/B) ⇒ α = tan^{-1} (27 cm / 30 cm) ⇒ α = 42 deg. Knowing α, we can solve for β using α + β + γ = 180 degrees ⇒ 42 deg + β + 90 deg = 180 deg ⇒ β = 180 deg − 42 deg − 90 deg ⇒ β = 48 deg. Finally, we can use the Pythagorean theorem to determine the straight-line distance between the shoulder and wrist: C = √A^2 + B^2 ⇒ Shoulder to Wrist = √27cm^2 + 30cm^2 ⇒ Shoulder to Wrist = 40.4 cm.

For situations in which the triangle is non-right, it is still possible to find missing side and angle information, but the equations used are a little more complex. Two sets of "laws" will work for any type of triangle, right or non-right. Those laws are the **Law of Sines**, and the *law of cosines*.

The Law of Sines is stated as follows: A / sin(α) = B / sin(β) = C / sin(γ). You will only ever need two of the three relationships to solve for missing information. A possible stumbling block for using the Law of Sines exists in something called the ambiguous case. That is a situation in which no physical version of the triangle exists for the information provided. Remember, triangles are mathematical representations of structures that can be physically modeled in the real world. (For more information regarding the ambiguous case please refer here.

The **Law of Cosines** states that the sides of any triangle and the angles within the triangle are related as follows:

$$A^2 = B^2 + C^2 - 2BC\cos(\alpha)$$

$$B^2 = A^2 + C^2 - 2AC\cos(\beta)$$

$$C^2 = A^2 + B^2 - 2AB\cos(\gamma)$$

For example, if the flexion angle at the forearm of the same triangle discussed previously was changed from 90 to 110 degrees (Figure 4.13), what would be the values for α, β, and what would the straight-line length between the shoulder and wrist be?

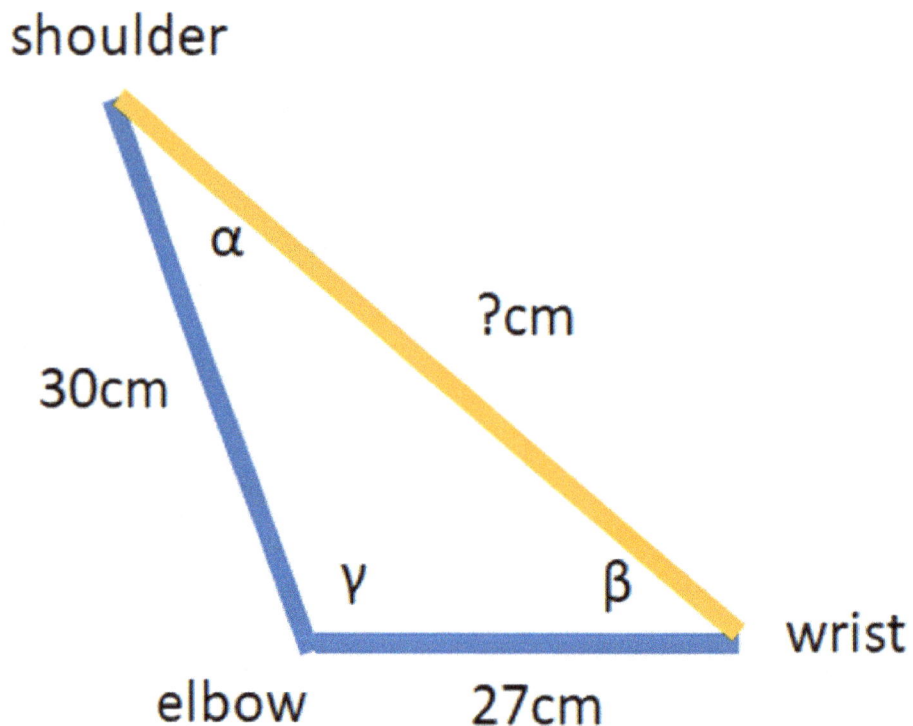

Figure 4.13   Upper body–labeled non–right triangle.

For this problem, we know the value of γ is 110 deg, and that side A is 27 cm and side B is 30 cm.

As far as the triangle sides are concerned, the only unknown side is the hypotenuse, side C. Choosing the relationship $C^2 = A^2 + B^2 - 2AB\cos(\gamma)$ will allow us to solve for the missing side:

$C^2 = (27\text{ cm})^2 + (30\text{ cm})^2 - 2(27\text{ cm})(30\text{ cm})\cos(110)$

$C^2 = 729\text{cm}^2 + 900\text{ cm}^2 - (1620\text{ cm}^2 * \cos(110))$

$C^2 = 2183.1\text{ cm}^2$

$C = 46.7\text{ cm} \Rightarrow$ Shoulder to Wrist

Now select $A^2 = B^2 + C^2 - 2BC\cos(\alpha)$ to solve for α:

$A^2 = B^2 + C^2 - 2BC\cos(\alpha)$

$A^2 - B^2 - C^2 = -2BC\cos(\alpha)$

$(A^2 - B^2 - C^2) / -2BC = \cos(\alpha)$

$\cos^{-1}[(A^2 - B^2 - C^2) / -2BC] = \alpha$

$\alpha = \cos^{-1}[(A^2 - B^2 - C^2) / -2BC]$

$\alpha = \cos^{-1}[((27\text{ cm})^2 - (30\text{ cm})^2 - (46.7\text{ cm})^2) / -2(30\text{ cm})(46.7\text{ cm})]$

$\alpha = 32.9$ deg

To solve for β, remember $\alpha + \beta + \gamma = 180$ deg.

$\alpha + \beta + \gamma = 180$ deg

32.9 deg + β + 110 deg = 180 deg – 32.9 deg – 110 deg

$\beta = 37.1$ deg

By modeling the human body as a group of motion segments, we can use trigonometry to find missing length and angle information, which will help us understand how the body is oriented when movement occurs around any joint.

Vectors

What happens when we need to know more than just the orientation of the body? What if we want to understand what happens when a force is applied to the body, or when two or more bodies collide? To solve such problems, we will use vector mathematics. Vectors are quantities that are fully defined based on their size (magnitude) and the direction in which they are acting. Values such as velocity and force are vector quantities (Figure 4.14).

8m/s

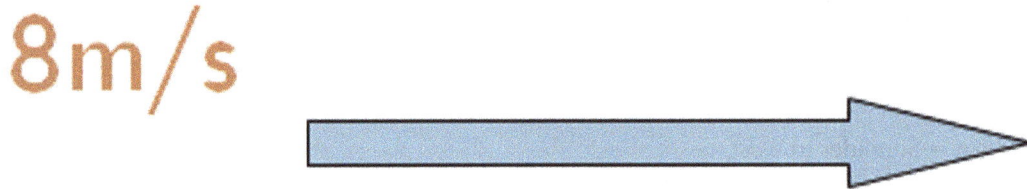

Figure 4.14   Velocity vector.

Vector algebra allows vectors to be added, and the resultant vectors generated by that addition can be determined. Vectors are depicted using arrows that indicate direction and, based on their size, the magnitude of the values they represent. The direction of a vector can be expressed in a number of ways, such as relative to the points on a compass rose. It is correct to describe direction as north, south, east, or west. It is also possible to use the terms up, down, right, or left when referring to the direction of a vector. When performing vector addition, it is best to indicate direction with an angle that indicates where the vector arrow is pointing. The convention we will use for vector direction will be the use of angles reported in units of degrees that could be easily mapped onto a 2D Cartesian coordinate system. The coordinate system will consist of 4 equal 90-degree quadrants. The right horizontal will be labeled as 0 degrees, and the angular value will increase in size in a counterclockwise direction such that straight up will equal 90 degrees, to the left horizontally will equal 180 degrees, straight down 270 degrees, and right horizontal 360 degrees.

Here is a quick summary of vectors: **Vectors** are quantities that possess both magnitude and direction. Vectors can represent a variety of kinematic and kinetic variables. Regardless of what variable the vector represents, it can be represented by an arrow. The arrow instantly provides the viewer with an understanding of the direction in which the vector is acting, and the size of the arrow relative to other vectors indicates its magnitude. Vectors can easily be mapped on a 2D Cartesian coordinate system, which gives them direction potentials from 0 to 360 degrees, starting at right horizontal increasing in a counterclockwise direction.

When vectors are drawn to scale it is possible to determine the resultant magnitude and direction of their sum by adding them graphically through the use of the "tip-to-tail" method of vector addition, which allows vectors to be added in any sequence as long as the "tip" or arrowhead of each successive vector added terminates at the "tail" or end of the arrow of the next vector being added. The building of the tip-to-tail chain of vectors ends when all vectors to be added are connected in an unbroken chain. To determine the resultant vector of tip-to-tail addition, a totally new vector is drawn from the tail of the first vector in the addition chain to the tip of the final vector added. That new vector accurately represents the resultant in both direction and magnitude. Figures 4.15 and 4.16 show an example.

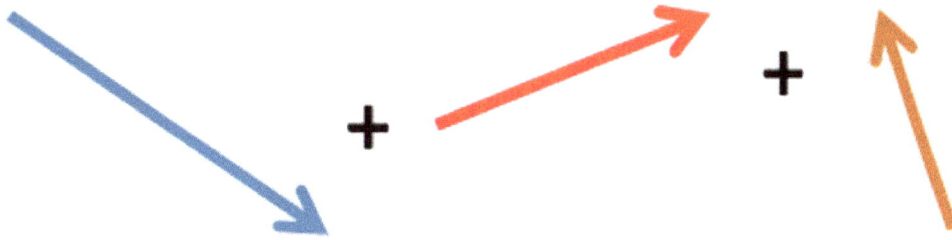

Figure 4.15   Three individual vectors.

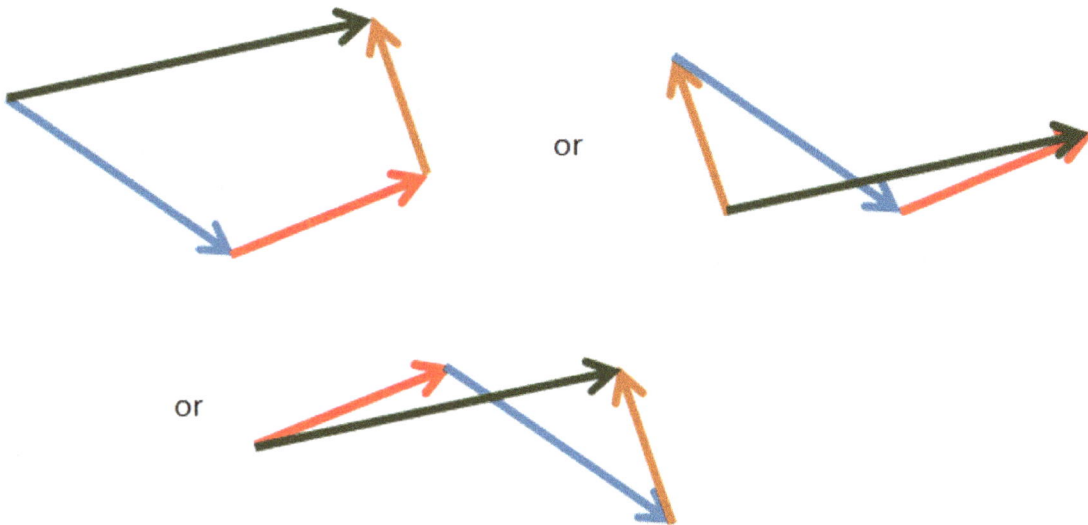

Figure 4.16   Vector addition plus resultant.

Regardless of the order of addition, the same green resultant vector is found when the tip-to-tail method is applied correctly. One important note to remember is that only vectors of similar units can be added or subtracted from one another.

Vector Resolution

Any vector that represents a variable in 2D space can be broken down into its vertical (y) and horizontal (x) components; this process is call **vector resolution**. Graphically, a vector can be resolved into its components by drawing two vectors, one horizontal and the other vertical, which can be added together via the tip-to-tail method in such a way that the original vector equals the result of the addition of those horizontal and vertical vectors. For example, resolve the vector in Figure 4.17 into its horizontal and vertical components.

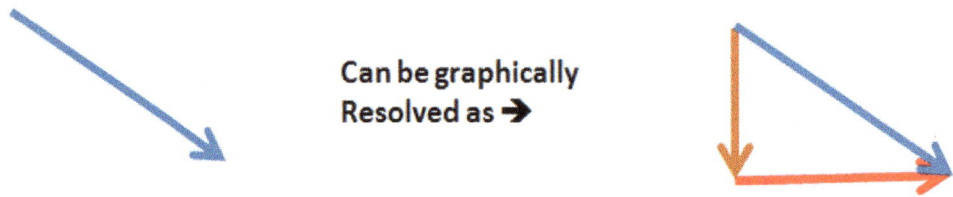

Can be graphically
Resolved as ➔

Figure 4.17   Vector resolution to show components.

What happens if you are not a great artist and your vector drawings are not always perfectly drawn to scale? How can you be sure that your values when resolving a vector are correct? By plotting all 2D vectors on a standard two-dimensional Cartesian coordinate system, it is possible to use the trigonometric functions of sine, cosine, and tangent to resolve any vector into its horizontal and vertical components. Assume that any vector that you wish to resolve into its components originates from the origin of the coordinate system and projects outward from that origin at some angle between 0 and 360 degrees. That means that if you had a velocity vector of 25 m/s directed at 35 degrees it could be visually expressed as Figure 4.18.

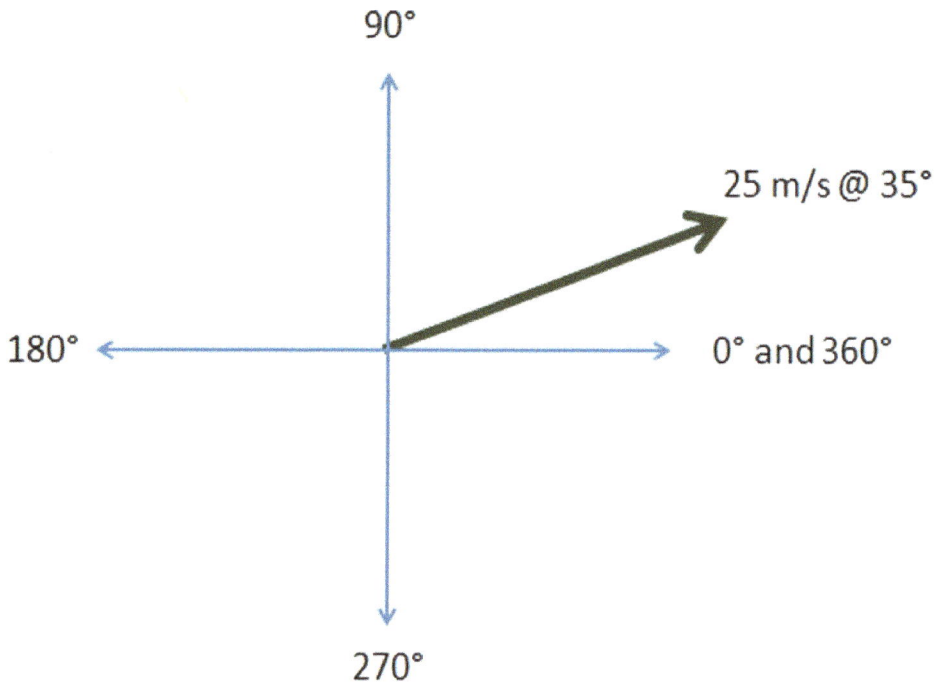

Figure 4.18 Vector mapped on 2D coordinate system.

To find the components of the vector, we need to complete the right triangle that has as its hypotenuse the velocity vector of 25 m/s directed at 35 deg.

The adjacent side of the right triangle can be found using the cosine function. The adjacent side also happens to be the horizontal component of the velocity vector:

Cos(35) = Adjacent / Hypotenuse

Cos(35) * Hypotenuse = Adjacent

Cos(35) * 25 m/s = Adjacent

20.48 m/s = Adjacent = Horizontal component of the velocity vector 25 m/s @ 35 deg.

The opposite side of the right triangle, or the vertical component of the velocity vector, can be found using the sine function:

Sin(35) = Opposite / Hypotenuse

Sin(35) * Hypotenuse = Opposite

Sin(35) * 25 m/s = Opposite

14.34 m/s = Opposite = Vertical component of the velocity vector 25 m/s @ 35 deg.

To confirm that the magnitudes of the vertical and horizontal components are correct, check using the Pythagorean theorem:

Magnitude of the original velocity vector = Sqrt (Magnitude of Horizontal component^2 + Magnitude of Vertical component^2)

25 m/s = $\sqrt{(20.48 \text{ m/s})^2 + (14.34 \text{ m/s})^2}$

25 m/s = 25 m/s $\Rightarrow$ Check!

Visually the result is shown in Figure 4.19.

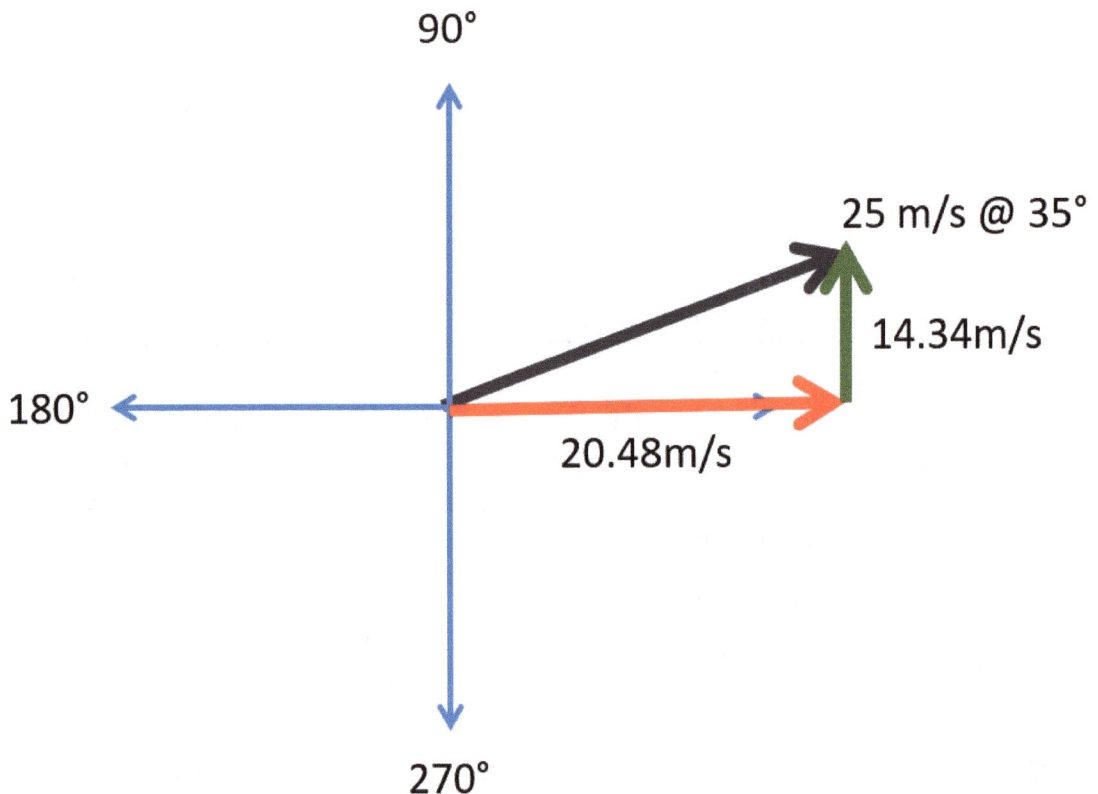

Figure 4.19   Vector mapped on 2D coordinate system and showing components.

Note that this process will work for resolving any vector mapped in the Cartesian coordinate grid. The magnitudes and directions of the horizontal and vertical components are provided by the sine and cosine functions. The directions indicate which way the vectors point. Positive is to the right (0 or 360 deg) for horizontal and negative to the left at 180 deg. For vertical components, positive indicates the component is oriented upward at 90 deg and negative or downward at 270 deg.

Sine and cosine values provide the following directions of vertical and horizontal components in the four quadrants of a 2D Cartesian coordinate grid. Both the values (+ or -) as well as the direction of the associated vector arrows are shown in Figure 4.20.

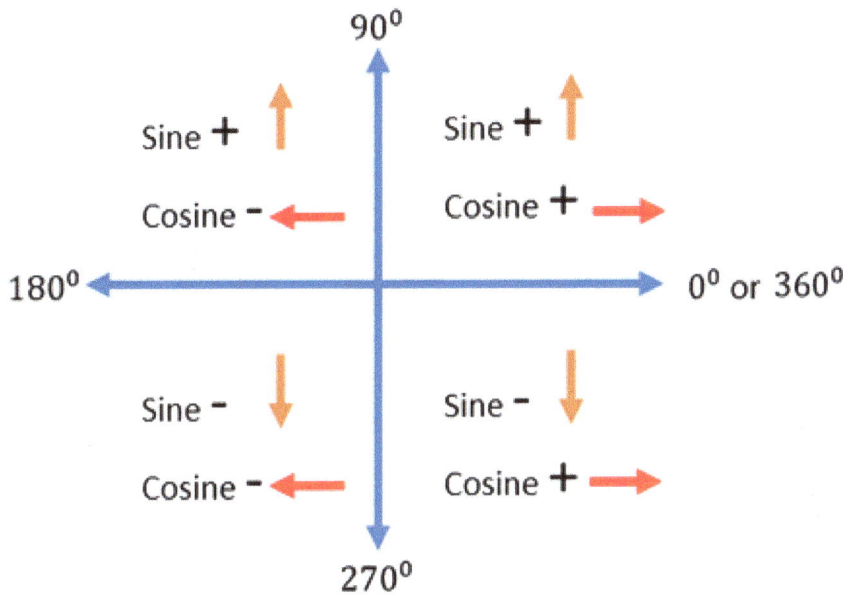

Figure 4.20   2D coordinate system with sine and cosine values.

Adding Vectors

We've seen how vectors can be added using the graphical tip-to-tail method, but since most of us are not perfect when drawing our vectors, this method often provides only a "good guess" as to the final resultant vector direction and magnitude when vectors are added. To find the exact answer to a vector addition problem we must rely on our understanding of how to resolve vectors into horizontal and vertical components and a little trigonometry.

The following represents a method of solving for vector addition that will always work for any combination of vectors that can be accurately graphed on a 2D Cartesian coordinate system with the right horizontal being equal to zero or 360 deg. For example, what is the resultant force vector formed by the addition of the following individual force vectors?

15N @ 210 deg, 22N @ 40 deg, and 12N @ 305 deg

Step 1: Draw the vectors individually on their own Cartesian grid (Figures 4.21–4.23).

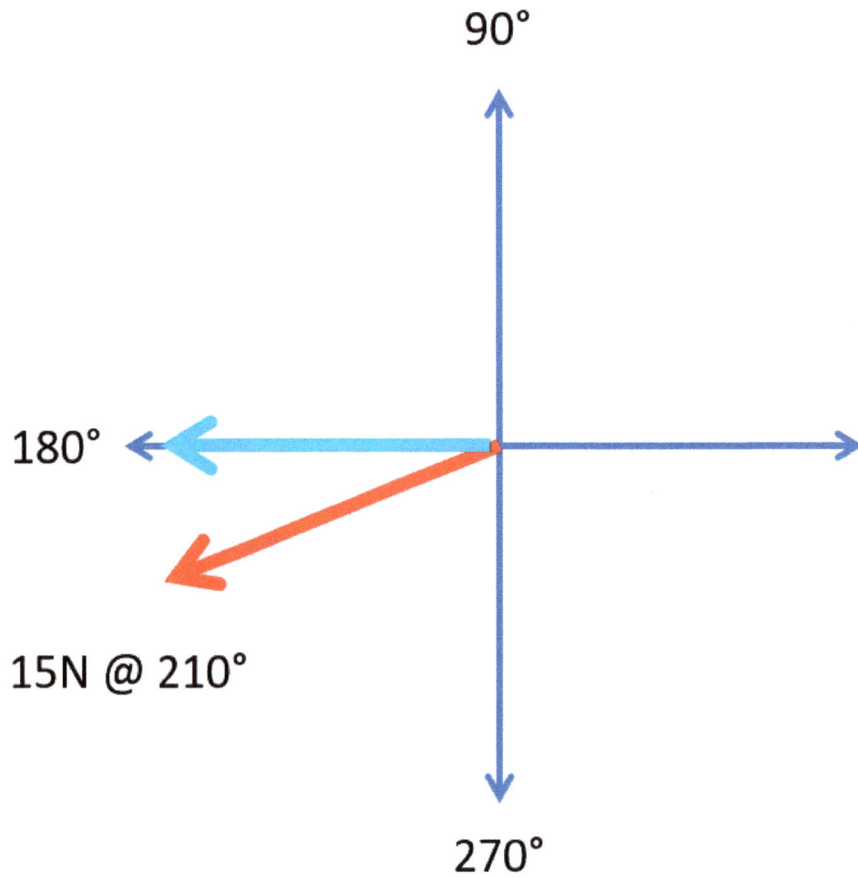

90°

180°

15N @ 210°

270°

Figure 4.21   Vector 1.

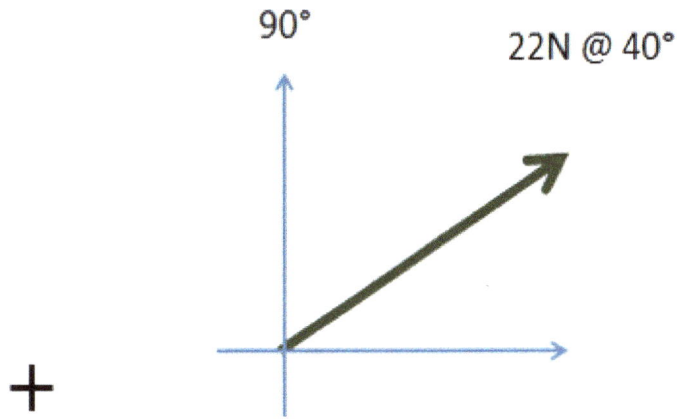

+

Figure 4.22   Vector 2.

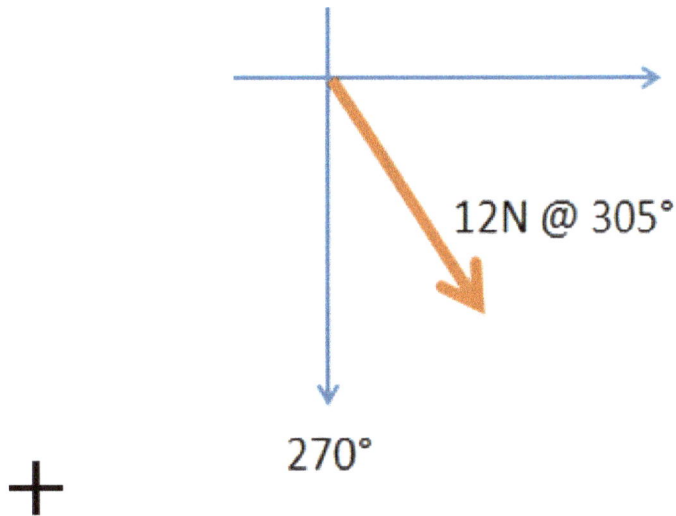

+

Figure 4.23   Vector 3.

Step 2: Use the tip-to-tail method to estimate your final answer (Figure 4.24).

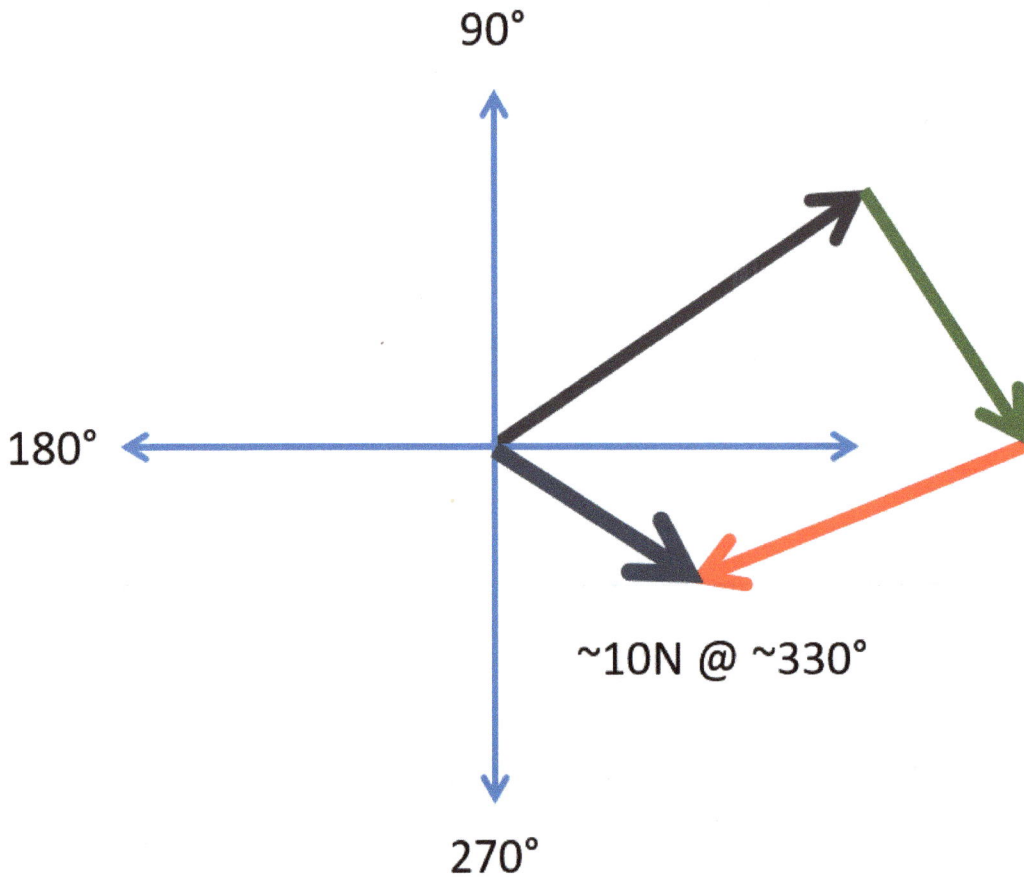

90°

180°

270°

~10N @ ~330°

Figure 4.24   Tip-to-tail addition with resultant in blue.

The graphical method estimates that the final result (the blue vector) will be approximately 10 N directed at 330 deg. Now let's see how to solve for the resultant using trig functions.

Step 3: Determine and add, first, all of the vertical components of the vectors, then all of the horizontal components.

Vertical components:

sin(210) * 15 N + sin(40) * 22 N + sin(305) * 12 N

-7.5N + 14.14N + -9.83N

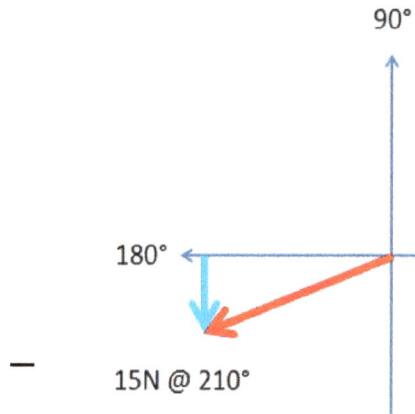

Figure 4.25   Vertical component of vector 1.

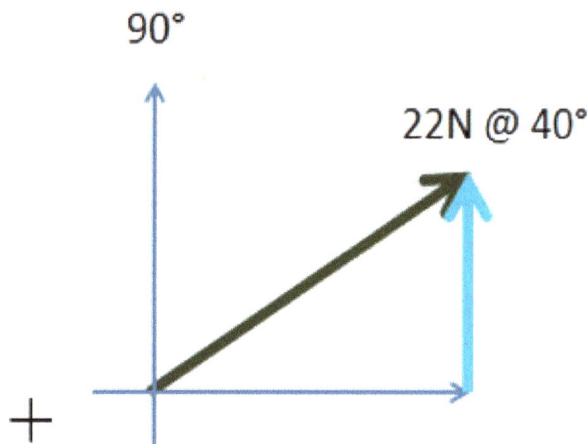

Figure 4.26   Vertical component of vector 2.

Sum of vertical components = -3.19 N

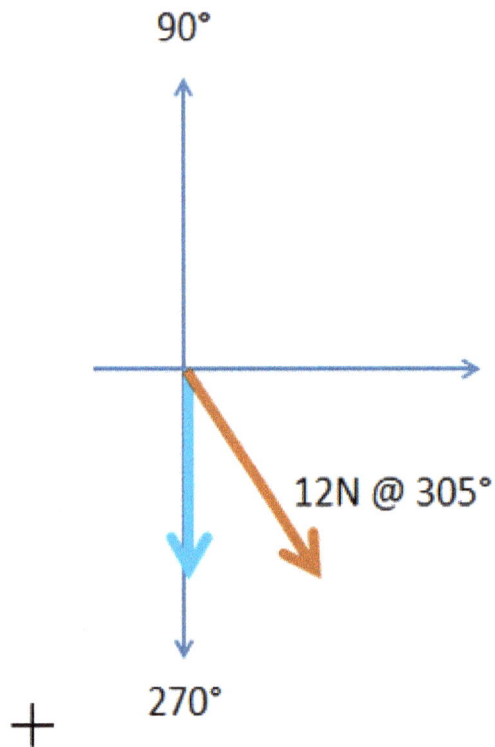

Figure 4.27   Vertical component of vector 3.

Horizontal components:

cos(210) * 15 N + cos(40) * 22 N + cos(305) * 12N

-12.99N + 16.85N + 6.88N

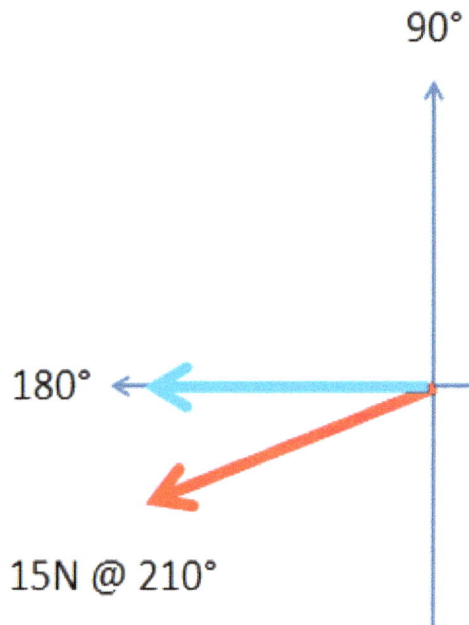

Figure 4.28   Horizontal component of vector 1.

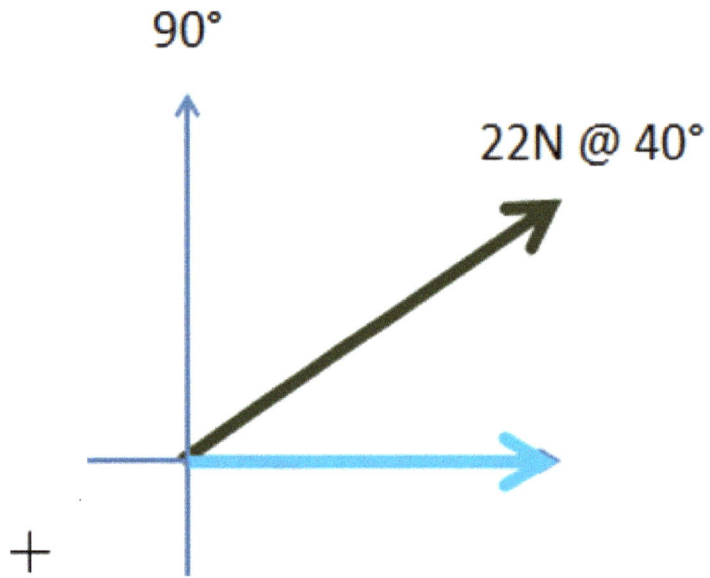

Figure 4.29   Horizontal component of vector 2.

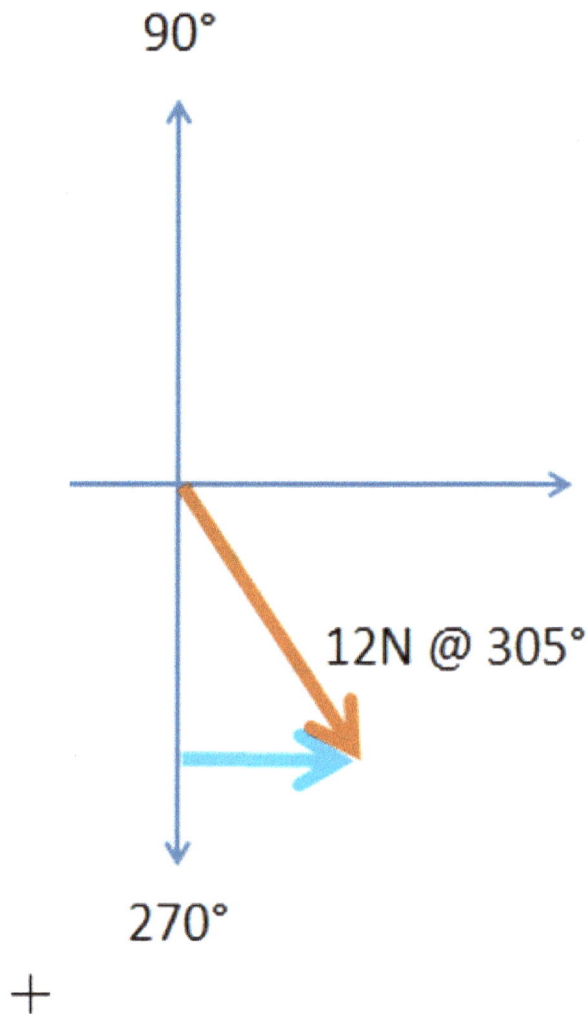

90°

270°

12N @ 305°

+

Figure 4.30   Horizontal component of vector 3.

Sum of horizontal components = 10.74 N

Step 4: Using the tip-to-tail method, add the sum of the vertical components to the sum of the horizontal components from step 3 and use the Pythagorean theorem to determine the magnitude of the hypotenuse of the new right triangle you created.

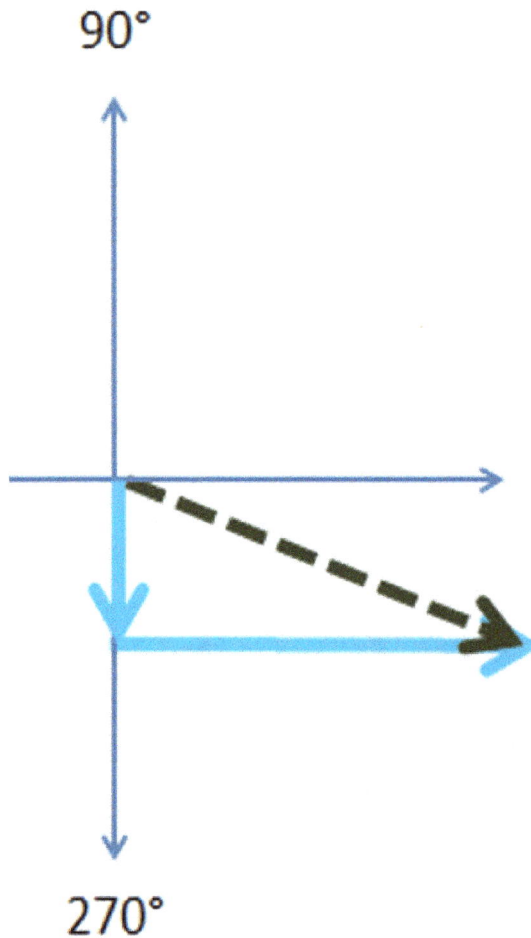

Figure 4.31   Resultant of vertical and horizontal components.

$C^2 = A^2 + B^2$

$Resultant^2 = Vertical^2 + Horizontal^2$

$Resultant^2 = -3.19\ N^2 + 10.74\ N^2$

$Resultant^2 = 10.18\ N^2 + 115.35\ N^2$

$Resultant^2 = 125.53\ N^2$

$Resultant = \sqrt{(125.53\ N^2)}$

Resultant = 11.2 N	(which represents the magnitude of the resultant vector)

Step 5: Use the tangent function to determine the angle Ɵ.

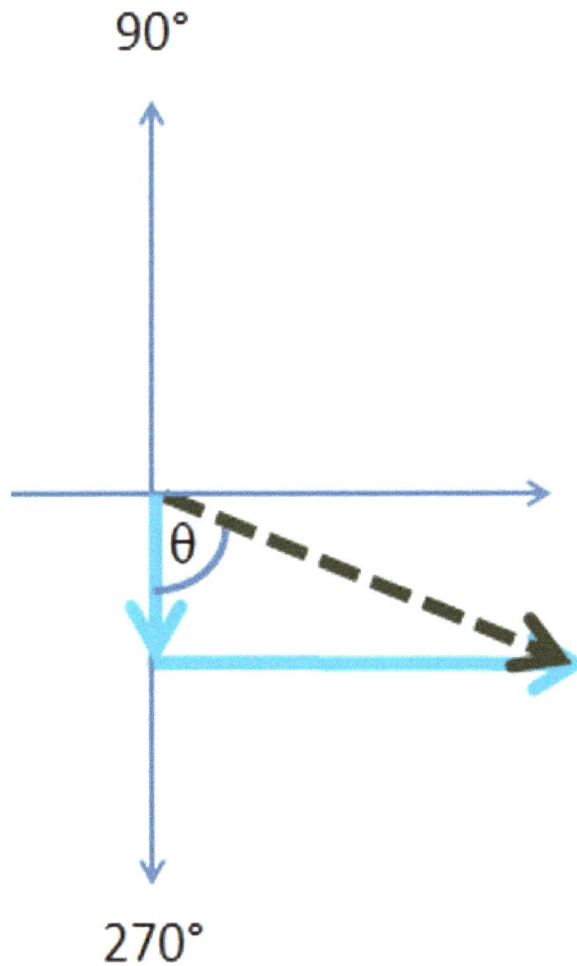

Figure 4.32   Resultant angle.

Tan(Ɵ) = Opp / Adj

Tan(Ɵ) = 10.74 N / 3.19 N	Note: Use the magnitude of the vectors, which results in

$\Theta = \tan^{-1}(10.74 \text{ N} / 3.19 \text{ N})$ any negative signs being dropped from the equation.

$\Theta = 73.46 \text{ deg}$

Now, measuring from 0 deg horizontal, determine the final angle of the resultant vector. In this case, you will measure from 0 to 270 deg, then add the angle Θ to arrive at your final angular direction (Figure 4.33).

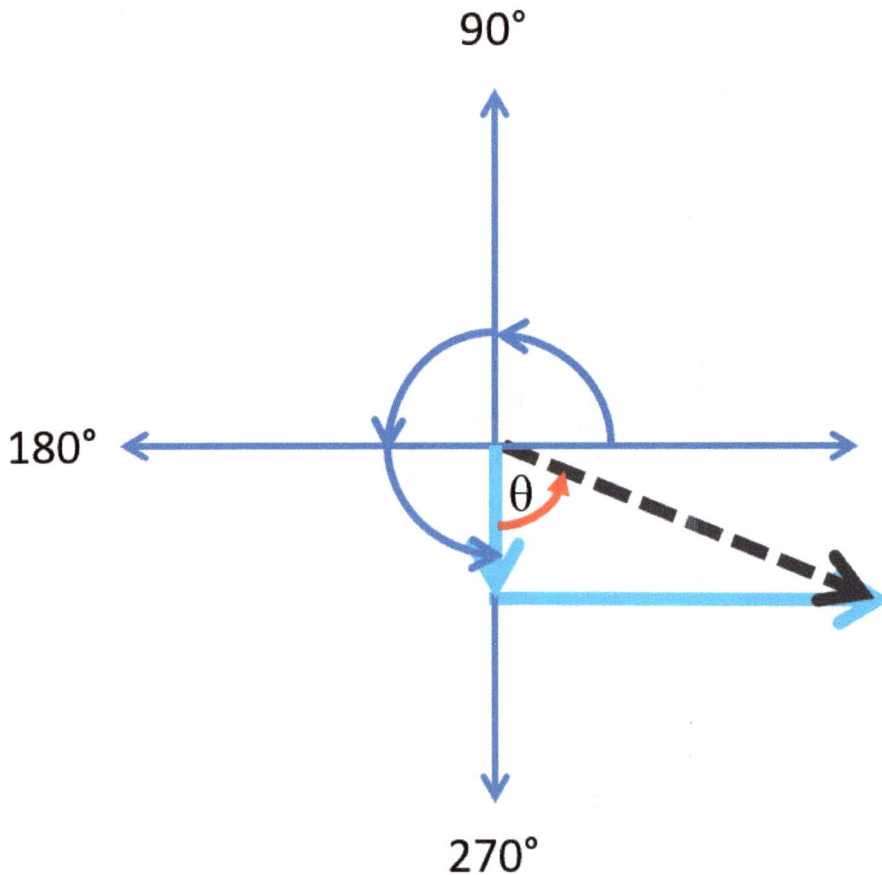

Figure 4.33   Determining final resultant angle.

The final angle is 270 deg + Θ ⇒ 270 deg + 74.46 deg = 344.46 deg.

Therefore, the resultant vector resulting from the addition of the three force vectors is 11.2 N @ 344.46 deg. In step 2, we estimated the final answer to be approximately 10 N @ 330 deg, and while it is not as exact as our computed value, it did give us a reasonable estimate, putting the final vector in the fourth quadrant and helping us feel confident that our computed answer was, in fact, correct. Following this five-step process for solving vector addition problems will allow you to accurately determine the result of any vector addition problem you may encounter.

Summary

Problem Solving

In the past two chapters, a number of different types of problems have been described, and some of the tools used by biomechanists have been presented. Whether specialized equipment is used to measure/record/analyze data related to human movement or stick figures/trigonometry/vectors provide the tools needed to answer our questions, the keys to problem solving are understanding the problem and being able to select the correct tools needed to arrive at the correct solution.

The question to be answered may be qualitative or quantitative, or a combination of both. Solving a problem may require the use of prior knowledge and experience, specialized equipment, the application of mathematics, and collaboration with others. Regardless of how simple or complex the problem is, you must identify the intended outcome. Is it to help an elderly person walk without the fear of falling, determining the velocity of a baseball, or identifying when certain muscles are active when bending over to pick up an object? All are reasonable examples of questions in the field of biomechanics.

Developing and applying the skills necessary to tackle questions about human movement requires effort, but being able to understand more about what it is to be human, with our incredible range of movement possibilities, is well worth the effort!

Example of Problem Solving in Action

A middle-aged woman playing in a local soccer league plants her foot while turning, feels something "pop" in her knee, and falls to the ground in pain (qualitative assessment of the injury indicates the knee is unstable and hurts when use is attempted). After a medical evaluation, it is determined that she has ruptured her ACL (qualitative assessment based on the Lackman test and subsequent MRI, kinematic evaluation).

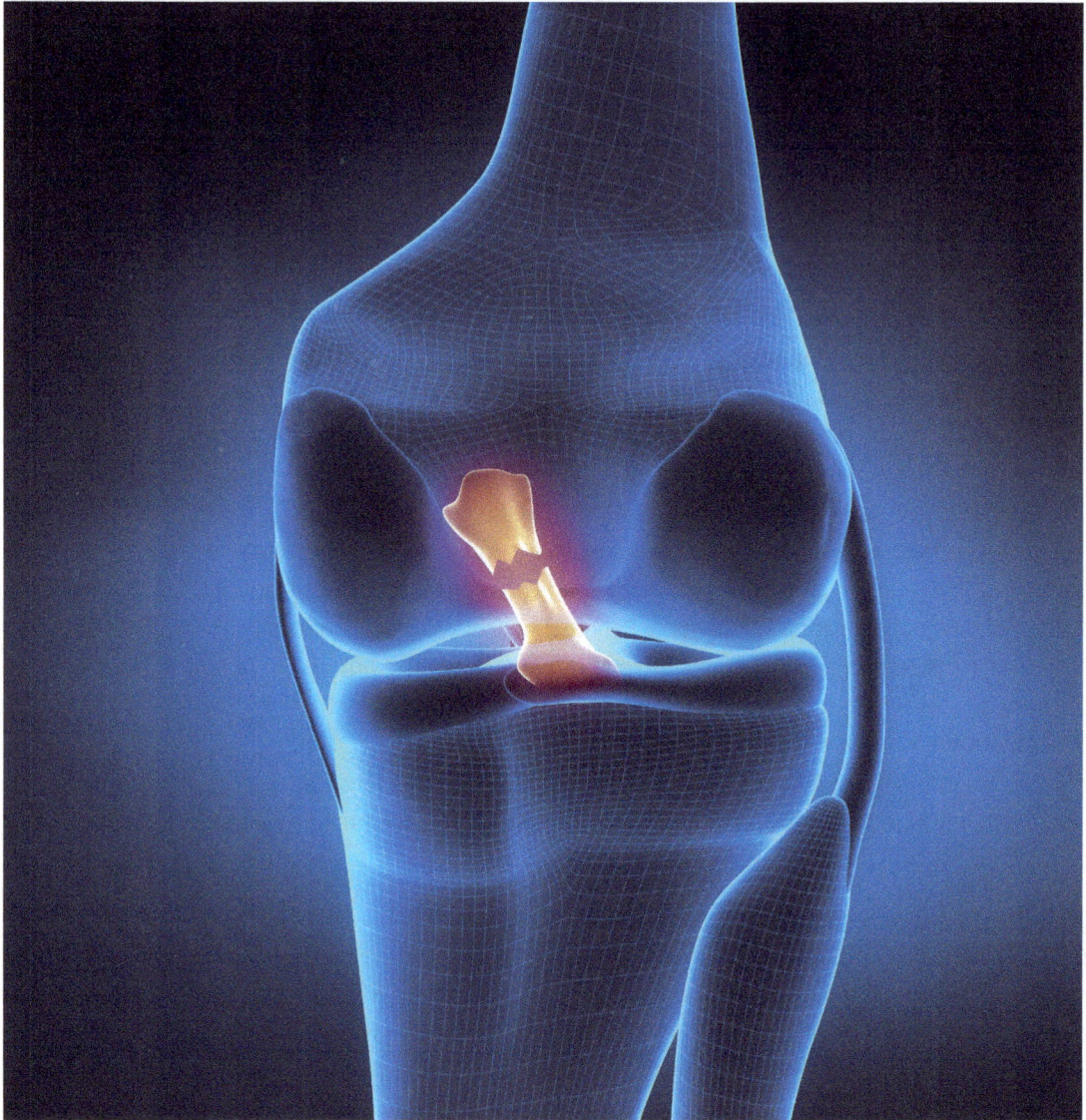

Figure 4.34   ACL tear.

Rehab begins immediately after ACL reconstructive surgery. Baseline data related to range of motion (quantitative kinematic data captured using an electro-goniometer) and flexion/extension strength are recorded (quantitative kinetic data captured using a knee dynamometer). Baseline data indicates a 6-month plan for rehabbing the knee that includes training in balance (qualitative and quantitative self and medical care assessment) and strength training (qualitative and quantitative self and medical care assessment).

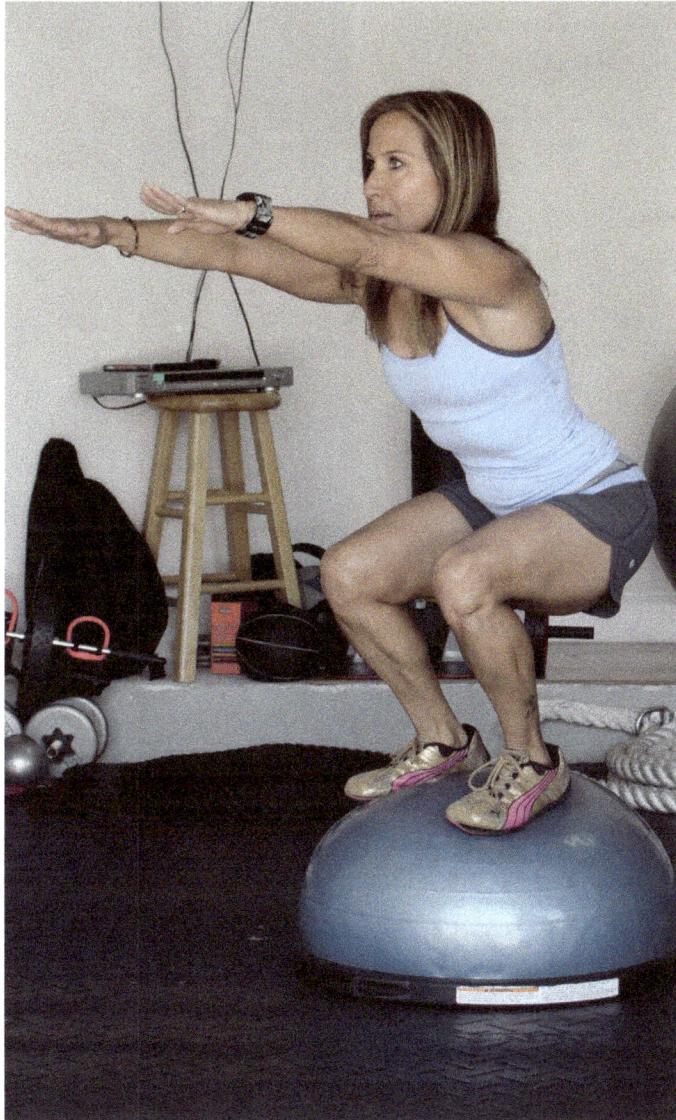

Figure 4.35   Balance training.

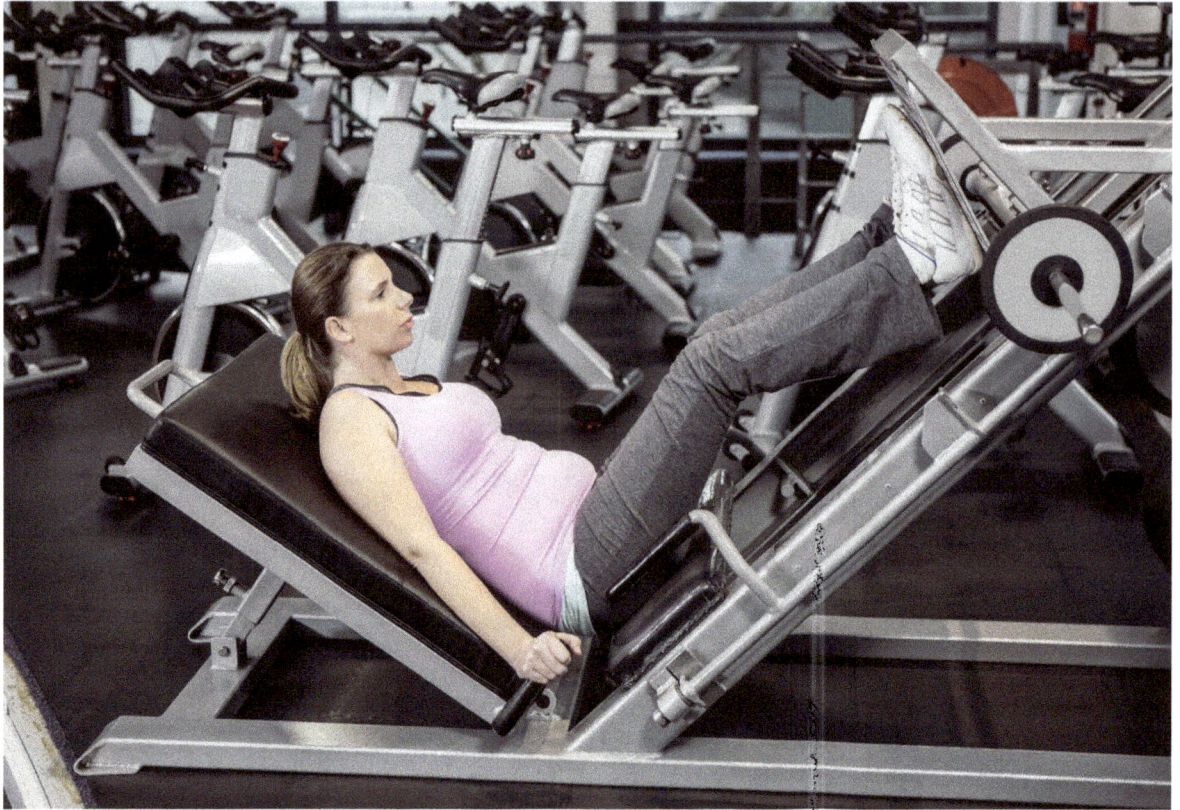

Figure 4.36   Strength training.

At each stage, from injury through the completion of rehab, the human machine is evaluated and given its state of movement potential. Both qualitative and quantitative questions are asked and answered through an understanding of human anatomy, the physics of motion, and an interpretation of the data being recorded. This is a real-world example of the application of biomechanics with the goal to improve performance while assisting a person overcome a significant injury.

List of Key Takeaways

1. The human body can be thought of as a group of motion segments, each comprised of two body segments connected at a joint.
2. Stick figures are line drawings that show body segments and joint locations.
3. Using arrows to depict a vector provides a simple visual way of indicating both the magnitude (size of the arrow) and the direction (where is it pointed) of the vector.
4. Only vectors with similar units can be added together.
5. The tip-to-tale method is a graphical way of adding vectors.
6. By following a standard convention for the directions of vectors, it is possible to follow five steps

to solve any vector addition problem.

Image Credits

Fig. 4.34: Copyright © 2013 Depositphotos/CLIPAREA.
Fig. 4.35: Copyright © by Teran61 (CC BY-SA 3.0) at https://commons.wikimedia.org/wiki/File:Bosu.jpg.
Fig. 4.36: Copyright © 2016 Depositphotos/Wavebreakmedia.

Chapter 5

Linear Kinematics

Preparing to Learn: *Watch*

Movement comes in many forms, but all require both position change and time. When watching the following videos notice the path that both objects and people follow when moving; then think about what the shape of that path tells you. Finally, note that differences in age and health status often result in the adoption of adapted movement patterns to accomplish the desired position changes.

One or more interactive elements has been excluded from this version of the text. You can view them online here: https://pb.cognella.com/83647-1b/?p=51#oembed-4

Please refer to the interactive ebook in Cognella Active Learning for interactive/media content.

One or more interactive elements has been excluded from this version of the text. You can view them online here: https://pb.cognella.com/83647-1b/?p=51#oembed-5

Please refer to the interactive ebook in Cognella Active Learning for interactive/media content.

Preparing to Learn: *Respond*

Directions: Based on what you saw in the video, respond to the following questions:

1. Did you notice different phases of motion related to the actions shown in the videos?
2. What was a similar feature of the beginning of each motion related to how

fast the motion was performed?

3. What was the approximate time needed to accomplish each of the movements?

Introduction to the Chapter

All motion requires that a person, object, or part of a system change their position during a period of observation. Force must be present for motion to occur, but motion can be studied and explained without knowing anything specific about force through the use of kinematics. Kinematics is a way of describing motion through information about time and space in which the motion occurs. The track, or path a motion follows, provides the knowledgeable observer with a great deal of information about the activity.

In this chapter we will introduce the various linear kinematic parameters and equations that allow us to better understand the wide range of position change options for people, objects, and systems. Time is an essential component of motion, and how it is used to determine some of the most useful kinematic parameters will be demonstrated. A variety of examples will be presented to help quantify linear motion for both earth-bound and objects in free fall.

Learning Objectives

After completing this chapter, students should be able to do the following:

- Define linear kinematics
- Know the different scalar and vector parameters commonly associated with linear kinematics
- Know the primary units for each kinematic parameter
- Solve kinematic rectilinear, curvilinear, and projectile problems
- List and describe the path shape of the four types of projectile motion
- Solve any of the four types of projectile motion problems
- Identify the type of activity and predict the likelihood of motion success based on motion paths

Defining Linear Kinematic Variables

Motion, by definition, requires some amount of time to accomplish and a position change that is observable and/or measurable. *Kinematics* encompasses the terms and definitions that allow us to describe the temporal (time) and spatial (position) changes a body experiences during movement.

One or more interactive elements has been excluded from this version of the text. You can view them online here: https://pb.cognella.com/83647-1b/?p=51#oembed-1

Kinematics describes motion by noting changes in position while measuring the time required for the motion. Video technology is an ideal method of recording and analyzing kinematic motion data. The cause (force) of motion is not directly measurable using kinematic techniques.

The temporal part of kinematics is time, and it is a scalar. A scalar is a value that has magnitude but no direction. The basic unit of time is the second. Depending on the situation, seconds can be divided into finer increments such as tenths, hundredths, thousandths, and smaller fractions to best represent the duration of a movement. Time can also be aggregated into larger bundles such as minutes, hours, days, or years.

Table 5.1 **Time Units**

Time Unit	Seconds(s)
Year	31536000
Month (4 weeks)	2419200
Week	604800
Day	86400
Hour	3600
Minute	60
Second	1
Decisecond	0.1
Centisecond	0.01
Millisecond	0.001
Nanosecond	0.000000001

When reporting most dynamic human actions such as striking a ball with a bat, time is represented in seconds or smaller fractions of a second. Longer duration activities such as running a marathon often require the event time to be represented using several units of time, such as hours, minutes, and seconds, to avoid confusion and help people immediately grasp the scale of the time involved.

For example, the first place male finisher of the 2015 Boston Marathon finished the race in 2:09:17, or 2 hours, 9 minutes, and 17 seconds. His amazing feat is easily understood by most runners who are accustomed to having marathon times reported in that fashion. If his winning time was announced as 7,757 seconds, his accomplishment is no less amazing, but few who follow the sport could immediately appreciate where his time "fits" relative to other elite marathoners. Selecting and using the correct units for a variable related to an activity helps clarify what the value means in the context of real-world experiences for someone reading or hearing the value.

When using video to determine the time of a movement, you have several options depending on the type of software you are using. Since video is captured at a constant frame rate, you can use that information to determine the time between each of the individual frames of the video. For example, if the video was captured at 30 fr/s, the time between any two consecutive still images from the video is equal to 1 sec/30 frames, or 0.033 s/fr. If a motion is captured that requires 18 frames of video to show the movement from start to finish, then the time for the movement is 18 frames * 0.033 s/fr = 0.594 s, or just under 6 tenths of a second.

The faster the frame capture rate of the video, the smaller the interval between adjacent images, and the more precise the measurement of time. Video captured at 60 fr/s provides time measurement precision to 0.017 s, 120 fr/s $\Rightarrow$ 0.008 s, and so on.

If the movement being performed or observed results in an object changing position such that its movement path is a straight or curved line, then the movement is *linear*. Linear motion is a type of movement in which the COM of a body tracks along a straight (rectilinear; e.g., a person skateboarding) or curved (curvilinear; e.g., skier cutting back and forth down a hill) path. Linear motion is also sometimes called translational motion. It is possible for a body made up of segments, such as the human body, to perform whole body linear or translational movement of its COM while the segments that make up the body move in a nonlinear fashion (e.g., person cycling]) It is rare that a person performs a true rectilinear or curvilinear movement since for their body to perform such a motion, all of their body segments must move in the same direction at the same rate of speed. Can you think of any examples in which a person performs a true linear movement?

Not all motion is linear, however, and if the motion is the result of one or more levers rotating about an axis, rotational or angular motion is present. Articulation about any of the joints of the human body can be described as angular motion. The flexion and extension that occur during a biceps curl is an example of angular motion, with the upper and lower arms rotating around the joint axis of the elbow (Figure 5.1).

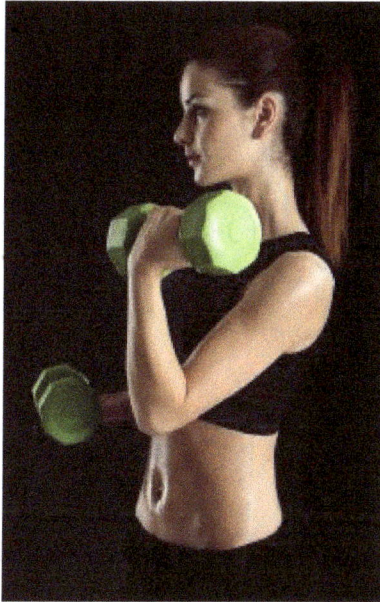

Figure 5.1   Biceps curl, example of angular kinematic motion.

General motion is motion that includes both linear and angular motion. General motion is the most common type of human motion and can be observed in actions such as walking, running, jumping, throwing, and lifting (Figure 5.2).

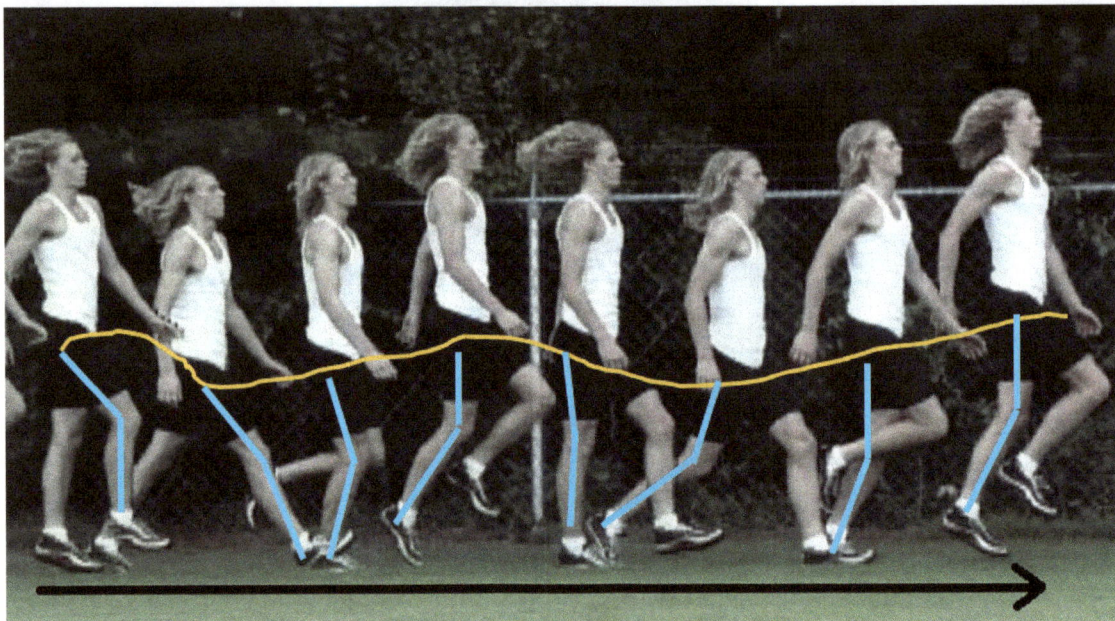

Figure 5.2   General motion, COM motion track during skipping.

The discussion of angular motion will be greatly expanded in the chapters focusing on angular kinematics and angular kinetics.

Distance

When the position of a body changes, the measured length of the position change represents the distance traveled during the movement. Distance (l) is a scalar, possessing magnitude but no direction. Distance can be reported in any units of length, such as mm, cm, m, km, inches, feet, yards, or miles. The accepted standard unit of distance is the meter (m). One meter is equivalent to 39.37 inches. Distance represents the total path length of the movement during a period of observation. At least two distinct points of reference are needed to describe the distance covered during a movement. For example, if you measured the path you followed from your home to your biomechanics class, the result would be a distance that reported in units of length such as meters, kilometers, feet, or miles. Distance encompasses the length of the path of motion regardless of how many twists or turns occurred during the position change (Figure 5.3).

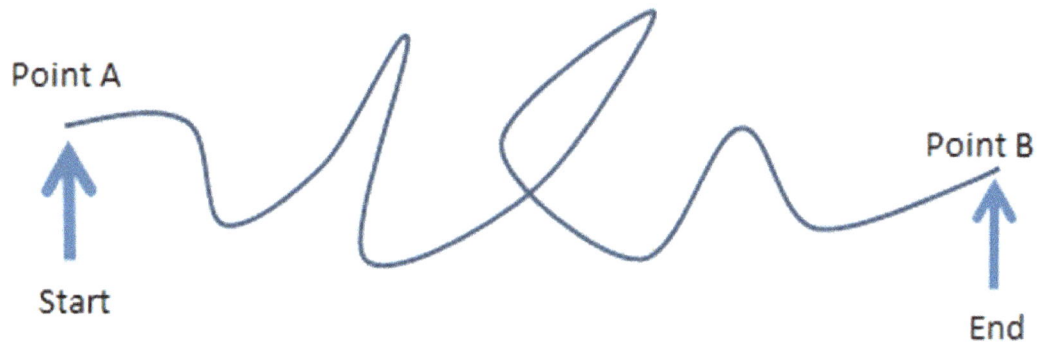

Overhead view of path travelled

Point A

Start

Point B

End

Figure 5.3   Distance, path traveled from point A to point B.

Displacement

The straight line (or rectilinear) distance a body covers during an action is called its displacement. Displacement is a vector. The units of displacement are the same as those of distance: mm, cm, m, km, inches, feet, yards, miles, and so on. The standard unit of displacement is the meter (m).

   The displacement of a movement ignores the actual path a body takes from point A to point B and reports only the straight-line distance between those points. That means that the body does not need to have traveled along that line of displacement during the movement for the displacement value to accurately describe the movement in vector form. In Figure 5.4 the orange line represents the displacement that occurred during the movement. Note that while the displacement arrow crosses the path of motion, it does not follow it. It simply shows where the path started and where it ended. It provides both a magnitude and direction related to the movement that can be used to better understand the motion kinematically.

Overhead view of displacement travelled

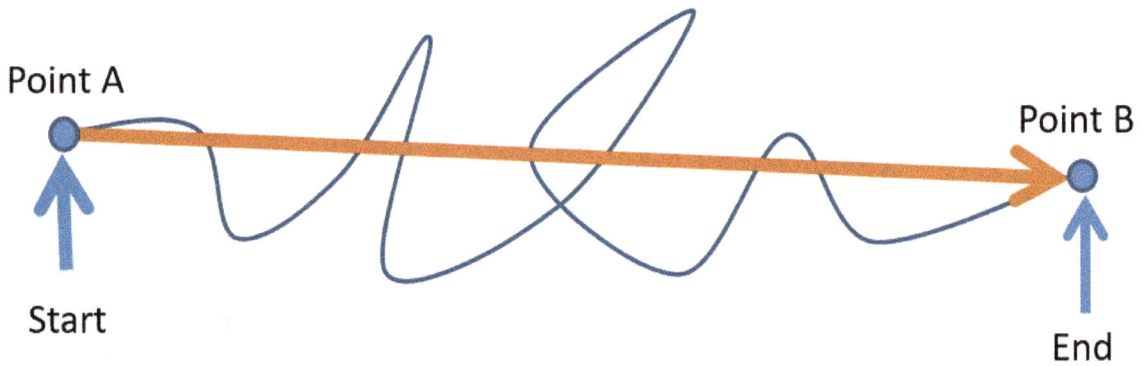

Figure 5.4   Path of displacement versus distance traveled.

Throughout this text we use standard conventions when illustrating and interpreting vectors. As such, 2D information will be graphed on a Cartesian coordinate system (Figure 5.5) with values directed to the right horizontally or up vertically being considered positive (+) and those to the left horizontally or down vertically as negative (-).

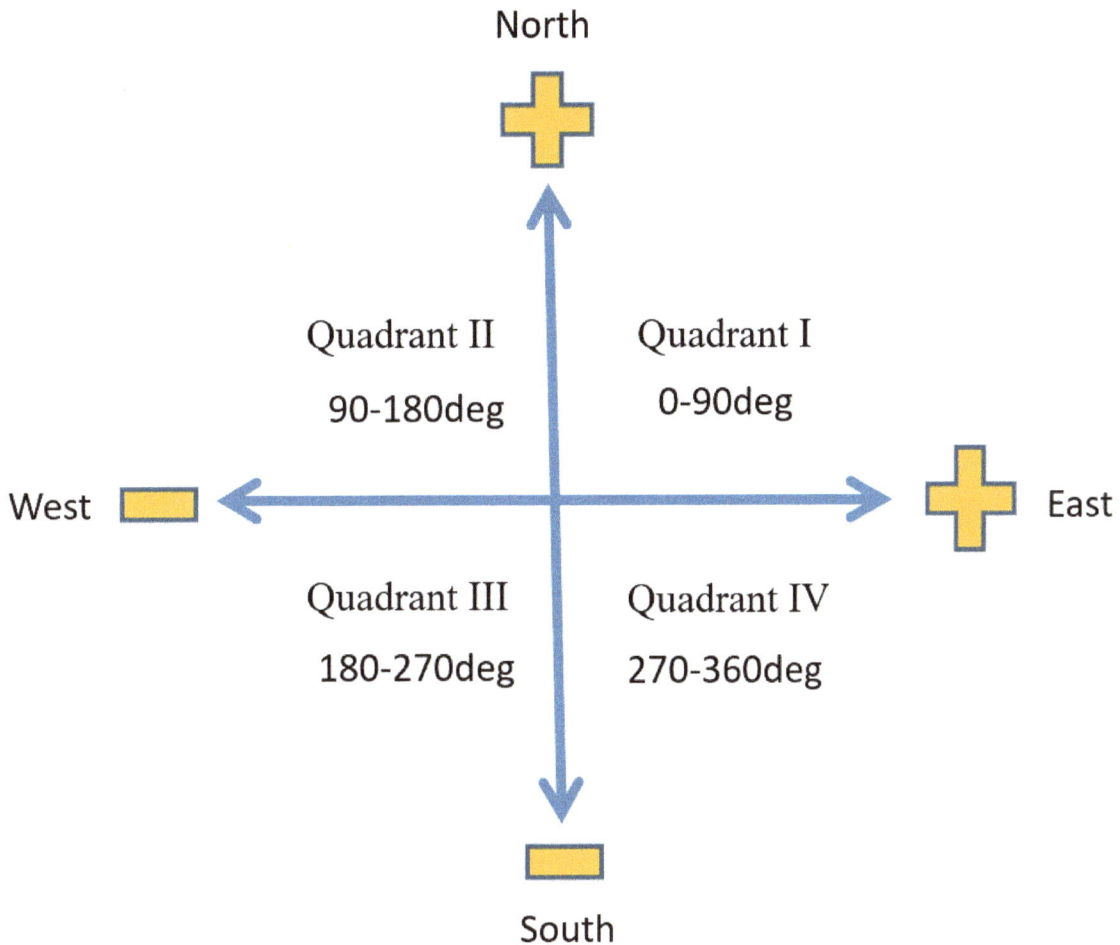

North

Quadrant II
90-180deg

Quadrant I
0-90deg

West

East

Quadrant III
180-270deg

Quadrant IV
270-360deg

South

Figure 5.5   Cartesian coordinate system.

Speed

Speed is the rate of distance covered by an object over a given period of time. Speed is determined by dividing the path length (or distance) traveled by the time it took to accomplish the movement. Speed(s) is a scalar quantity and is calculated as $s = \Delta\text{position} / \Delta\text{time}$. Note that the SI symbol for speed is recommended to be "v"; however, in an attempt to avoid confusion with the character "v" used for velocity we will use the symbol "s" to denote speed in this text. Speed can be correctly reported in units of mm/s, cm/s, m/s, km/s, km/hr, inches/s, feet/s, miles/hr, and so on. The standard acceptable units of speed are m/s. An example of an everyday sensor that calculates speed is the speedometer in a car, which accurately reports the speed of a moving vehicle without regard to the direction of movement.

Speed, and many other kinematic variables, can be determined as an average value for the entire movement or for an interval or instantaneous portion of the movement. The difference is based on the size of the time slice used to determine the resulting speed. For example, the speed of a sprinter in a 100-meter dash could be calculated as an average speed, interval speed, or instantaneous speed during the race.

Average, Interval, and Instantaneous Speed Calculations
100 m race values

Total race time = 10.45 s

10–20 m interval time = 1.21 s

10–10.2 m very small time = 0.033 s

Average race speed = 100 m/10.45 s $\Rightarrow$ 9.57 m/s

Interval speed 10–20m = 10 m/1.21 s $\Rightarrow$ 8.26 m/s

Instantaneous speed 10–10.2 m = 0.2 m/0.033 s $\Rightarrow$ 6.06 m/s

In the case of the speed reported by a bicycle's speedometer, the speed is considered *instantaneous* because it is updated based over a very small time period relative to the total time of the motion. The speed reported by the speedometer is typically updated after each rotation of the tires.

Often the average speed for a long activity is of interest to the observer. The average speed for a longer trip or activity may be calculated based on the total distance traveled divided by the total time of the trip or activity. Here's an average speed example: Driving from Pittsburgh, Pennsylvania, to Atlanta, Georgia, is a trip of 685 miles. If the trip takes the 9 hours and 51 minutes, as estimated by Google Maps, what would the average speed for the trip be?

Average speed = 685 miles /(9 hrs + 51 min)

Average speed = 685 miles / (9 hrs *60 min/hr + 51 min)

Average speed = 685 miles / (591 min)

Average speed = 1.159 miles/min or 1.159 miles/min * 60 min/1hr = 69.54 mph

Here's an interval speed example: During a 60 m race, times were recorded for a runner as they passed each 10-meter interval from 0 to 60 meters. The times are shown in Table 5.2.

Table 5.2 60 m Time and Position Values

Cumulative Time (s)	Interval Time (s)	Interval Start Position (m)	Interval End Position (m)
1.55	1.55	0	10
2.65	1.10	10	20
3.55	0.95	20	30
4.55	1.00	30	40

Table 5.2 60 m Time and Position Values

5.65	1.10	40	50
6.75	1.10	50	60

What was the fastest interval time and where in the race did it occur?

Interval speed = (Interval End Position – Interval Start Position)/Interval Time

Interval speed from 0 to 10 meters = (10 m – 0 m)/1.55 s ⇒ 6.45 m/s

10 to 20 meters = (20 m – 10 m) / 1.10 s ⇒ 9.09 m/s

20 to 30 meters = (30 m – 20 m) / 0.95 s ⇒ 10.53 m/s

Since no interval was covered in less than the 0.95s calculated between the 20- and 30-meter mark, that interval speed of 10.53 m/s represents the fastest interval speed achieved during the race.

Velocity

The vector equivalent of speed is velocity. Velocity contains information of both magnitude and direction of a body over a given time period. The equation for velocity is Velocity = Δdisplacement / Δtime. Velocity can be reported in the same units as speed: mm/s, cm/s, m/s, km/s, km/hr, inches/s, feet/s, miles/hr, and so on. The standard units of velocity are m/s. Often, velocity vectors are decomposed into vertical and horizontal components to assist in understanding what the body does in a given action.

For example, as a NASCAR driver rockets down the back straight away at Talladega speedway, he covers the 0.8-kilometer stretch in 9.12 s. What was his average velocity during that portion of the race?

Velocity = Δdisplacement / Δtime

Velocity = 800 m / 9.12 s

Velocity = 87.72 m/s, or over 196 mph!

From a performance standpoint, what appears to be a small change in velocity may result in a large change in a movement outcome. For example, when analyzing a 7.5 m long-jump performance (a classic projectile, which will be covered in more detail later in this chapter), it may be useful to the coach and athlete to know how close a takeoff velocity was to the athlete's optimal ability. If the takeoff velocity vector was determined to be 8 m/s @ 35 deg, the jumper was moving at 4.56 m/s vertically and at 6.56 m/s horizontally at takeoff. Flight time is based on the vertical component at takeoff, and this jumper will be airborne for 0.928 s. Using that information, the coach and athlete decide to focus on increasing the horizontal velocity component at takeoff.

+1m/s

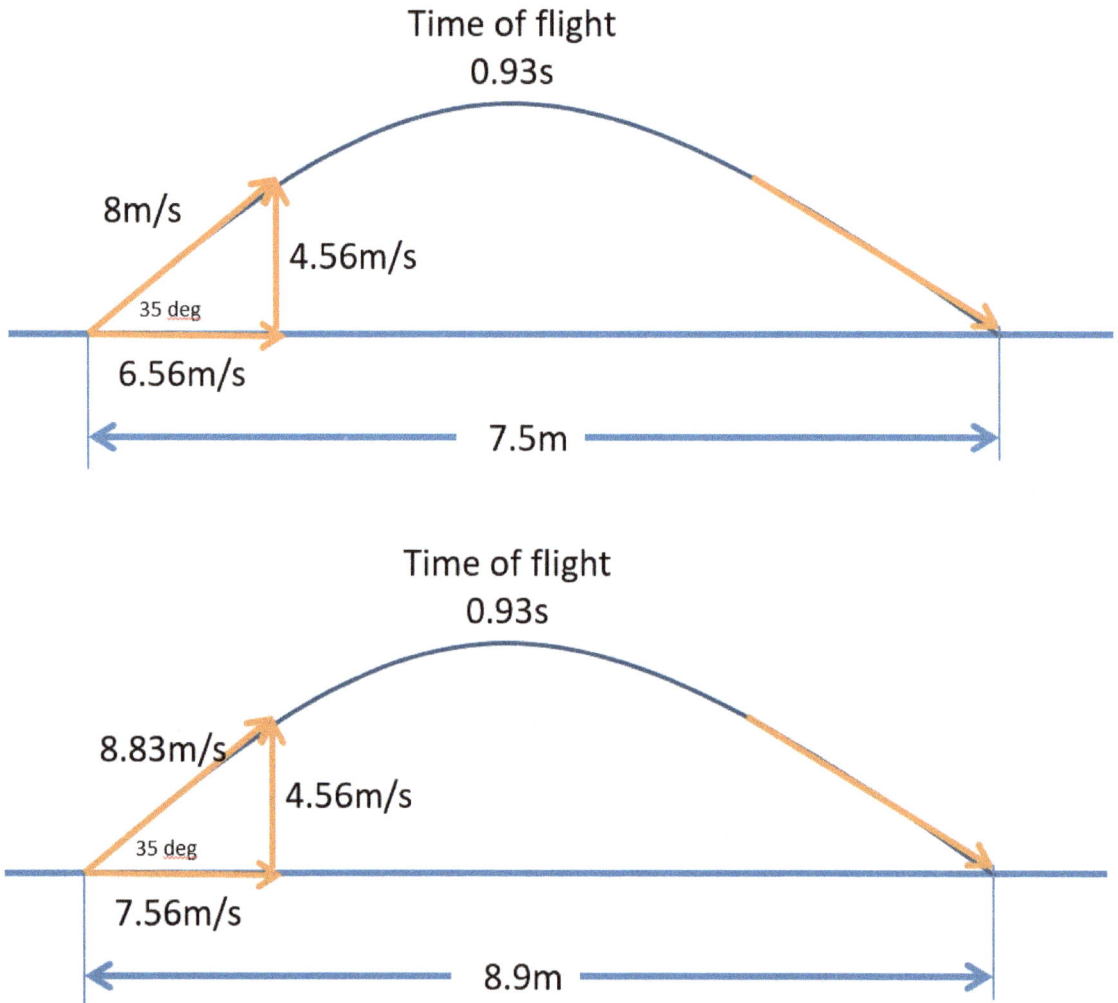

Figure 5.6   Effect of increasing horizontal long jump velocity by 1 m/s.

With no other changes, a 1 m/s increase in horizontal velocity at takeoff would result in a jump of 8.9 m. That difference of 1 m/s in the horizontal velocity changes the jump length from 7.5 m, which was less than the 1901 world record of 7.61 m set by Peter O'Connor of Ireland, to almost matching the current world record of 8.95 m set in 1991 by Mike Powell of the United States (Wikipedia, 2020).

Steps and Strides

One of the easiest ways to determine distance or displacement traveled while walking or running is to determine your average step and stride lengths. *Step length* is defined as the displacement from the toe-off or point of heel strike of the lead foot to the same point of contact of the trailing foot during normal gait.

One or more interactive elements has been excluded from this version of the text. You can view them online here:
https://pb.cognella.com/83647-1b/?p=51#oembed-2

Please refer to the interactive ebook in Cognella Active Learning for interactive/media content.

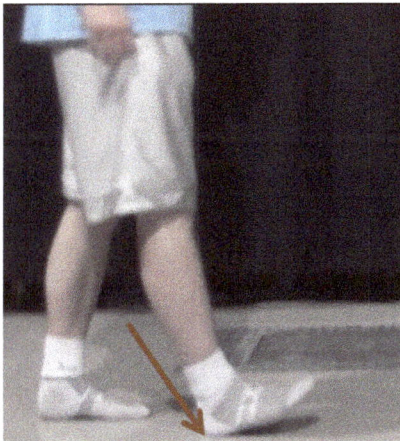

→ → →
Step length based on heel strike

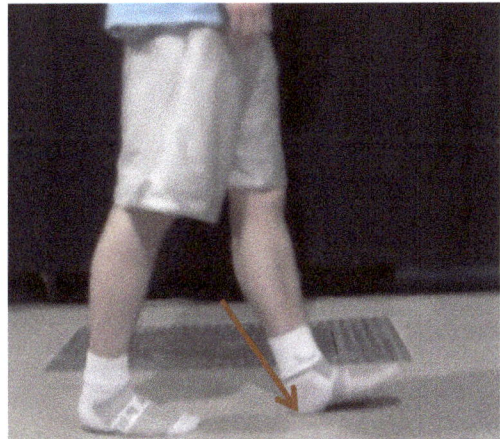

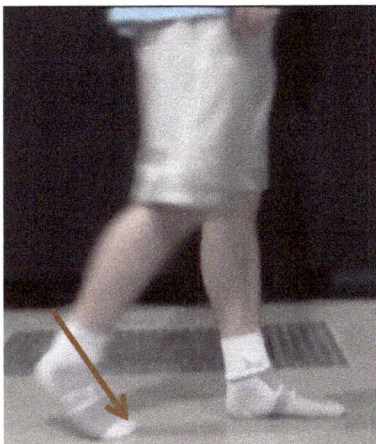

→ → →
Step length based on Toe-off

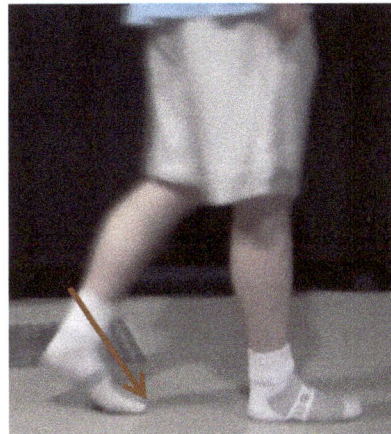

Figure 5.7   Illustration of step length recorded using heel or toe contact.

Stride length, which is always a larger value than step length for the same person, is defined as the displacement between successive ground contact locations of the same part of the same foot during normal gait.

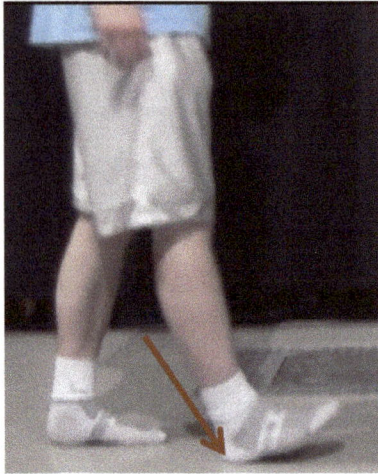

Stride length
based on
heel strike of
the right foot

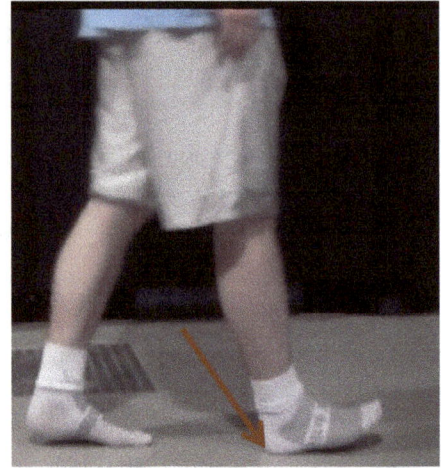

Figure 5.8   Stride length measured using heel strike location.

Step rate and stride rate, as the terms imply, provide information of the number of steps or strides taken over a given time interval, typically 1 second. Step rate = number of steps / Δtime, and stride rate = number of strides / Δtime. Since both steps and strides are measures of length, they are reported in units of meters. That means that both step rate and stride rate have units of m/s.

Example 5.1: What was the running velocity of a jogger with a step rate of 2.6 steps/s if she had a step length of .84 m per step?

Velocity = Step rate * step length

Velocity = 2.6 steps/s * 0.84 m/step

Velocity = 2.18 m/s

Example 5.2: How far did a hiker travel during his 5 hr, 27 min, 43s extreme hike, if his stride length was 1.31 m and stride rate was 1.2 strides/s?

Distance = hiking speed * hiking time

Distance = (stride rate * stride length) * hiking time

Distance = (1.2 strides/s * 1.31 m/stride) * (5 hr * 3,600 s/hr + 27 min * 60 s / min + 43 s)

Distance = 1.572 m/s * 19663 s

Distance = 30,910.24 m, or 30.91 km

Acceleration

When an object increases or decreases its velocity, acceleration occurs. Acceleration is based on a change in velocity over time. The equation for acceleration is Acceleration = Δvelocity / Δtime. Units for acceleration are mm/s^2, cm/s^2, m/s^2, $inches/s^2$, $feet/s^2$, and so on. The standard units are m/s^2. Acceleration is a vector. The most common acceleration we are exposed to is gravity, which has a value of -9.81 m/s^2. For objects close to the surface of the earth, gravity can be considered a constant. The negative sign indicates that gravity always acts in a downward direction. The acceleration of gravity is always assumed to act directly through an object's COM.

Acceleration is unique in that it does not have a scalar partner of similar magnitude such as the relationship that distance and speed have to displacement and velocity. Some argue that "slowing down" or "speeding up" is the scalar partner of acceleration, but those terms will not be used for describing a "scalar equivalent of acceleration" in this text.

Another unique attribute to acceleration is that it does not always conform to our conventions for determining the direction of vectors, as shown in Figure 5.5. The expanded equation for acceleration is acceleration = $(V_{final} - V_{initial}) / (t_{final} - t_{initial})$. Accelerations can be tricky since the direction of motion does not, in itself, provide you with the sign (+ or -) of the acceleration.

For example, an object that is increasing velocity while moving in a positive direction results in a positive (+) acceleration. If the same object, still moving in a positive direction, decreases in velocity, it experiences a negative (-) acceleration.

How It Works

A slap shot in a junior hockey league contest results in a stationary puck changing its velocity from 0 m/s to 27.4 m/s in 0.21 s. If the direction of the puck was right horizontal or 0 degrees, what is the acceleration experienced by the puck?

Acceleration = $(V_{final} - V_{initial}) / (t_{final} - t_{initial})$

Acceleration = (27.4 m/s − 0 m/s) / (0.21 s − 0.0s)

Acceleration = + 130.48 m/s^2

If the exact same shot was taken in the opposite direction (180 degrees), which would be in a negative (-) direction according to the motion graphed on a Cartesian coordinate grid, the resulting acceleration would be as follows:

Acceleration = $(V_{final} - V_{initial}) / (t_{final} - t_{initial})$

Acceleration = (-27.4 m/s − 0 m/s) / (0.21 s − 0.0 s)

Acceleration = -130.48 m/s^2

The puck shot at 0 degrees decreases in velocity from 27.4 m/s to 20 m/s over 1.14 s as it slides across the ice. The resulting acceleration of the puck moving in a positive (+) direction would be as follows:

Acceleration = $(V_{final} - V_{initial}) / (t_{final} - t_{initial})$

Acceleration = $(20.0 /s - 27.4 m/s) / (1.14s - 0.0 s)$

Acceleration = $-6.49 m/s^2$

The puck shot at 180 degrees decreases in velocity from -27.4 m/s to -20 m/s over 1.14 s as it slides across the ice. The resulting acceleration of the puck moving in a negative (-) direction would be as follows:

Acceleration = $(V_{final} - V_{initial}) / (t_{final} - t_{initial})$

Acceleration = $(-20.0 /s - -27.4 m/s) / (1.14 s - 0.0 s)$

Acceleration = $+6.49 m/s^2$

Projectile Motion

A good way to learn about the interactions between kinematic variables is to study projectile motion. For this discussion, we will define projectiles as objects that take off and fly for relatively short distances close to the surface of the earth. Projectiles are nonpowered, meaning that they have no internal or external means of propulsion after becoming airborne. Projectiles are objects in freefall, only affected by gravity and air resistance. Examples of projectiles are the many types of sport objects, such as balls, pucks, arrows, flying discs, or javelins while in flight. People also act as projectiles by launching themselves into space when jumping for a rebound in basketball, sailing above a half pipe on their snowboard, or hopping from one roof top to another during a parkour run.

There are several terms you should know that will be useful in correctly describing and understanding projectiles. The path that a projectile follows during its flight is called the *trajectory*. Each projectile must have a *takeoff point*, which is the point at which the object leaves contact with the ground or the object such as a bat or racket that launches the projectile. All projectiles end their flight at a *landing point*. At some point during the trajectory of each projectile, the object reaches its highest point relative to its takeoff point, called the *apex*. Projectiles may change position vertically, horizontally, or both during their flight. Change in vertical position is referred to as *instantaneous height or vertical displacement* as it is measured in a straight line from the location of the projectile up or down to a reference plane, most often the ground. The *apex height* is a special instantaneous height that indicates the vertical displacement from the level of takeoff to the apex of the flight. The measurement of the horizontal displacement of a projectile related to a reference plane as the result of its flight is called the *range or horizontal displacement* of the projectile.

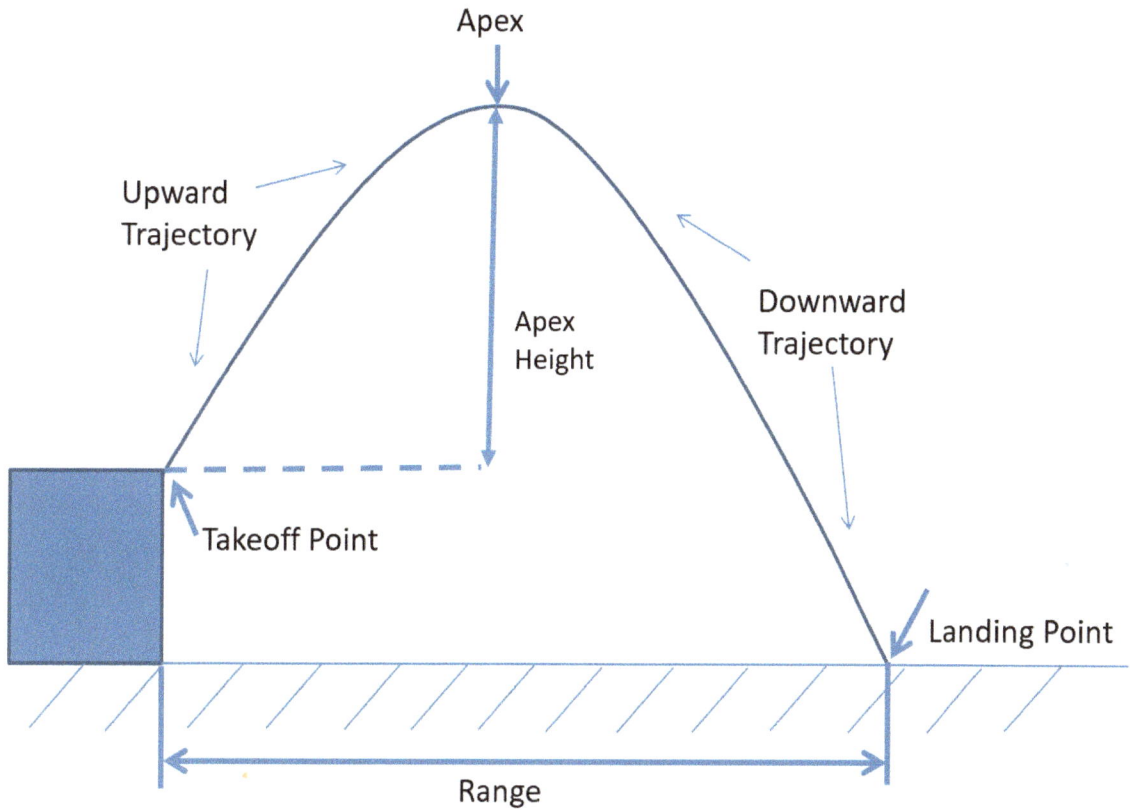

Figure 5.9   Projectile motion diagram and terms.

The flight of a projectile can be accurately predicted if the *takeoff angle*, *takeoff height* relative to landing height, and *takeoff speed* are known. Often, a takeoff velocity is provided or can be determined for a projectile. A *takeoff velocity* combines both the takeoff angle and takeoff speed in a single term, so the only other value needed is the takeoff height to calculate a projectile's flight. Note that most projectiles contain both an upward and downward phase of flight. The upward phase of flight ends at the apex of the trajectory, which in turn signals the beginning of the downward phase of the projectile's trajectory.

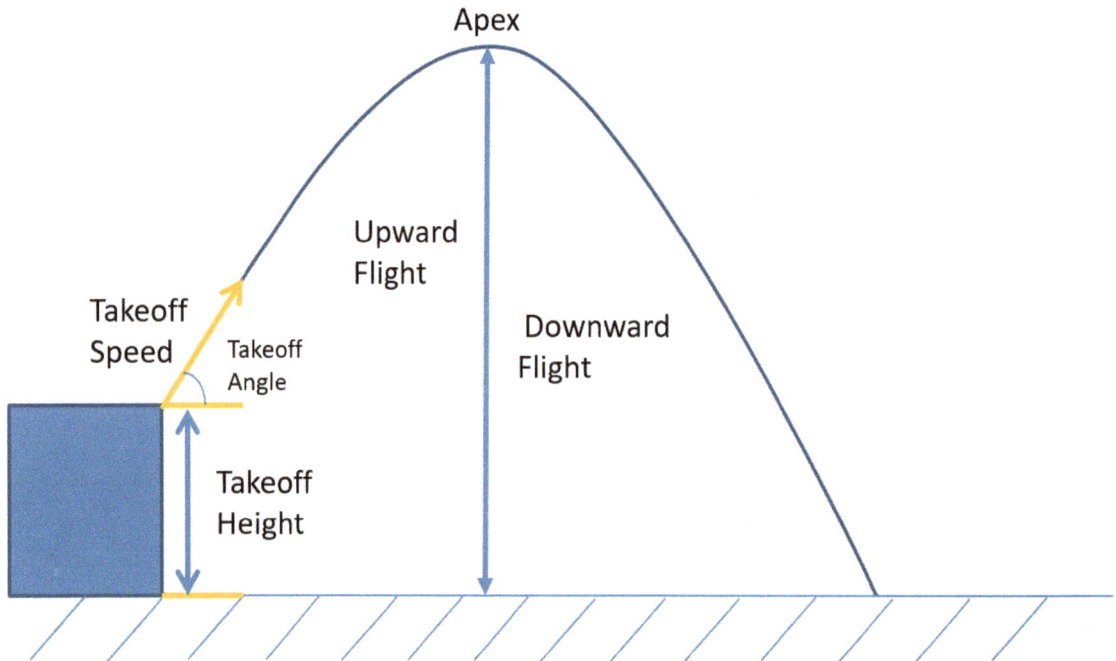

Figure 5.10   Projectile takeoff parameters and flight phases.

All projectiles can be placed into one of four categories of motion. It is of great benefit to those solving projectile motion problems to be able to correctly categorize the type of projectile motion that they are dealing with. Each of the categories provides a variety of known projectile relationships that can greatly reduce the time needed to solve the problems and ensure that the outcomes match real-world results.

The four categories of projectiles are vertical, horizontal, classic, and general. Each of the categories represents a particular trajectory associated with the flight of the projectile.

One or more interactive elements has been excluded from this version of the text. You can view them online here:
https://pb.cognella.com/83647-1b/?p=51#oembed-3

Please refer to the interactive ebook in Cognella Active Learning for interactive/media content.

Vertical Projectile

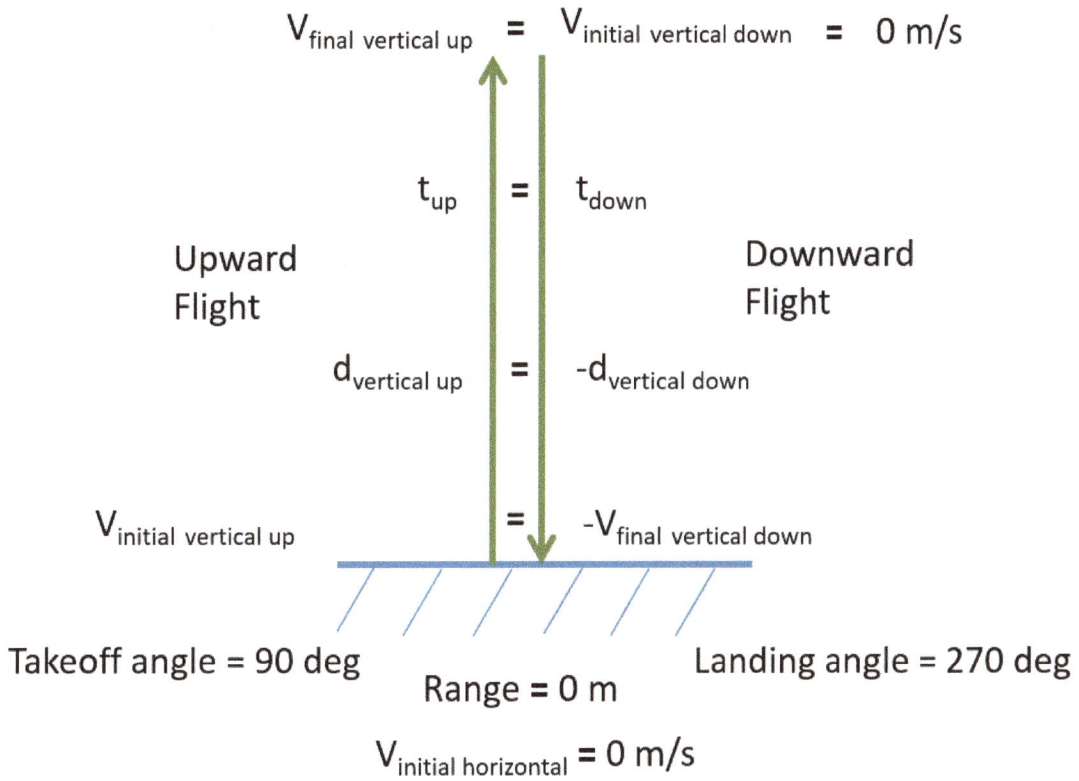

$V_{\text{final vertical up}}$ = $V_{\text{initial vertical down}}$ = 0 m/s

t_{up} = t_{down}

Upward Flight   **Downward Flight**

$d_{\text{vertical up}}$ = $-d_{\text{vertical down}}$

$V_{\text{initial vertical up}}$ = $-V_{\text{final vertical down}}$

Takeoff angle = 90 deg   Landing angle = 270 deg

Range = 0 m

$V_{\text{initial horizontal}}$ = 0 m/s

Horizontal Projectile

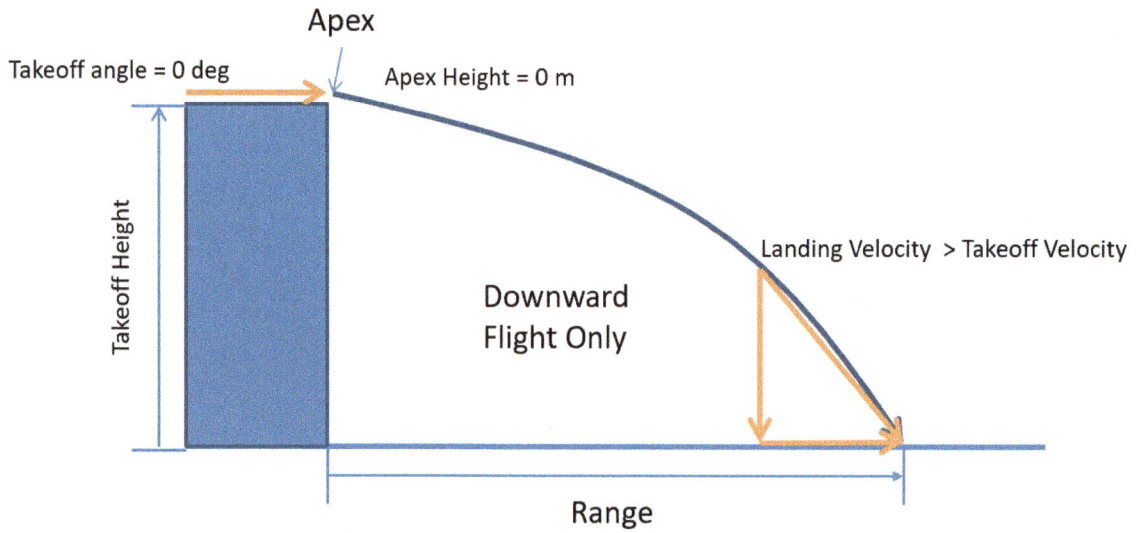

Apex

Takeoff angle = 0 deg

Apex Height = 0 m

Takeoff Height

Landing Velocity > Takeoff Velocity

Downward Flight Only

Range

Classic Projectile

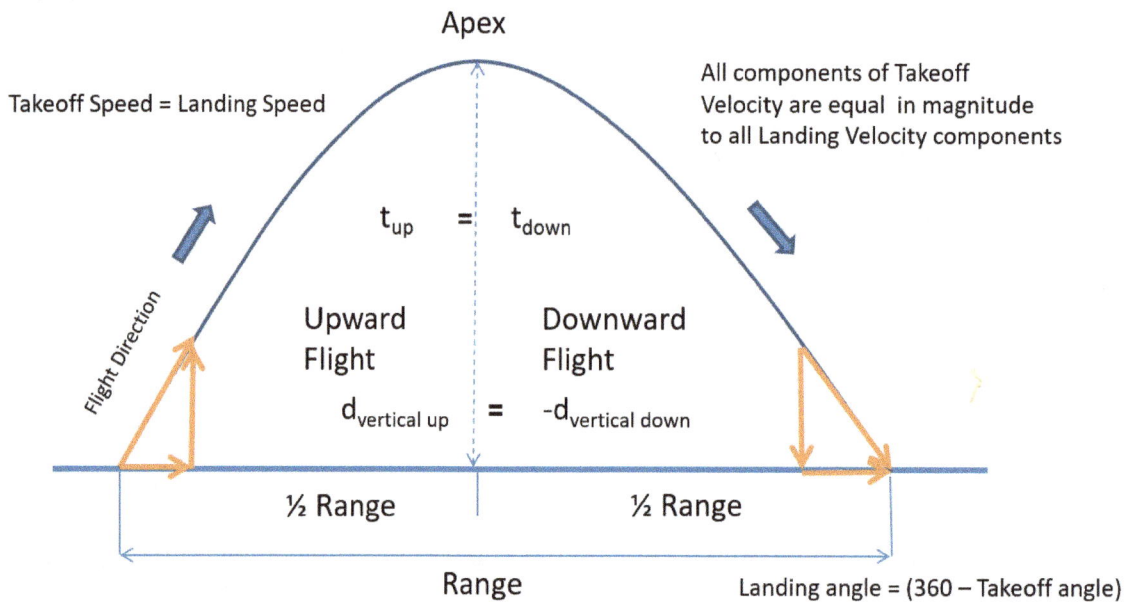

Apex

Takeoff Speed = Landing Speed

All components of Takeoff Velocity are equal in magnitude to all Landing Velocity components

t_{up} = t_{down}

Flight Direction

Upward Flight

Downward Flight

$d_{vertical\ up}$ = $-d_{vertical\ down}$

½ Range

½ Range

Range

Landing angle = (360 – Takeoff angle)

General Projectiles

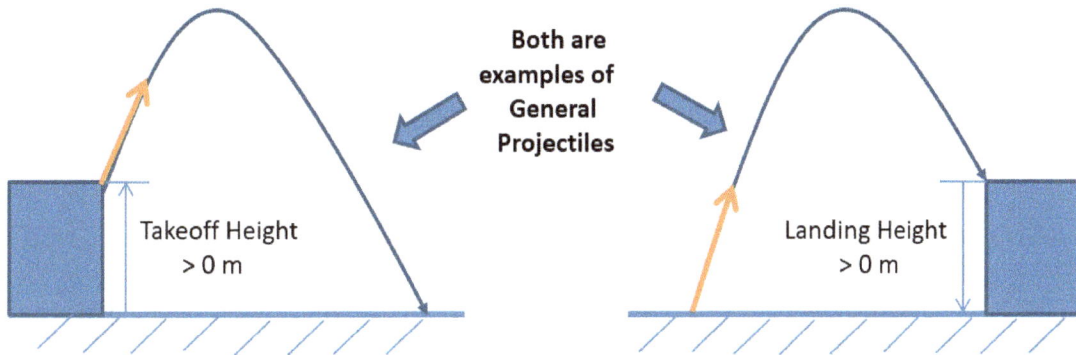

Both are examples of General Projectiles

Takeoff Height
> 0 m

Landing Height
> 0 m

Figure 5.11   Annotated diagrams of each of the four types of projectiles.

Can you identify the type of projectile seen in the following video clip?

One or more interactive elements has been excluded from this version of the text. You can view them online here:
https://pb.cognella.com/83647-1b/?p=51#oembed-6
Please refer to the interactive ebook in Cognella Active Learning for interactive/media content.

It is a horizontal projectile. The motorcycle takes off at an angle of approximately zero degrees so it has no upward phase of flight but does have a downward phase of flight and a range greater than zero.

For many short-duration, close-to-earth projectile events, it is possible to simplify our analysis and the mathematics used to describe the motions if the effect of air resistance is ignored. This assumption does not significantly change the difference between real-world findings and mathematical predictions for many human-powered projectile activities. Sir Isaac Newton initially made the assumption of zero air resistance when studying projectiles. As a result, he was able to establish a group of equations that could be used to accurately predict the flight and landing characteristics of projectiles. Newton called his equations "equations of constant acceleration" because all of the accelerations used were equal to the gravitational acceleration constant of -9.81m/s^2. The equations of constant acceleration for projectiles assuming zero air resistance are as follows:

$$V_{Final} = V_{Initial} + at \qquad d = V_{Initial}t + 1/2\ at^2 \qquad V_{Final}^2 = V_{Initial}^2 + 2ad$$

where V_{Final} and $V_{Initial}$ are vertical or horizontal components of projectile velocity during the upward or downward phase of flight; "d" is the horizontal or vertical displacement of a projectile; and "a" represents the constant acceleration of gravity. Note that when using the equations, you must keep the direction of the values constant within an equation. That is, if you use the equation: $d = V_{Initial}t + 1/2at^2$, use the same directional terms for all variables. If you use the "d" equation to determine the vertical displacement to the apex of a trajectory, $V_{Initial}$ represents the initial vertical component of the takeoff velocity. If you use the "d" equation to determine horizontal displacement (range), $V_{Initial}$ represents the initial horizontal component of the takeoff velocity. This pattern must be followed when using any of the equations of constant acceleration.

All projectile problems can be solved following essentially the same series of steps. (Hint: Solve the problem in the direction of the motion, that is, from takeoff to landing.)

1. Draw a diagram of the motion of the projectile and determine the category of motion that it represents.
2. Determine the takeoff vertical and horizontal components of motion.
3. Label your diagram with all known information.
4. Determine the time up of the flight, which is the time from takeoff to the point the object reaches the apex of the trajectory.
5. Determine the vertical displacement from takeoff to the apex.
6. Determine the vertical displacement down from the apex to the landing height.
7. Calculate the time down from the apex to the landing point.
8. Determine the range the projectile travels.
9. Calculate the landing values of landing angle, the magnitude of the landing velocity, and final vertical and final horizontal components of velocity.

Projectile Motion Example

If a world-class athlete jumped straight up with a vertical takeoff speed of 4.5 m/s what could be determined about his projectile motion?

1. Diagram the movement:

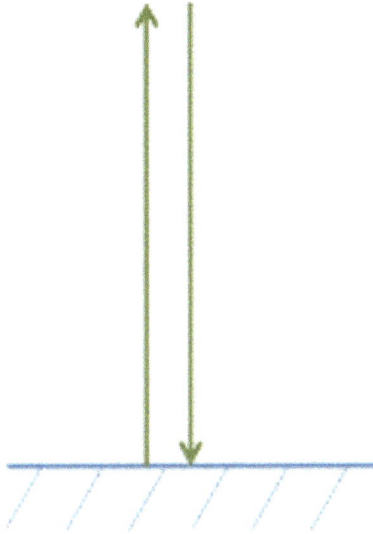

Image 5.1

Based on the diagram we are talking about a vertical projectile.

2. Mathematically: The vertical component of takeoff is $V_{Initial\ Vertical} = \sin(90) * 4.5$ m/s $\Rightarrow + 4.5$ m/ s

The horizontal component at takeoff is $V_{Initial\ Horizontal} = \cos(90) * 4.5$ m/s $\Rightarrow 0.0$ m/s

3. Graphically: Since we know the motion was straight up, all of the velocity was directed up vertically, and the magnitude was given as 4.5 m/s. Since there was no horizontal motion, the value of the horizontal component at takeoff was 0.0 m/s. These values are known because it is a vertical projectile. Label your diagram:

Vertical Projectile

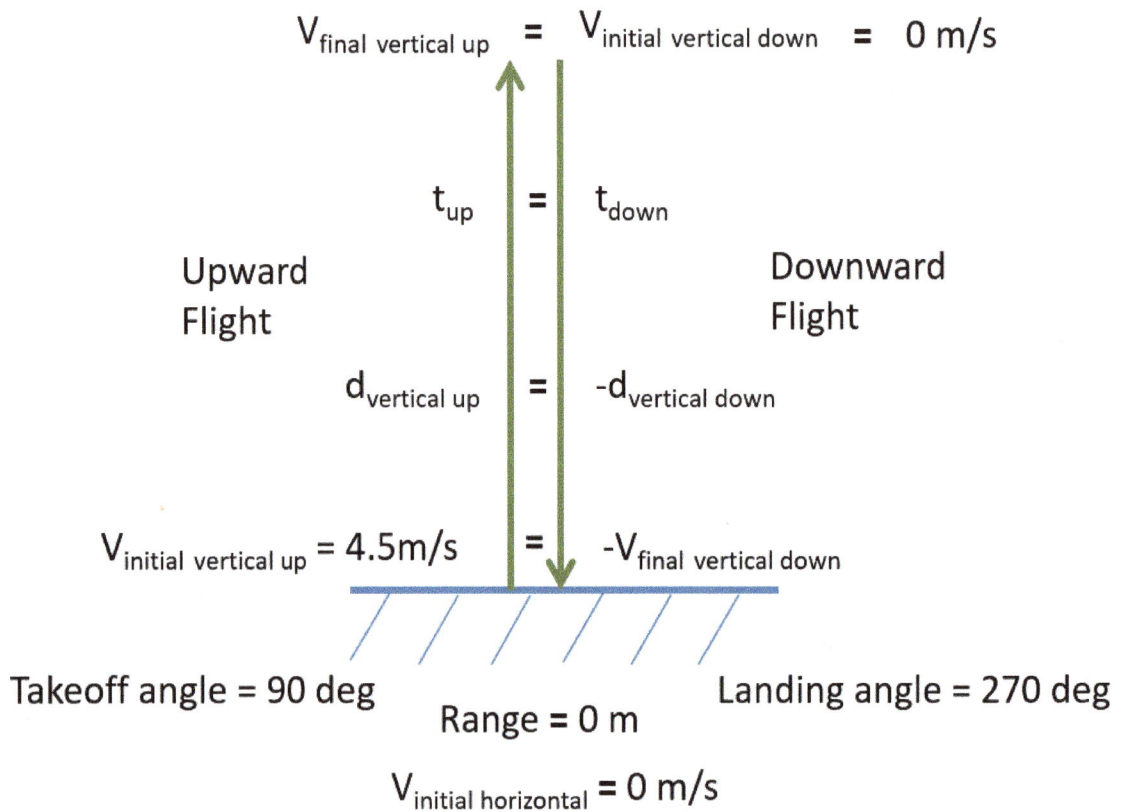

$V_{\text{final vertical up}}$ = $V_{\text{initial vertical down}}$ = 0 m/s

t_{up} = t_{down}

Upward Flight

Downward Flight

$d_{\text{vertical up}}$ = $-d_{\text{vertical down}}$

$V_{\text{initial vertical up}}$ = 4.5m/s = $-V_{\text{final vertical down}}$

Takeoff angle = 90 deg

Landing angle = 270 deg

Range = 0 m

$V_{\text{initial horizontal}}$ = 0 m/s

Image 5.2

4. Time up:

$V_{Final} = V_{Initial} + at$

$0 \text{ m/s} = 4.5 \text{ m/s} + (-9.81 \text{ m/s}^2) * t_{up}$

$-4.5\text{m/s} = (-9.81 \text{ m/s}^2) * t_{up}$

$(-4.5\text{m/s}) / (-9.81 \text{ m/s}^2) = t_{up}$

$0.46\text{s} = t_{up}$

5. Vertical displacement to the apex:

$$d_{\text{vertical to apex}} = V_{\text{Initial vertical up}} \cdot t_{up} + 1/2\ at_{up}^2$$

$$d_{\text{vertical to apex}} = (4.5\ \text{m/s} \cdot 0.46\ \text{s}) + \tfrac{1}{2}\ (-9.81\ \text{m/s}^2 * (0.46\ \text{s})^2)$$

$$d_{\text{vertical to apex}} = 1.04\ \text{m}$$

6. Vertical displacement down to the ground:

Since vertical displacement up equals negative vertical displacement down for vertical projectiles, then

vertical displacement down = -1.04 m.

7. Since time up equals time down for vertical projectiles, then t_{down} = 0.46s. (Remember that time is a scalar and always a positive number.)
8. Since there is no horizontal velocity associated with a vertical projectile, range = 0 m.
9. For a vertical projectile, the following is true for its landing parameters:

Landing angle = 270 deg (The body is traveling straight down at landing)

$$V_{\text{Final Vertical at Landing}} = -V_{\text{Vertical Initial at Takeoff}}$$

$$V_{\text{Final Vertical at Landing}} = -4.5\ \text{m/s}$$

Note on scalars and vectors: Any value that is calculated using only scalar terms will itself be a scalar. If any of the terms used to calculate a value are vectors, then the resulting term will also be a vector.

Table 5.3 Linear Kinematic Variables and Their Units

Variable Equation and Symbol	Units	Vector or Scalar	Comments
Distance (l) = path length	Meters (m)	Scalar	
Displacement (d) = straight-line distance from point A to point B	Meters (m)	Vector	
Speed(s) = Δdistance / Δtime	Meters/sec (m/s)	Scalar	
Velocity (v) = Δdisplacement / Δtime	Meters/sec (m/s)	Vector	

Acceleration (a) = Δvelocity / Δtime	Meters/sec/sec (m/s^2)	Vector	
$V_{Final} = V_{Initial} + at$			For use with constant acceleration projectiles only
$d = V_{Initial}t + 1/2at^2$			For use with constant acceleration projectiles only
$V_{Final}^2 = V_{Initial}^2 + 2ad$			For use with constant acceleration projectiles only

Summary

- Kinematics is the description of motion based on time and position change information. Kinematic parameters often come in scalar and vector pairs, such as distance and displacement and speed and velocity. Force is not factored into kinematic equations used to describe motion.
- An important category of kinematic problems is projectile motion. Projectiles represent the motion of a body in freefall, only affected by air resistance and the pull of gravity. Equations of constant acceleration, which assume no air resistance, have been identified to accurately predict the time, displacement, velocity, and acceleration of projectile motion.
- Being able to correctly identify the type of projectile (vertical, horizontal, classic, or general), based on takeoff values of speed, angle, and height, and its subsequent trajectory, greatly reduces the amount of work needed to solve a projectile problem.

Think of It This Way: Projectile Motion Example

There are limits to the amount of vertical velocity a person can generate and the time they can stay airborne as a projectile when jumping. Once those values are known you can use that knowledge to quickly check your calculations to see if your answers fall within the possible range of human performance.

Since a vertical jump of approximately 1 meter is considered an elite performance, we know that 1 meter is about the maximum a human can project themselves into the air. The total time a person can stay in the air is about 1 second (flight time = $t_{up} + t_{down}$ or 0.46s + 0.46s = 0.92s). Also, we know that the maximum vertical velocity a person can generate is about +4.5 m/s.

Being able to draw a simple diagram of the motion path of an object under observation often provides the problem solver with important visual information regarding the success or failure of the motion (Figure 5.12). Additionally, a good drawing provides confirmation of the values calculated using the various linear kinematic equations presented in this chapter.

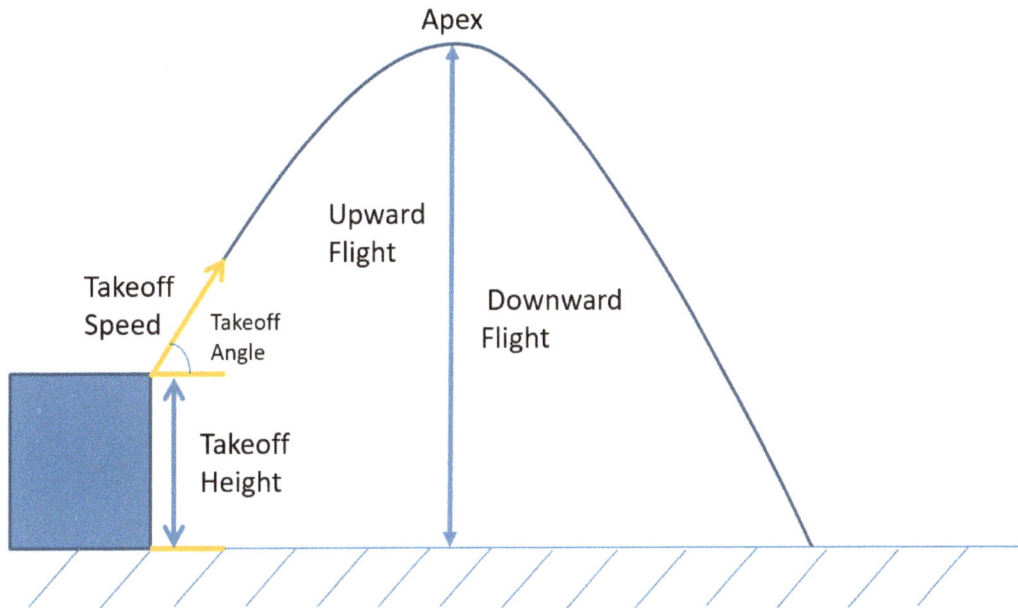

Figure 5.12   Motion path of an object.

Such a drawing immediately indicates you are working with a general projectile that takes off at a height above its landing height and has a time down greater than the time up and a landing speed greater than its takeoff speed. It also indicates that the final vertical velocity at landing is greater than the initial vertical velocity at takeoff and that the range is greater than zero!

List of Key Takeaways

The formulas and units of kinematic parameters, such as distance, displacement, speed, velocity, and acceleration, provide us with tools to solve problems and understand the relationship an object has to position change and time as it moves.

When attempting to solve a kinematic problem, it is important to take the time to draw the movement path followed by an object. Being able to draw simple diagrams of object motion is a way of proving you know what the motion looked like. An accurate diagram of motion can also quickly lead you to identify the category of the motion and which equations should be used to solve questions related to the motion.

References

Wikipedia. (202, November 23). Long jump world record progression. https://en.wikipedia.org/wiki/
Long_jump_world_record_progression

Image Credits

Fig. 5.1: Copyright © 2012 Depositphotos/sumners.

Chapter 6

Angular Kinematics

Preparing to Learn: *Watch*

Angular motion is found within almost every type of human movement. From crawling to walking, to running, and jumping, the complex motions that we perform every day require the transformation of angular movements into linear outcomes. The following videos will provide a small sample of how complex linear motion is linked to an angular event that can be described and better understood through the tools associated with angular kinematics.

One or more interactive elements has been excluded from this version of the text. You can view them online here: https://pb.cognella.com/83647-1b/?p=53#oembed-10
Please refer to the interactive ebook in Cognella Active Learning for interactive/media content.

See Video: Down a Ramp in a Wheelie: SCI Empowerment Project Wheelchair Skills Video 10 at: https://www.youtube.com/watch?v=kv0rnb-eAOE

Preparing to Learn: *Respond*

Directions: Based on what you saw in the videos, respond to the following questions:

1. Did body position change the rate of rotation for the Simon's flips, twists, and summersaults?
2. Why do a wheelie down a ramp in a wheelchair? Why might it be safer than the normal four-wheel contact associated with wheelchair use?

Introduction to the Chapter

Angular motion often is present during the linear motion of a body or its segments. Angular motion is the result of one, two, or more levers rotating about an axis. The human knee, a hinge joint, is a perfect example of a system that may generate purely angular motion, such as as when performing leg extension (Figure 6.1) exercises on a weight bench, or a combination of angular and linear motion, such as during leg flexion (Figure 6.2) during a squat.

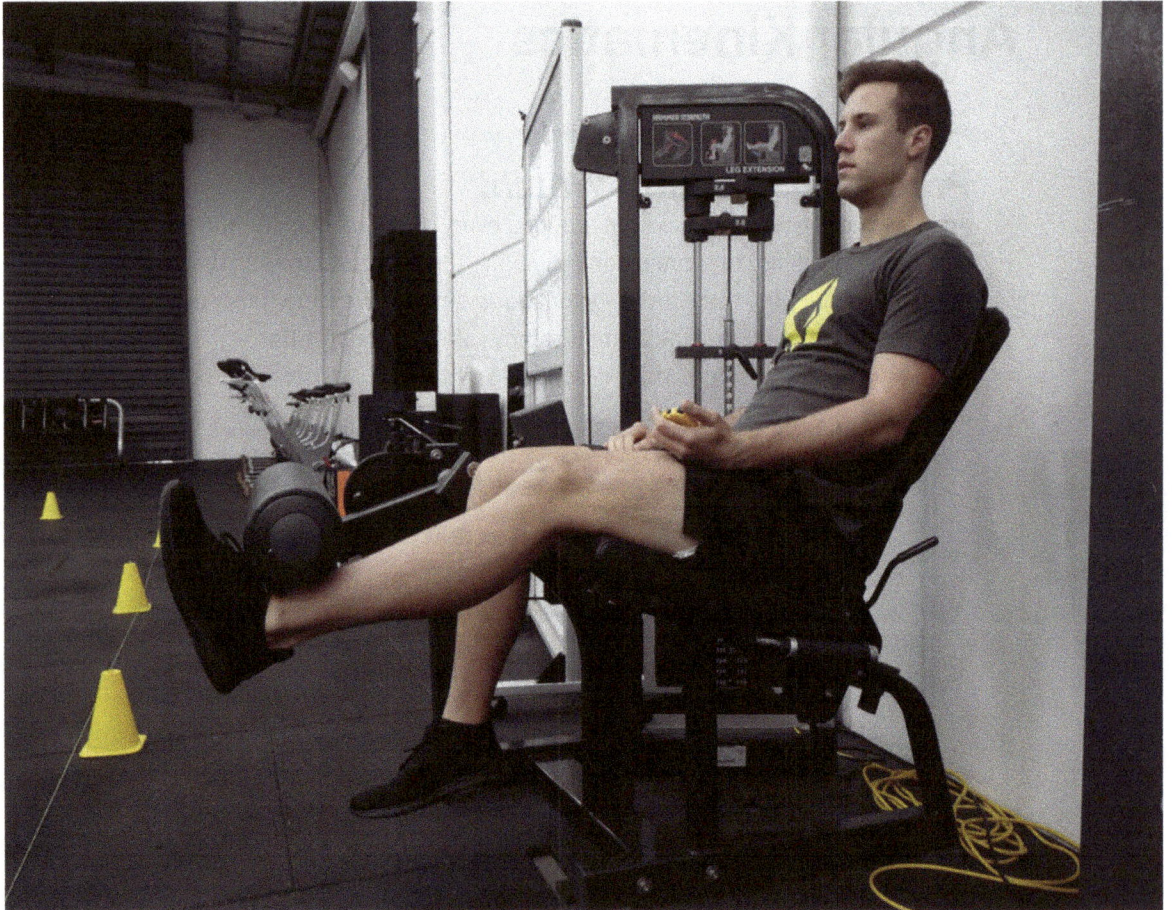

Figure 6.1   Leg extension.

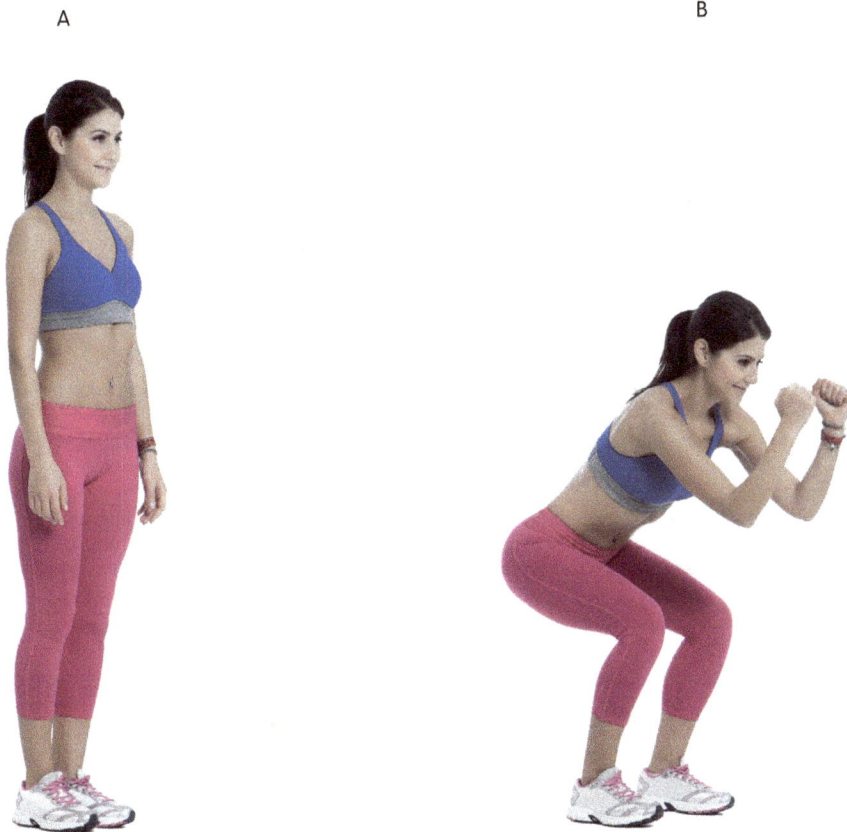

A   B

Figure 6.2   Knee flexion.

Angular kinematics describes angular motion based on space and time values but does not consider the underlying forces necessary for angular motion. Both scalars and vectors make up the parameters that are used in kinematic equations designed to explain or predict the outcome of rotating systems. Angular and linear kinematics are closely related with the radian, the standard unit of angular measurement in the SI system, holding the key to mathematically converting between values of angular and linear measurements.

Learning Objectives

After completing this chapter, students should be able to do the following:

- Define angular kinematics
- List the parts of a rotating system
- Calculate angular kinematic scalar and vector values

- Report angular values in degrees, radians, or revolutions
- Convert between linear and angular kinematic values

Understanding Angular Kinematics

At first glance this chapter may appear somewhat shorter than previous chapters, but it is not because the material is any less important; it is simply that many of the concepts and definitions, such as scalars, vectors, distance, displacement, speed, velocity, and acceleration, have already been defined previously. Now we will use all of those same concepts but apply them to rotating bodies.

📄 *One or more interactive elements has been excluded from this version of the text. You can view them online here:* *https://pb.cognella.com/83647-1b/?p=53#oembed-1*

Please refer to the interactive ebook in Cognella Active Learning for interactive/media content.

📄 *One or more interactive elements has been excluded from this version of the text. You can view them online here:* *https://pb.cognella.com/83647-1b/?p=53#oembed-2*

Please refer to the interactive ebook in Cognella Active Learning for interactive/media content.

In Chapter 5 it was stated that all motion requires a measurable change in the position of a whole body or one or more of its segments, and that position change requires some amount of time to occur. The same holds true for rotational or angular motion. When a body or its segments rotate about an internal (joint) or external axis, an angular position change occurs, and that position change requires time. In fact, all of the values associated with linear motion, such as distance, displacement, speed, velocity, and acceleration, are again found in the discussion of angular kinematics. There are both angular scalar values (angular distance, angular speed, and time) and angular vector values (angular displacement, angular velocity, and angular acceleration) used to describe rotational motion.

Angular Direction and the Right Hand Rule

Before we can fully understand how angular motion works, we must quickly review a little basic geometry. Circles are round, two-dimensional objects in which all of the points that make up the circumference (boundary) are located at an equal distance from its center. If circles are graphed on a 2D Cartesian coordinate system, the center of the circle is located at the origin of the x, y axis grid. Motion along a circular path is considered positive (+) if the motion is counterclockwise and negative (-) if clockwise. It is possible to use the "right hand rule" to determine the direction of motion of an object following a circular path. To use the right hand rule, curl the fingers of the right hand in the direction of the motion. If your right thumb points up from the plane of the rotation, the direction of the motion is considered positive (+). If the right thumb points down onto the plane of rotation, the motion is in a negative (-) direction (Figure 6.3).

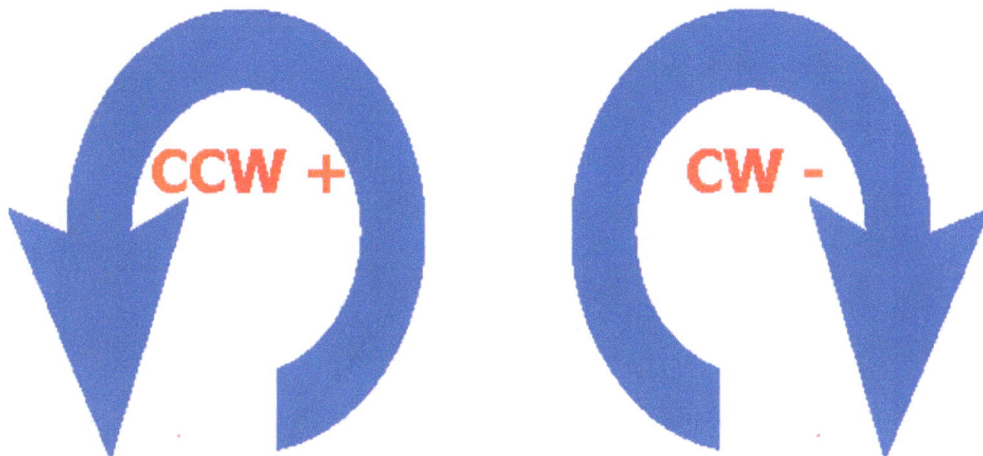

Figure 6.3   Angular direction.

The units of angular position can be thought of as the size of a slice of apple pie. If you want to talk about a whole pie, then using the unit of revolutions is easiest. One revolution equals the path length associated with the circumference of one complete circle. If you want very small slices of pie, you could cut your apple pie into 360 equal sections, 1 degree in width each. The units of radians may be less familiar than those of degrees as an angular measure to most, but radians have an advantage over degrees as a mathematical gateway that can be used to easily convert kinematic values back and forth between linear and angular measures. A radian is the equivalent of a slice of pie that has the length of the arc of the pie measured along the circumference of the circle, equal in length to the length of its radius. The value of a radian is defined as the size of the angle subtended at the center of a circle by an arc equal in length to the radius of the circle (Figure 6.4).

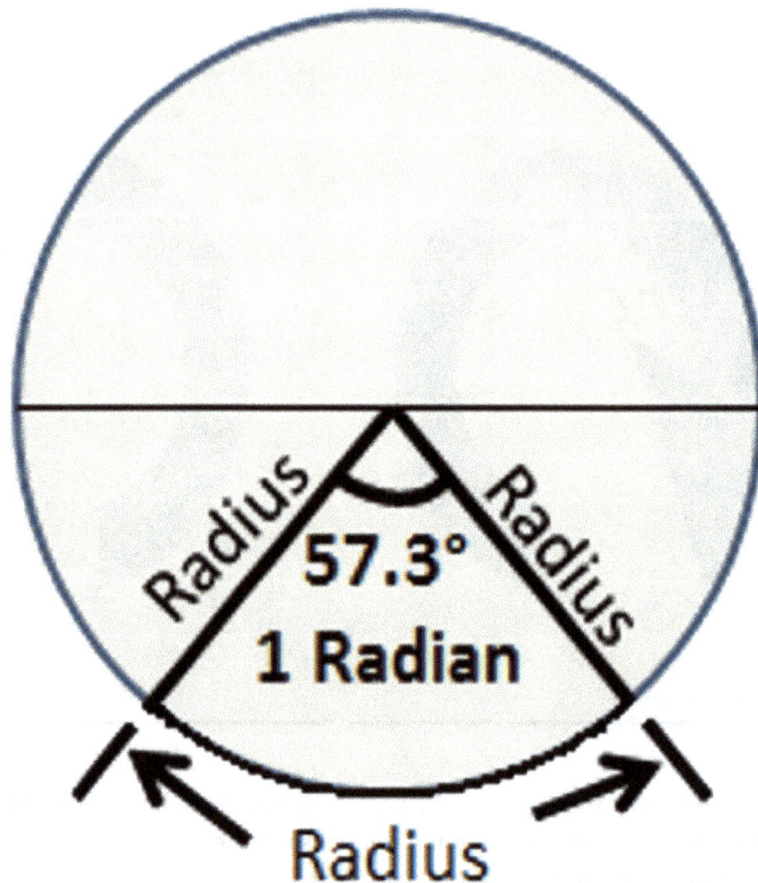

Figure 6.4   Radian and radius.

If the ratio of the arc length was divided by the radius length of that piece of pie, you would have a value of 1. One radian is equivalent to 57.3 deg or ~0.16 rev for circles of any size. A uniquely helpful property of a radian is that technically, since it is ratio, it has no units even though the term rad is attached to angular values that represent the result of an arc length divided by the radius of a given circle. That allows the unit placeholder of "rad" to be added or subtracted as needed when performing calculations. This feature is especially useful when converting between angular and linear values. This concept will be discussed in more depth later in this chapter.

Relative and Absolute Angles

Angles are referred to as **relative** or **absolute**, and often both are required to fully understand the orientation and rotational movement of an object. *Relative angles are angles formed between the longitudinal axes of adjacent body segments* (Figure 6.5). Human joints such as the knee or elbow are good examples of anatomical-based systems whose movement or orientation can be reported using relative angular measurement.

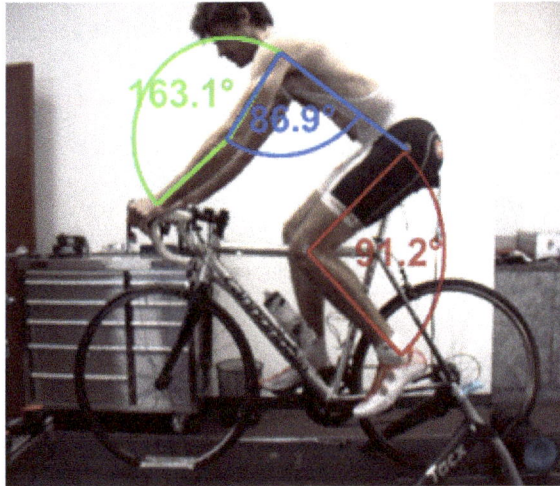

Figure 6.5   Relative angular measurements.

While relative angles provide information about how two adjacent segments relate to one another in space, they do not provide information about the orientation of the segments relative to external reference planes. To understand how segments are oriented relative to the surface of the earth or another plane of reference, the absolute angles of the segments must be measured. *An absolute angle is the measure that provides the angular orientation of a body segment with respect to a fixed line of reference (Figure 6.6)*. The fixed line of reference is often aligned with that of the vertical and horizontal axes of a 2D Cartesian coordinate system.

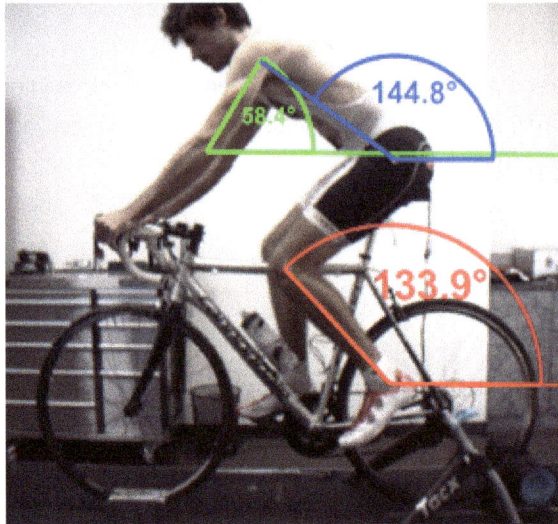

Figure 6.6   Absolute angular measurements.

A relative angle provides the orientation of two adjacent segments while an absolute angle describes the orientation of one segment at a time.

In practice, it is difficult to measure the angular orientation of human body segments exactly since the exact location of the distal and proximal endpoints of bones are seldom available. In addition, the exact location of the axis around which bones rotate varies throughout the range of motion of most joints. Finding the instant center (Figure 6.7), the precisely located center of rotation of a joint, is a problem that has plagued biomechanics from the beginning of angular kinematic analysis.

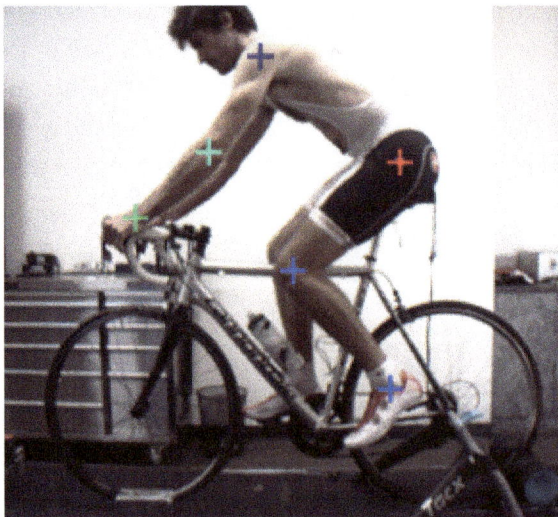

Figure 6.7   Joint center locations.

Joint motion is often simplified to allow estimates of angular motion to be computed. The knee joint, for example, may be referred to as acting like a hinge, yet a hinge has a fixed axis of rotation, while the knee moves through anterior/posterior translation, flexion/extension, and internal/external rotation during a movement such as a knee bend. Students should be aware of the difficulty of making exact angular measurements of human motion and take care to be as accurate as possible when assigning a joint center to the analysis of a movement.

Angular Units

Angular position is reported in units of degrees (deg), radians (rad), or revolutions (rev). **Angular distance** (**Φ**) represents the total angular position change from the beginning to end of an observation. Angular distance is a scalar.

The following are examples of how the magnitude of angular distance accumulates over the course of a movement. The angular distance traveled by the minute hand on a clock over the course of 24 hours is equal to -24 rev, -48pi rad, and -8,640 deg. All values would be considered negative since the direction of the motion of the minute hand is clockwise. Angular distance continues to increase in magnitude even if the direction changes during the motion. For example, while running a woman flexes, extends, and hyperextends the hip of her right leg 157 times as she completes one circuit of a 400-meter track (Figure 6.8). Each hip movement generates an angular distance of 48 deg, for a total of 7,536 deg of angular distance.

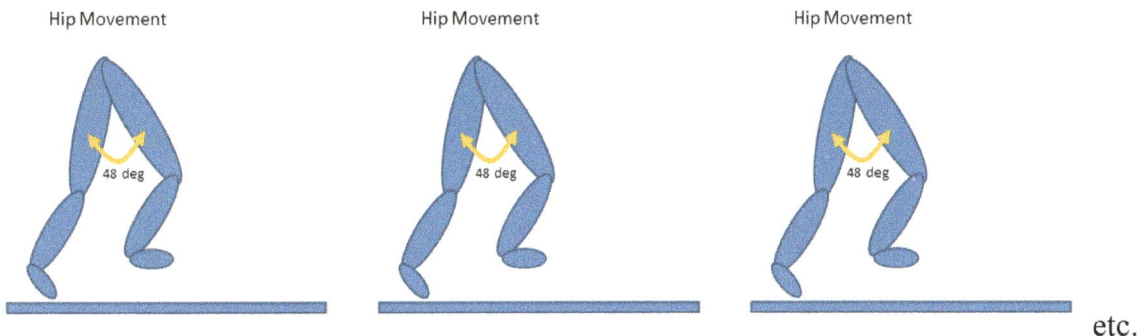

etc.

Figure 6.8   Repeated hip movement.

One or more interactive elements has been excluded from this version of the text. You can view them online here:
https://pb.cognella.com/83647-1b/?p=53#oembed-3
Please refer to the interactive ebook in Cognella Active Learning for interactive/media content.

One or more interactive elements has been excluded from this version of the text. You can view them online here: https://pb.cognella.com/83647-1b/?p=53#oembed-4

Please refer to the interactive ebook in Cognella Active Learning for interactive/media content.

Angular Displacement

Angular displacement is similar to angular distance in that it can be accurately reported in degrees, radians, and revolutions and the sign of the direction of angular displacement can be correctly determined using the right hand rule. **Angular displacement (Θ)**, however, is a vector and represents the difference between the angular position of an object at the beginning and end of the movement sequence (Figure6.9). *Angular displacement is the change between the initial (Θ_1) and final position (Θ_2) of a point of interest over a given time interval.* Angular displacement $\Delta\Theta = \Theta_2 - \Theta_1$. If both angular positions, Θ_2 and Θ_1, are angles that represent the location of a body as it travels along the arc of a circle, then the maximum value for angular displacement cannot be greater than 360 degrees. The direction is determined by the initial direction of the angular position change.

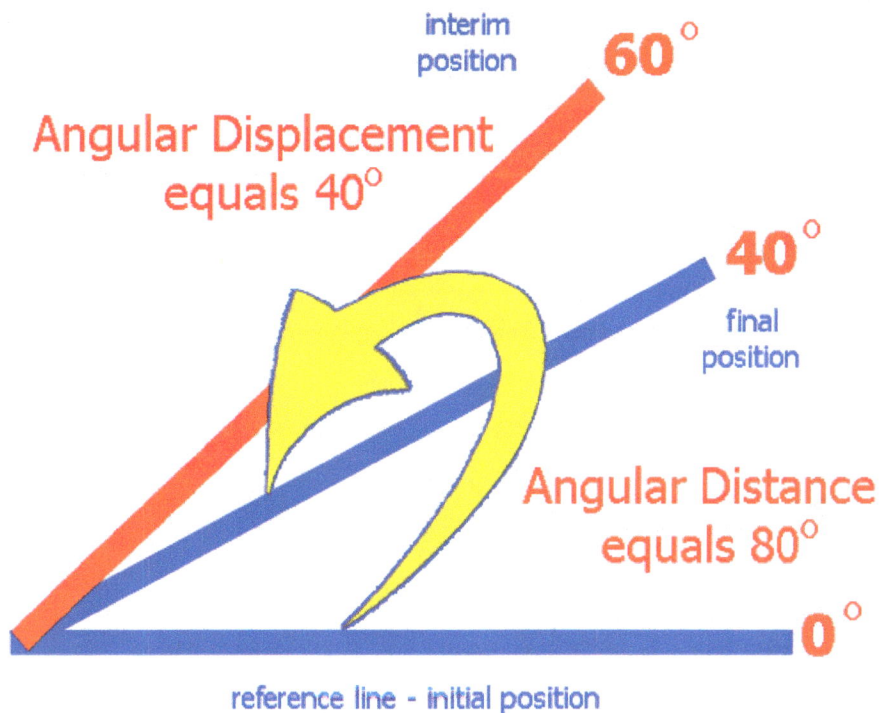

Angular Displacement equals 40°

interim position **60**°

40°

final position

Angular Distance equals 80°

0°

reference line - initial position

Angular Distance v. Displacement

Figure 6.9   Angular distance versus displacement.

The following video illustrates changes in angular distance and the displacement of markers on a wheel. Note how the distance and displacement values relative to the green tape will change based on the selected time interval of observation.

One or more interactive elements has been excluded from this version of the text. You can view them online here:
https://pb.cognella.com/83647-1b/?p=53#oembed-5

Please refer to the interactive ebook in Cognella Active Learning for interactive/media content.

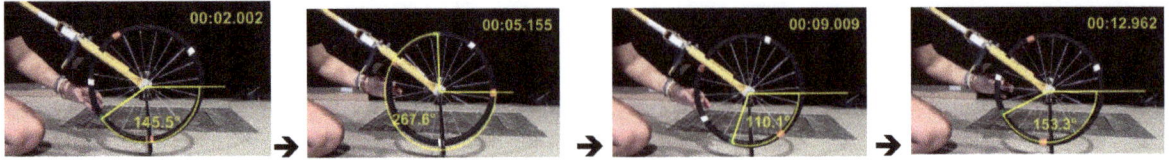

Figure 6.10   Displacement measurement sequence.

As a person performs a series of biceps curls to failure, the flexion angle decreases from 70 to 20 degrees. What is the angular displacement between the initial starting position and the flexion angle reached during the final attempted curl? The movement sequence is illustrated in Figure 6.11.

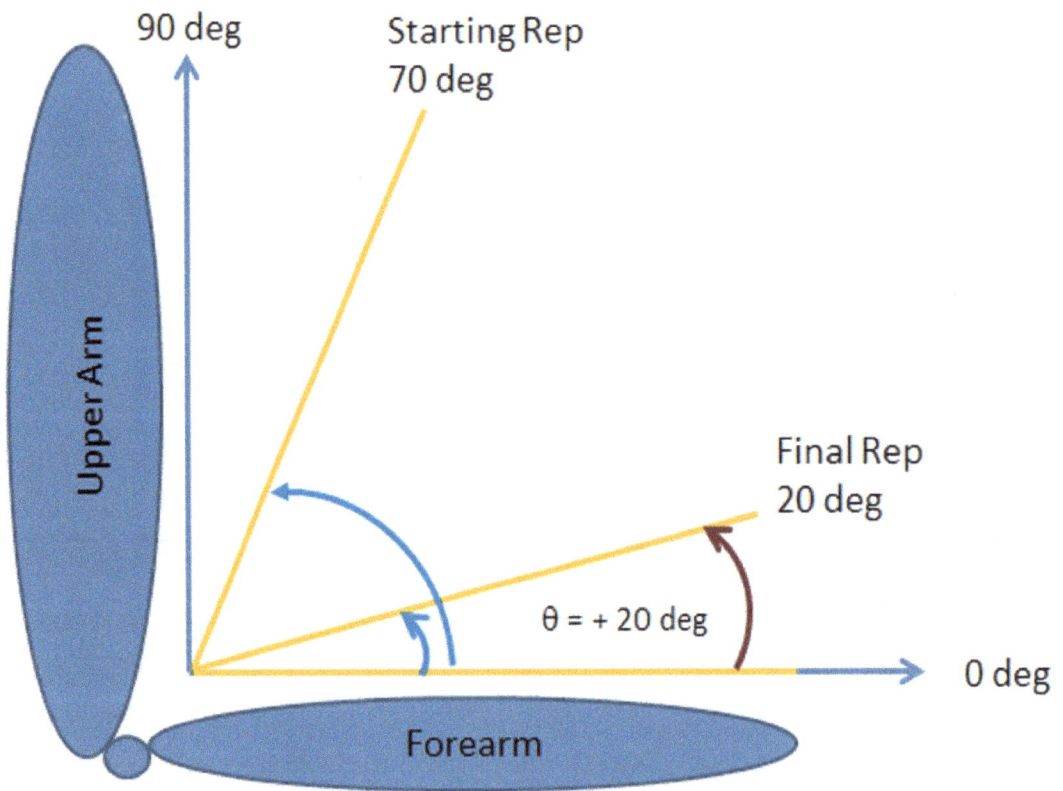

Figure 6.11   Arm displacement during biceps curl.

The result is an angular displacement of the forearm, from beginning to failure of the exercise, at +20 degrees. Note that for this example angular distance would be a much larger number and the angular displacement would be 0 degrees if measured between the initial orientation and the final horizontal resting position of the forearm.

Angular Speed

Angular speed (σ) *describes the angular distance change over a given time period.* Angular speed = ΔΦ / Δt and is a scalar quantity. The units for angular speed are deg/s, rad/s, or rev/s. The greater the angular speed of an object, the greater its linear speed, and if attached to a lever, such as a long bone in the human body, the faster the lever rotates.

Angular Velocity

Angular velocity (ω) *represents a change in angular displacement over time.* Angular velocity = ΔΘ / Δt and is a vector. The units for angular velocity are the same as those for angular speed, deg/s, rad/s, or rev/s. For a given motion it is possible for the angular velocity to equal the angular speed of an object, but it will not exceed it. Angular velocity provides a direction as well as rate of angular position change of a rotating object or lever.

An American football player, when punting a ball, swings his kicking leg through 170 deg of angular motion during the kicking phase of the motion in 0.45s. The action is completed 0.58s later when the kicker brings his kicking leg back down to its starting position and his foot contacts the ground. Determine the angular distance, displacement, speed, and velocity for the kick in units of degrees, radians, and revolutions for both the phases of the motion.

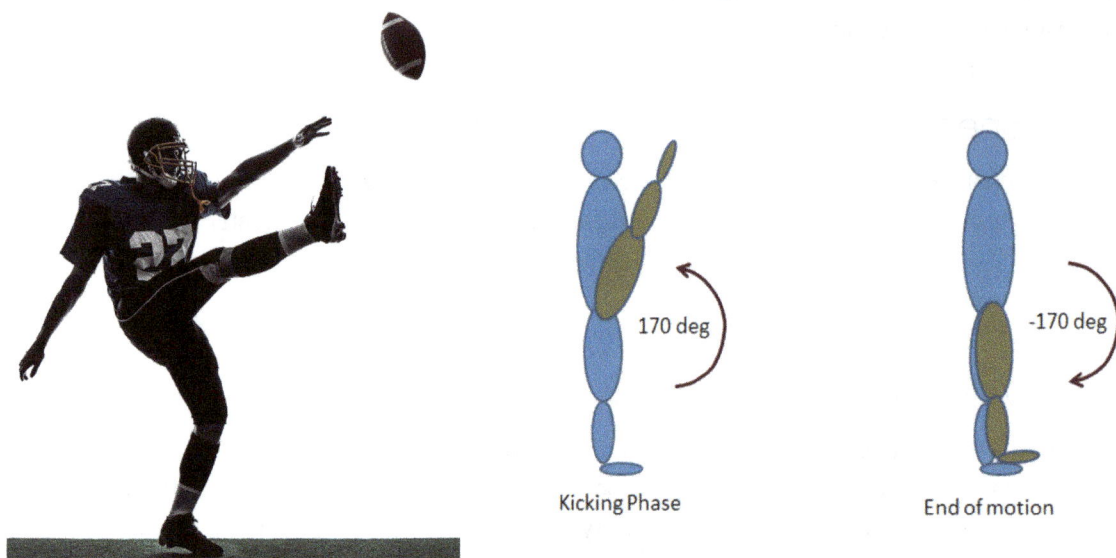

Figure 6.12   Leg displacement during football punting.

From the start to the end of the kicking phase of the motion, angular distance and angular displacement are equal:

Φ = Θ = 170 deg

Since angular distance and displacement are equal during the kicking phase of the motion, angular speed and angular velocity are equal:

σ = ω = 170 deg / 0.45s = 388.89 deg/s

σ = ω = 388.89 deg/s * 1 rad / 57.3 deg = 6.79 rad/s

σ = ω = 388.89 deg/s * 1 rev / 360 deg = 1.08 rev/s

From the end of the kicking phase of the motion until the kicking leg returns to its original location on the ground, the player's leg moves through -170 deg of angular position change:

Φ = 170 deg + | -170 deg | = 340 deg

Φ = 340 deg * 1 rad / 57.3 deg = 5.93 rad

Φ = 340 deg * 1 rev /360 deg = 0.94 rev

Θ = 170 deg + -170 deg = 0°

Θ = 0 deg * 1 rad / 57.3 deg = 0.0 rad

Θ = 0 deg * 1 rev / 360 deg = 0.0 rev

Angular speed and angular velocity are calculated over the entire time of the action. Δt = 0.45s + 0.58s = 1.03s for the complete motion:

σ = (340 deg / 1.03s) = 330.1 deg/s

σ = 330.1 deg/s * 1 rad / 57.3 deg = 5.76 rad/s

σ = 330.1 deg/s * 1 rev / 360 deg = 0.92 rev/s

Θ = (0 deg / 1.03 s) = 0.0 deg/s

Θ = 0.0 deg/s * 1 rad / 57.3 deg = 0.0 rad/s

Θ = 0.0 deg/s * 1 rev / 360 deg = 0.0 rev/s

Keep in mind that values of zero for vectors such as angular displacement and angular velocity do not mean that no motion took place; it may be the result of a motion beginning and ending at the same angular location.

Angular Acceleration

When angular velocity increases or decreases an angular acceleration is present. *Angular acceleration expresses the change in angular velocity over a given time period.* **Angular acceleration (α)** = Δω / Δt or $\alpha = (\omega_{Final} - \omega_{Initial}) / (t_{Final} - t_{Initial})$. Angular acceleration is a vector and is described with units of deg/s^2, rad/s^2, or rev/s^2. The direction (+ or -) of the acceleration is based on the outcome of difference and direction of the relationship ($\omega_{Final} - \omega_{Initial}$).

Angular acceleration is a key value for the determination of injury for biological systems such as humans. For example, it is the combination of angular and linear acceleration that is used to predict the severity of concussions.

When describing the biomechanical factors necessary for mild traumatic brain injury (concussion), it has been suggested that a peak linear head acceleration of 165 g, a Head Injury Criteria score (HIC) of 400, and a peak angular head acceleration of 9,000 rad/s^2 can result in a concussion of the average adult human (Funk, 2007). The HIC equation is shown in Figure 6.13.

$$HIC^* = (t_2 - t_1) \left[\frac{1}{t_2 - t_1} \int_{t_1}^{t_2} a(t)dt \right]^{5/2} \qquad GSI = \int_{0}^{T} a(t)^{2.5} dt$$

where a(t) = linear acceleration of the head center of gravity

$t_2{-}t_1 <= 15$ ms

* HIC can be calculated over any duration of time. Throughout this paper HIC is calculated over a 15 ms window.

Figure 6.13   HIC equation.

Angular acceleration can actually be thought of as several different types of accelerations acting on a body simultaneously as an object rotates. We've just seen how angular acceleration can be calculated based on changes in angular velocity, but rotating bodies contain more than just angular acceleration.

- There are two linear components of acceleration that are present in a rotating system. **Tangential acceleration** is the linear component of angular rotation directed along a tangent to the path of motion that indicates change in linear speed (Figure 6.14). Radial acceleration is the linear component of angular rotation directed toward the center of curvature that indicates change in direction (Figure 6.15) with the total linear acceleration based on the tangential and radial accelerations is shown in Figure 6.16.

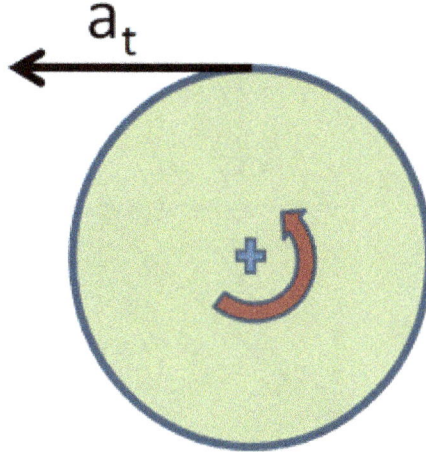

Figure 6.14   Tangential acceleration.

Tangential Acceleration

Tangential acceleration is the same as for linear accelerations: $a_t = (v_f - v_i) / \Delta t$.

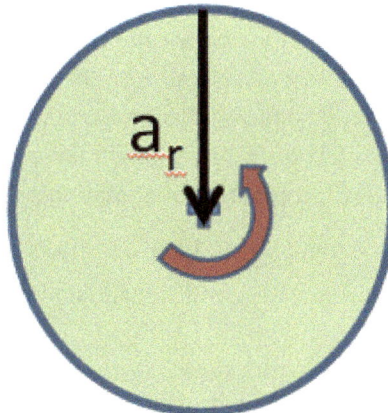

Figure 6.15   Radial acceleration.

Radial Acceleration

Radial acceleration is $a_r = v^2/r$.

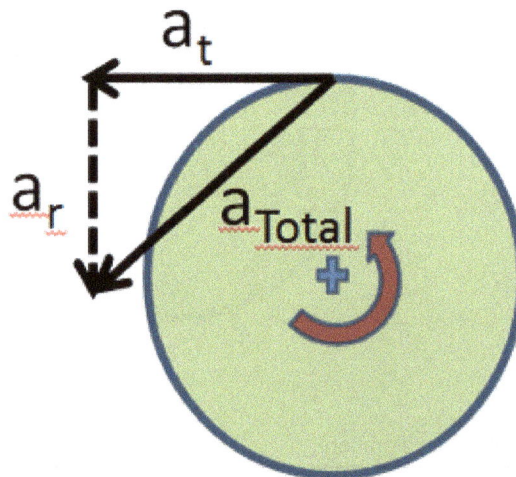

Figure 6.16   Total acceleration.

Total Linear Acceleration of a Rotating System

- The total linear acceleration of a rotating body can be determined by adding the linear tangential and linear radial acceleration vectors associated with the rotating body. Using the tip to tail method of vector addition, the Pythagorean theorem, and the arctan function it is possible to calculate the magnitude and direction of the resultant linear acceleration vector of a rotating system. The new value, **the total acceleration of a rotating system**, can be determined as $a_{total} = (a_t^2 + a_r^2)$ with a direction of arctan (a_r / a_t). Table 6.1 shows the one to one relationship and equation form similarities between linear and angular kinematic variables.

Table 6.1 Linear and Angular Kinematic Variable Equations

distance (l), displacement (d)	angular distance (Φ), angular distance (Θ)
Speed (s), velocity (v) $a = (d_2 - d_1) / (t_2 - t_1)$ $v = (d_2 - d_1) / (t_2 - t_1)$	angular speed (σ), angular velocity (ω) $\sigma = (\Phi_2 - \Phi_1) / (t_2 - t_1)$ $\omega = (\Theta_2 - \Theta_1) / (t_2 - t_1)$

Table 6.1 Linear and Angular Kinematic Variable Equations

Acceleration (a)	angular acceleration (α)
$a = (v_2 - v_1) / (t_2 - t_1)$	$α = (ω_2 - ω_1) / (t_2 - t_1)$

With all of the similarities between the equations of linear and angular kinematics, wouldn't it be great if we could tie them together mathematically as easily as we bundle linear and angular motion together for many of our most common movements such as walking or picking up an object?

Radius of Rotation

A simple term called the radius of rotation provides the bridge we need mathematically, along with some help from the concept of radians, to easily move back and forth between linear and angular kinematic relationships. The **radius of rotation** is the distance from the axis of rotation to a point of interest on a rotating body of a lever. It represents a linear distance and has units of mm, cm, m, and so on. The most common unit is m.

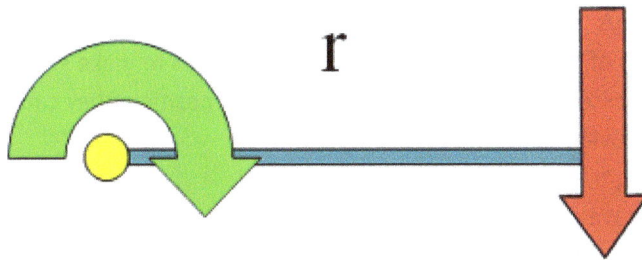

Figure 6.17   Radius of rotation.

Does Figure 6.17 remind you of anything? How about pedaling a bicycle or lowering a weight in a biceps curl? The world is full of examples of the radius of rotation making our lives better.

Angular ⇔ Linear

Once the radius of rotation for an action is known, it is simple to change a linear kinematic vector value to an angular one, or vice versa using the following relationships:

- $d = rΘ$
- $v = rω$
- $a = rα$

- Θ, ω, α must be in units using radians
  - rad, rad/s, rad/s^2

One or more interactive elements has been excluded from this version of the text. You can view them online here: https://pb.cognella.com/83647-1b/?p=53#oembed-6

Please refer to the interactive ebook in Cognella Active Learning for interactive/media content.

When converting from linear to angular or angular to linear values *it is necessary to have all angular units represented in radians* since the use of radians acts as a placeholder in equations and as such can be added or removed as needed to assist in solving problems using angular measures.

For example, if you wish to find out the linear velocity of the head of a tennis racket with a radius of rotation of 75 cm rotating at an angular velocity of 2578.5 deg/s, you can use the relationship v = rω to solve the problem:

- v = rω
- v = 0.75m * 2578.5 deg/s
- v = 1933.88 m deg/s
- But what are units of m deg/s? We need the units to be m/s to make sense of the solution.
- Since radians are essentially a placeholder in the unit's position, they can be added or removed as necessary to provide the correct unit result.
- v = 1933.88 m deg/s * (1rad / 57.3deg)
- v = 33.75 m rad/s We don't need rad to hold a unit's place, so it may simply be deleted.
- v = 33.75 m/s With the correct units of linear velocity, our solution is complete.

The following video illustrates the time associated with the phases (preparation, execution, and follow-thorough) of a golf swing. You may wish to use the time values to assist in calculating angular and linear values related to the movement.

One or more interactive elements has been excluded from this version of the text. You can view them online here: https://pb.cognella.com/83647-1b/?p=53#oembed-7

Please refer to the interactive ebook in Cognella Active Learning for interactive/media content.

One or more interactive elements has been excluded from this version of the text. You can view them online here: https://pb.cognella.com/83647-1b/?p=53#oembed-8

Please refer to the interactive ebook in Cognella Active Learning for interactive/media content.

One or more interactive elements has been excluded from this version of the text. You can view them online here: https://pb.cognella.com/83647-1b/?p=53#oembed-9

Please refer to the interactive ebook in Cognella Active Learning for interactive/media content.

Summary

Angular kinematics is the study of how rotating objects change position over time. The general forms of movement exhibited by people are an example of the combination of linear and angular movement. All of the linear kinematic variables discussed in Chapter 5 having matching analogs in angular kinematics. Angular changes can be correctly reported in values of degrees, radians, or revolutions. The right hand rule provides a mechanical method of determining the directional sign of rotating systems. When converting between linear to angular or angular to linear values, all angular units must be converted to radians.

List of Key Takeaways

- Angular kinematics describes rotational motion based on spatial and temporal parameters.
- There is a one-to-one correspondence between angular and linear parameters used to describe motion.
- Angular and linear kinematic variables are connected based on the values of radians and radius of rotation.

In table 6.2 you will find all of the names, symbols, units, and type (vector or scalar) of the angular kinematic variables described in this chapter.

Table 6.2 Angular Kinematic Variable and Equations Summary

Variable and Equation	Units	Vector or Scalar	Comments
Angular distance (Φ)	°, rad, or rev	Scalar	
Angular displacement (Θ)	°, rad, or rev	Vector	

Table 6.2 Angular Kinematic Variable and Equations Summary

Angular speed (σ) = $\Delta\Phi$ / Δt	°/s, rad/s, or rev/s	Scalar	
Angular velocity (ω) = $\Delta\Theta$ / Δt	°/s, rad/s, or rev/s	Vector	
Angular acceleration (α) = $\Delta\omega$ / Δt	°/s^2, rad/s^2, or rev/s^2	Vector	
Tangential acceleration (a_t) = (v_f - v_i)/Δt	m/s^2	Vector	
Radial acceleration (a_r) = v^2/r	m/s^2	Vector	
Total acceleration (a_{total}) = (a_t^2 + a_r^2)	m/s^2	Vector	
Linear displacement to angular displacement $d=r\Theta$	m, m*rad	Vector	Θ must be in units using radians
Linear velocity to angular velocity $v=r\omega$	m/s, m*rad/s	Vector	ω must be in units using radians
Linear acceleration to angular acceleration $a=r\alpha$	m/s^2, m*rad/s^2	Vector	α must be in units using radians

Reference

Funk, J. R. (2007). Biomechanical risk estimates for mild traumatic brain injury. Annals of Advances in Automotive Medicine, 51, 343–361.

Image Credits

Fig. 6.1: Copyright © by Core Advantage Pty Ltd (CC BY-SA 4.0) at https://commons.wikimedia.org/wiki/File:Osgood_Schlatters_Exercise_Isometric_Leg_Extensions.jpg.
Fig. 6.12a: Copyright © 2013 Depositphotos/STYLEPICS.
Fig. 6.2: Copyright © 2016 Depositphotos/blanaru.

Chapter 7

Linear Kinetics

Preparing to Learn: *Watch*

Forces are responsible for creating and altering movement. In sports, the player who can exert and overcome forces better than their opponent has a definite competitive advantage.

> One or more interactive elements has been excluded from this version of the text. You can view them online here: https://pb.cognella.com/83647-1b/?p=55#oembed-13
>
> Please refer to the interactive ebook in Cognella Active Learning for interactive/media content.

Every day we rely on forces generated by our muscles to accomplish routine activities such as sitting, standing, and walking.

> One or more interactive elements has been excluded from this version of the text. You can view them online here: https://pb.cognella.com/83647-1b/?p=55#oembed-14
>
> Please refer to the interactive ebook in Cognella Active Learning for interactive/media content.

Preparing to Learn: *Respond*

Directions: Based on what you saw in the videos, respond to the following questions:

1. Explain the goals of football in terms of how players use force to their advantage.

2. Does it make sense to think of the musculoskeletal system as a machine powered by the forces generated when muscles are active?

Introduction to the Chapter

In this chapter you will learn the definition of force and how to use a variety of equations that will allow you to solve problems involving force and energy.

One or more interactive elements has been excluded from this version of the text. You can view them online here: https://pb.cognella.com/83647-1b/?p=55#oembed-15

Please refer to the interactive ebook in Cognella Active Learning for interactive/media content.

No, not that force! We will discuss the different forms of pushes and pulls that exist in the real world!

Force is a necessary component of all motion. How it is generated, applied, resisted, and accommodated by individuals and objects determines its effect on motion. **Force** is a vector quantity that pushes or pulls on an object, resulting in an acceleration of the object's mass. Forces can originate internally or externally but must be applied to an object to have an effect. **Kinetics** is the study of force, with linear kinetics specifically focusing on how force application may cause an object to respond by resisting and/or changing its position following a straight or curvilinear path.

There are two types of force: contact and noncontact. Contact forces include ground reaction forces, friction, and air resistance, to name a few. An example of a noncontact force is the effect of gravity, which is considered an acceleration that pulls an object toward the center of the largest nearby mass. We will focus our discussion primarily on contact forces. **Contact forces** require a physical point of application on an object to have an effect.

Learning Objectives

After completing this chapter, students should be able to do the following:

- Define linear kinetics
- List the common types of contact forces and the necessary components of a contact force vector
- List and explain Newton's laws of linear motion
- Explain how friction works and distinguish between kinetic and static friction
- Define mechanical energy and list the various forms of energy used during human movement
- Solve problems using the equations presented in this chapter

Linear Kinetics concepts and variables

Linear kinetics helps us to understand why an object moves along a straight or curved path when acted upon by a force or forces.

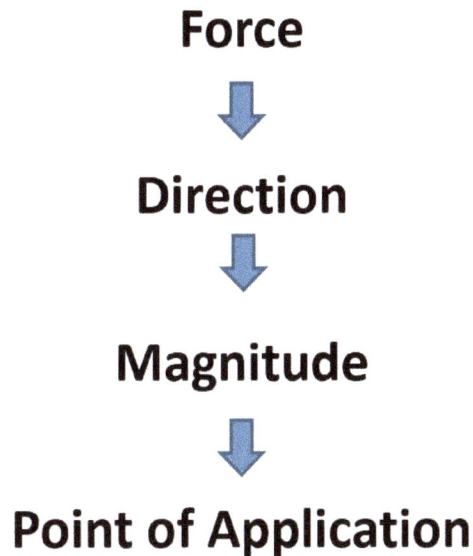

Force

⬇

Direction

⬇

Magnitude

⬇

Point of Application

Figure 7.1   Contact force.

In simplest terms, a force can be thought of as a push or a pull. Muscles within the human body generate tensile force when they seek to contract. An individual human muscle is only capable of generating a pulling force.

Forces are sometimes called loads when they act on an object. In the human body both internal and external forces interact with the structural frame, our skeleton, which supports all of the soft and hard tissue we are made of. The bones in our body are continually adapting to the needs we place on them through the forces we generate with our muscles, the mass we carry, and situations we place ourselves in during our daily lives. Bones actively remodel and get stronger when under some type of load. Forces that push down on our bones, whether generated dynamically by our muscles, passively by our weight, or through the application of external forces, are considered **compressive forces**. Compressive forces try to crush an object, reducing its length. Human bones require an almost constant state of compressive load to stay strong and healthy. This type of load is significantly reduced for astronauts in space, or bed-ridden patients, causing their bones to remodel into much more fragile versions of their prior form. Osteoporosis is a likely outcome in such cases. In general, human bones require compressive forces to keep them strong and healthy. Bones, particularly long bones, are well designed to handle compressive force.

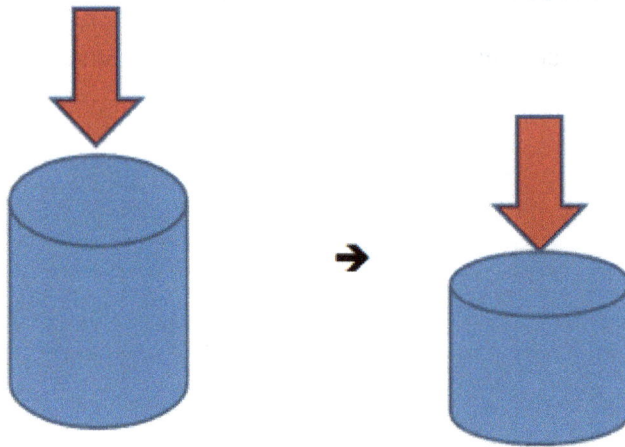

Figure 7.2   Compressive force.

One or more interactive elements has been excluded from this version of the text. You can view them online here: https://pb.cognella.com/83647-1b/?p=55#oembed-1

Please refer to the interactive ebook in Cognella Active Learning for interactive/media content.

Forces acting on an object in such a way that they try to pull the object apart are called **tensile forces**. Active muscles within the body generate tensile forces that load both bone and connective tissue such as tendons and ligaments. Human bones and connective tissue require frequent tensile force loading to remain strong and healthy. Bones and connective tissue are more likely to fail at a given tensile load than when under similar compressive loading.

The effect of tensile force

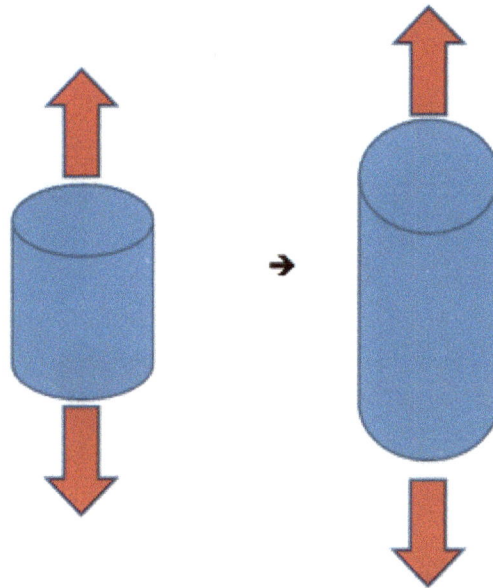

Figure 7.3   Tensile force.

One or more interactive elements has been excluded from this version of the text. You can view them online here:
https://pb.cognella.com/83647-1b/?p=55#oembed-2

Please refer to the interactive ebook in Cognella Active Learning for interactive/media content.

Bending is a combination of both tension and compression. Video 7.2 demonstrates bending force resulting in breaking a pencil. Tension is present on the top side of the pencil while compression exists on the bottom side.

The effect of shear force

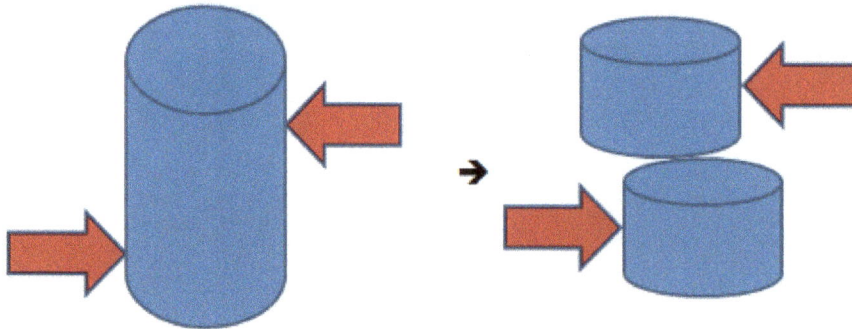

Figure 7.4   Shear force.

📽️ One or more interactive elements has been excluded from this version of the text. You can view them online here: *https://pb.cognella.com/83647-1b/?p=55#oembed-3*

Please refer to the interactive ebook in Cognella Active Learning for interactive/media content.

Forces acting perpendicular to the body of an object are called **shear forces**. Shear forces acting on the human skeleton can be created by internal muscle force or certain types of assumed body postures, but primarily occur from the body dealing with externally applied forces. Bones and connective tissue are much more likely to fail when experiencing shear forces than compressive or tensile forces of the same magnitude.

Before we can fully discuss and understand force, we must be able to understand how forces are created. In our chapters on kinematics we defined acceleration as the result of a change of velocity over time. It is that value of acceleration when multiplied by the mass of an object that defines force. Mass is the amount of matter or material that makes up an object. Common units for mass are grams, kilograms, ounces, or pounds. The recommended SI unit for mass is the kilogram or kg. Mass is a scalar quantity. The mass of an object is closely related to the concept of inertia. **Inertia** is the reluctance an object has to having its movement altered when a force is applied to the object. Inertia is directly proportional to the mass of the object. An object of low mass requires just a small amount of applied force to change its state of motion. The greater the mass, the greater the inertia and the larger the amount of force necessary to change its motion state.

To understand motion and the forces that cause it, one must understand the common properties of all motion. Sir Isaac Newton summarized several important "universal" truths about motion in his three laws of motion. **Newton's First Law of Motion** states that *an object at rest (not moving) stays at rest, and an object in motion will maintain its motion at a constant velocity unless acted upon by an unbalanced force*. The term unbalanced force indicates that the net force, the vector sum of all forces acting on the object, does not equal zero. As an example of how Newton's first law works, think of a chair. It is made up of matter and therefore has mass and inertia. The chair will sit motionless on the floor unless a force is applied to it, causing it to move. Now think of a much larger object, like the earth. It too is made of matter and obeys Newton's first law of motion. The earth is in a constant state of motion as it travels around the sun and moves through space as part of the Milky Way galaxy. Unless a sufficient unbalanced force acts upon the earth, it will continue along its celestial path forever. Remember that inertia is directly proportional to the mass of an object.

Newton's Second Law of Motion states that *when a force of sufficient magnitude is applied to a mass, it will cause a change in the velocity of the mass*. That change in velocity is a measurable acceleration. This allowed Newton to express the relationship between mass, force, and acceleration as $F = ma$. Force is proportional to and directed along the line of action of the acceleration of the mass:

$$F = ma \Rightarrow F = m_a \Rightarrow F = {}_m a$$

In honor of Sir Isaac and his contribution to the understanding of force, the SI unit (N) representing force was named for him. One Newton (N) is equivalent to 1kg accelerated at $1m/s^2$. Note that reporting the units of force as a value with units of $kg\ m/s^2$ is technically incorrect. The units of force in the English system are pounds (lbs).

Weight is a special type of force that is created by the acceleration of gravity ($-9.81m/s^2$) acting on a mass with the intent of pulling it toward the center of the earth. Any object with its mass close to the surface of the earth has weight, and its weight is the result of its mass times the acceleration of gravity. So, a 50kg rock has a weight of 490.5N. Weight can be thought of as $f_{weight} = m * a_{gravity}$.

Newton's Third Law of Motion deals with the forces associated with contact actions. It states that for every action there is an equal and opposite reaction. This is probably the least intuitive of the laws of motion. It is easy to see a rock sitting on the ground and understand that due to its inertia it will continue to sit motionless until or unless something disturbs it. It is also understandable that if someone pushes on the rock hard enough that the rock will move, meaning that it accelerated as a result of the applied pushing force. What is a little more difficult to grasp is that while the rock is sitting on the ground it is actually being held in place due to the upward ground reaction force countering its downward weight force, which is explained by the third law.

Newton's 1st Law

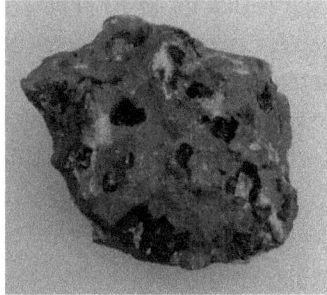

Motion ➜ Yes or No

The rock is stationary or moving at a constant velocity.

Large mass = Large inertia

Small mass = Small inertia

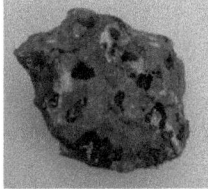

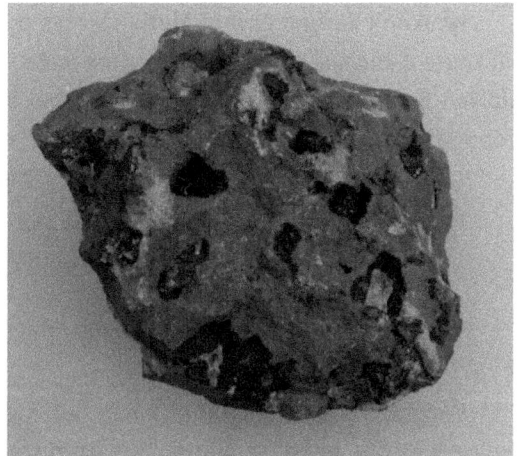

Figure 7.5   Newton's first law.

Newton's 2nd Law

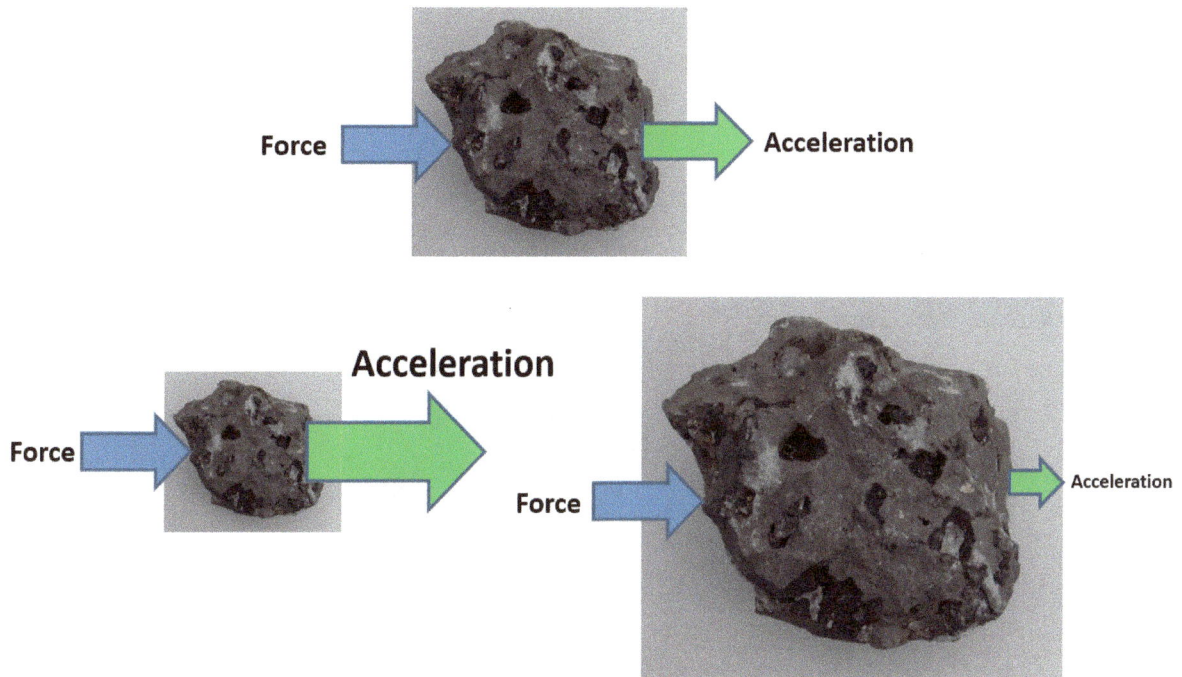

Figure 7.6   Newton's second law.

Newton's 3rd Law

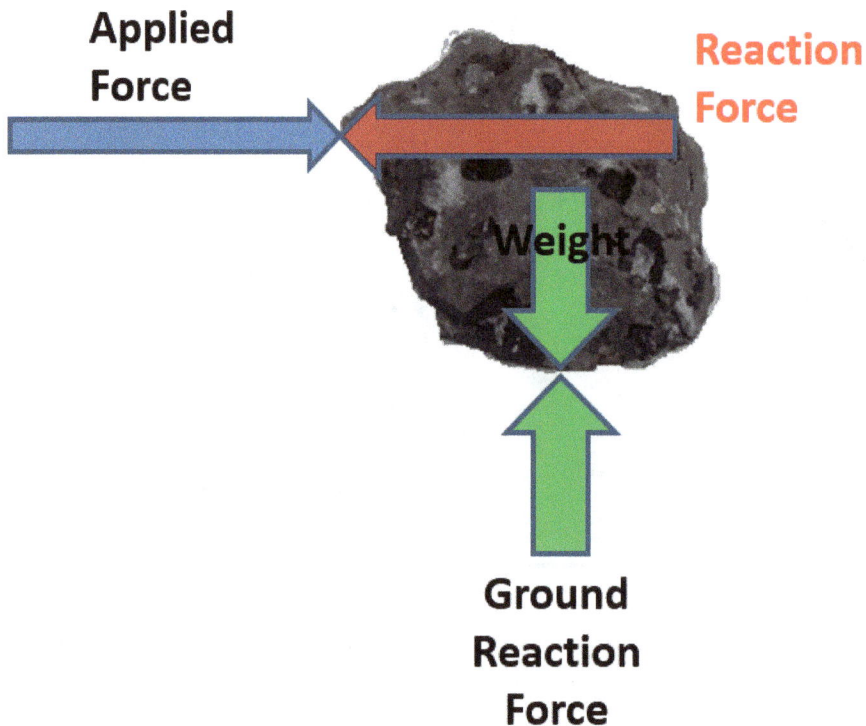

Applied Force **Reaction Force** **Weight** **Ground Reaction Force**

Figure 7.7   Newton's third law.

Newton's third law initiates us to the concept of force couples. A force couple is a pair of forces that are acting in direct opposition of one another. There are many examples of force couples that exist all around us. When you lift your arm, you are generating a muscular force to overcome the weight force resulting from the mass of your arm accelerated by gravity. When you stand quietly on the ground, the ground reaction force creates a net force equilibrium with your body's weight force.

Quiet Standing

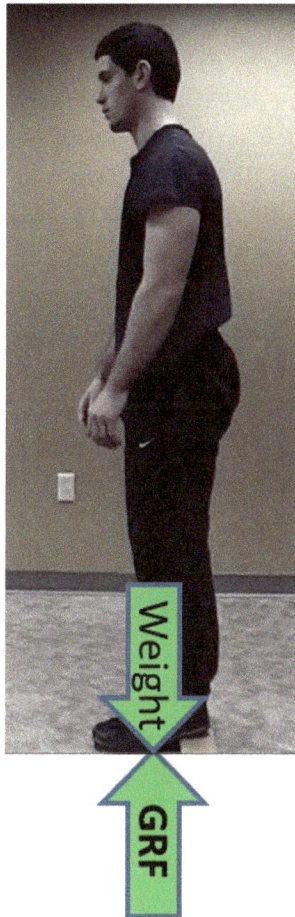

GRF + Weight = 0 N

Net Force = 0 N

Figure 7.8   Ground reaction force.

Did you ever wonder why when a car strikes a parked car, both cars are damaged? It is because at the instant of impact the parked car strikes back at the moving car with exactly the same force that the moving car exerts on it.

Not only does an airbag protect a person by increasing the area of impact, it also extends the contact time. **Impulse (Imp)** is the relationship between force and time and can be written Imp = F * t, where F is the applied force and t the duration of force application. Impulse is a vector with units of Ns. The time a force is applied to an object or person greatly affects the outcome of the applied force. The values for impulse are sometimes misunderstood by students. A large impulse doesn't necessarily mean the value is "good" or "bad." In the case of an airbag impact, often the larger the impulse for a given crash force, the lower the likelihood of injury for the person involved in the crash. Can you give examples of relatively small impulse situations that could be dangerous to a person?

Force is a vector quantity and can be broken into vertical and horizontal components, should those values be needed. It can be categorized as internal or external to the body. From a biomechanical perspective, muscles are responsible for active force generation within the body. When muscle is active it attempts to contract or shorten its overall length. If successful, the type of action generates is considered concentric. Should a muscle be actively trying to contract but due to other forces it actually elongates or lengthens, it is considered to be undergoing an eccentric muscle action. A muscle's length may also stay unchanged or static when it is actively trying to shorten; this is considered an isometric muscle action. Isokinetic muscle action results when a muscle generates a constant amount of muscle force throughout a movement. Should muscle action result in a movement performed at a constant rate of speed, the action is considered isotonic. It is likely that during complex human movement some of our muscles may be involved in concentric, eccentric, and isometric actions simultaneously.

The area over which a force is applied defines pressure (P): $P = F/A$, where F is an applied force and A represents the area of force application. Pressure is a vector with units of Pascals or the preferred units of biomechanists, which are N/cm^2. For a given force, an increase or decrease is directly proportional to the increase or decrease of the pressure. Pressure is a valuable measure when evaluating the possible injurious effects of external forces to the body. Stress (σ) is an internal equivalent of pressure. Its equation is $\sigma = F/A$ and has the same units as pressure.

For example, the average pressure across the plantar surface of an 825N man standing on both feet is tolerable for him. Assuming the surface contact area of each foot is 120.5 cm^2 and that his weight is equally spread across the surface of each foot, the average pressure he experiences when standing on two feet is

$P = F/A$

$P = (825N)/(120.5 \ cm^2 \ *2)$

$P = 3.42 \ N/cm^2$

The resulting value is low and is very unlikely to cause pain or injury.

However, if the same person were to step on a tack with its pointed surface area of 0.01cm^2, the resulting pressure would be

$P = F/A$

$P = (825N)/(0.01cm^2)$

$P = 82500 \ N/cm^2$

This value is equivalent to the force of full-sized elephant pushing the point of a tack into his foot! That will hurt!

Internally, the same thing occurs when a person damages the cartilage of the knee, resulting in bone-on-bone contact. The stress values at the bone-on-bone contact point will increase substantially, likely leading to damage to the bones and joint.

This same concept of increasing or decreasing surface area of force application in an attempt to change the outcome of an applied force is used in many everyday situations. As mentioned previously, airbags in cars are a good example of how manipulating pressure can be used to decrease injuries. Given the same car crash, a person is much less likely to be injured or killed if they hit an airbag with their head and torso than if they impact the much smaller area of a steering wheel and dashboard. Combative athletes may inflict much more damage to opponents by striking with feet or fists as compared to tackling their opponent, which would result in the impact forces being spread over a much larger surface area.

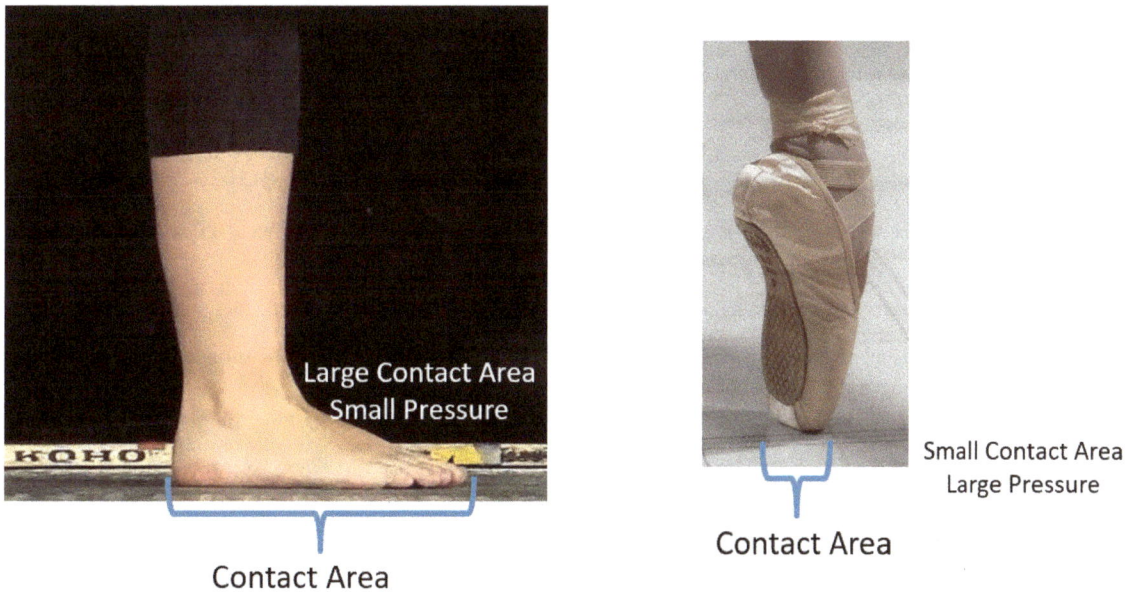

Figure 7.9   Contact area.

Impacts or collisions are events of large forces applied over a short time period. The terms large forces and short time are somewhat ambiguous, and it is up to the analyst to determine what large and short mean in the context of their work. For a geologist discussing the impact of an asteroid on earth, the force may be in trillions of Newtons occurring over minutes or hours of time. For a scientist studying the impact of a club head with a golf ball, the impact force may be hundreds or thousands of Newtons being applied in less than 1 ms.

All impacts or collisions fall somewhere between being perfectly plastic to perfectly elastic. A perfectly plastic collision is a collision in which all velocity present between the objects prior to colliding is dissipated during the collision. The net velocity at the conclusion of such an impact is zero. On the other end of the collision spectrum is the perfectly elastic collision, which is a situation in which none of the initial velocity of the colliding bodies is lost as a result of the collision. Can you provide examples of perfectly plastic and elastic collisions?

One or more interactive elements has been excluded from this version of the text. You can view them online here: https://pb.cognella.com/83647-1b/?p=55#oembed-4

Please refer to the interactive ebook in Cognella Active Learning for interactive/media content.

One or more interactive elements has been excluded from this version of the text. You can view them online here: https://pb.cognella.com/83647-1b/?p=55#oembed-5

Please refer to the interactive ebook in Cognella Active Learning for interactive/media content.

One or more interactive elements has been excluded from this version of the text. You can view them online here: https://pb.cognella.com/83647-1b/?p=55#oembed-6

Please refer to the interactive ebook in Cognella Active Learning for interactive/media content.

One or more interactive elements has been excluded from this version of the text. You can view them online here: https://pb.cognella.com/83647-1b/?p=55#oembed-7

Please refer to the interactive ebook in Cognella Active Learning for interactive/media content.

One or more interactive elements has been excluded from this version of the text. You can view them online here: https://pb.cognella.com/83647-1b/?p=55#oembed-8

Please refer to the interactive ebook in Cognella Active Learning for interactive/media content.

Ground Reaction Force

Ground reaction force (GRF) is a special reactive force that is essential for basic human locomotion. GRF is the normal or perpendicular ($\perp$) component of the reactive force present any time we contact the ground.

In a static condition the GRF may equal your weight. In dynamic situations it often is equal to multiple times your body weight (BW).

To accurately calculate ground reaction force it is necessary to determine if the object being studied is stationary or moving. The equation for ground reaction force states that GRF = $f_{vertical}$ + | $m_{object}a_{gravity}$ |, where $f_{vertical}$ = $m_{object}(\Delta v/\Delta t)$ or the mass of the object accelerated vertically + | $m_{object}a_{gravity}$ |, which represents the absolute value of the static weight of the object.

How It Works

What is the GRF of a stationary 75kg object resting on the ground? The stationary object has a ground reaction force equal to the sum of its mass accelerated by gravity plus the product of its mass times any other vertical acceleration present at the time. For a stationary object the only acceleration acting is that of gravity:

Therefore, GRF = $f_{vertical}$ + $m_{object}a_{gravity}$

GRF = $75kg(0m/s^2)$ + 75kg * $(-9.81m/s^2$

GRF = 0.0N + 735.75N

GRF = 735.75N

Now suppose that the object happened to be a person of mass of 75kg and that person performed a vertical jump such that he moved vertically from 0m/s to 4.1m/s in 0.28s. What is the GRF?

GRF = $f_{vertical}$ + | $m_{person}a_{gravity}$ |

GRF = $m_{person}(\Delta v/\Delta t)$ + | $m_{person}a_{gravity}$ |

GRF = [75kg * ((4.1m/s − 0.0m/s)/0.28s)] + | [75kg * $(-9.81m/s^2)$] |

GRF = 1098N + 735.75N

GRF = 1833.75N

This is equivalent to an average force of 2.43 BW.

What happens to GRF when a person is standing or walking up an incline? Remember that GRF represents the normal or perpendicular contact force generated by the weight of an object. To determine exactly what proportion of the overall weight is responsible for the GRF requires breaking the weight into components that act normal to the plane of action and along the plane of action.

Since the contact force generated by an object on an incline is not always given with an angle relative to a full 360° Cartesian grid, it may be necessary to generate a diagram to help understand how forces are acting on an object. For example, determine the GRF of a 62kg woman standing on a 20-degree slope.

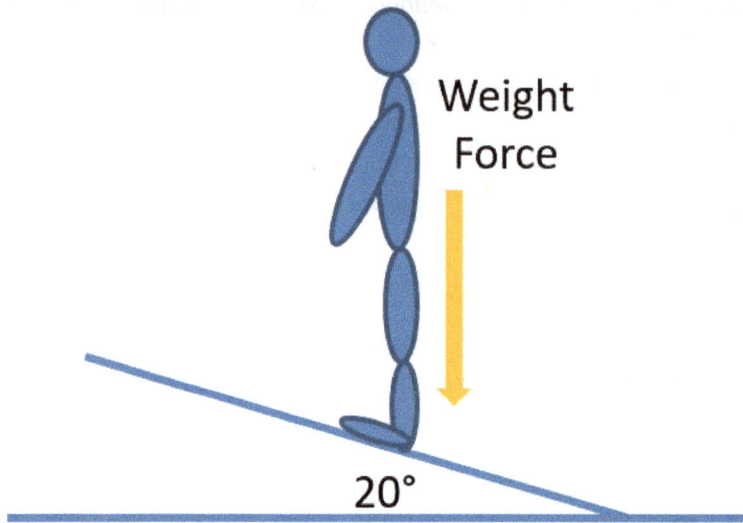

Figure 7.10   Standing on incline.

Figure 7.11 is what the free body diagram of the system looks like.

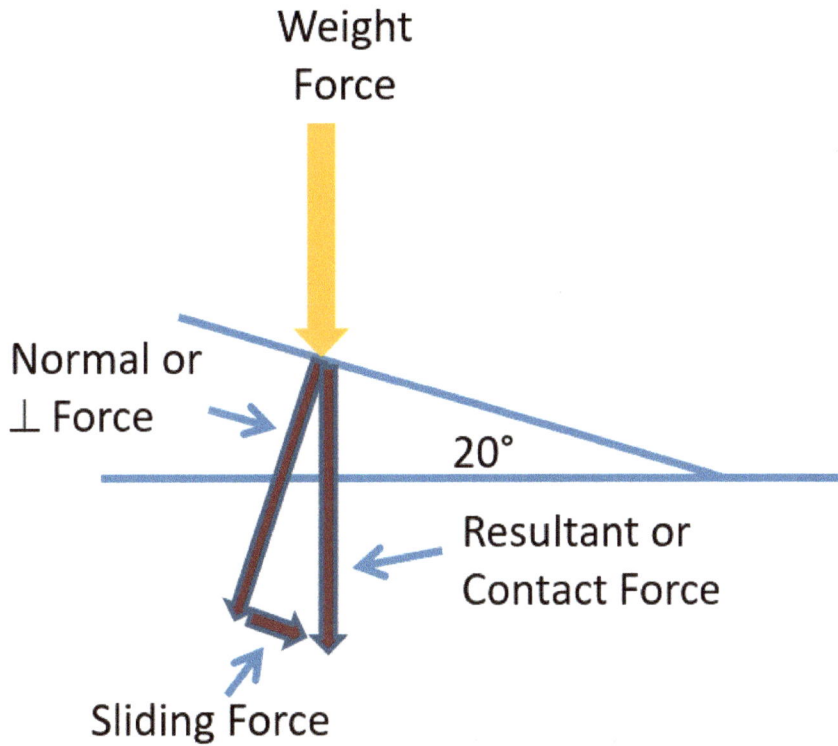

Figure 7.11   Free body diagram standing on incline.

Using geometry and trigonometry, solve for the normal and sliding components of the contact force.

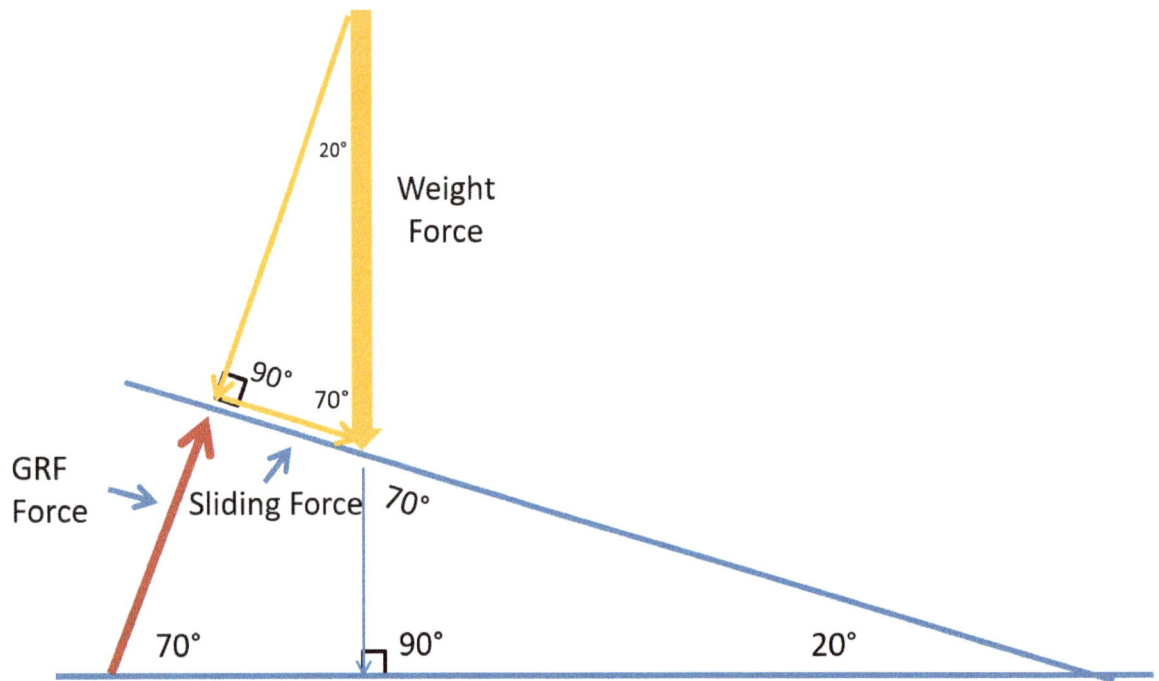

Figure 7.12   Geometry underlying free body diagram standing on incline.

It is now possible to determine the size and the angle at which the GRF force is acting. Her weight is $62kg*-9.81m/s^2 \Rightarrow -608.22N$ and represents the hypotenuse of the yellow right triangle formed by her weight vector. The smallest side of the weight triangle is the sliding force and is equal to

sin(20) = opp/hyp

sin(20) = sliding force / -608.22N

sin(20) * -608.22N = sliding force

sliding force = -208.02N

The remaining side is the normal contact force of the weight triangle and is equal to

cos(20) = adj/hyp

cos(20) = normal force / -608.22N

cos(20) * -608.22N = normal force

normal force = -571.54N

Remember that the GRF is in the opposite direction of the normal force, so it is equal to 571.54N.

Note that since all interior angles of the weight vector triangle were known, the same results for the sliding and normal forces could have been found by various appropriate combinations of the cosine and tangent functions and/or the Pythagorean theorem.

It is the normal force that generates the GRF reaction force, so according to Newton's Third Law the GRF force must equal 571.54N. According to our diagram of the vectors involved in this problem, the GRF can be expressed as a force vector of magnitude 571.54N @ 70° above the horizontal.

Friction

Another important everyday force was hinted at in the last example. The force of friction is a reaction force that is always in opposition of the motive force when objects in contact attempt to slide over one another. In the last example the friction force is equal in magnitude but opposite in direction of the sliding force. The equation for friction is $F = \mu R$, where F represents friction force, μ is the coefficient of friction, and R is a normal force. Mu (μ) is a value that represents the stickiness or slipperiness of a material and a surface it is contacting. As a coefficient, μ is a unitless value.

For most of us, friction is only noticed when either there is not enough or too much as we try to move. If you've ever slipped on ice or injured yourself because your foot stuck when playing a game, you realize just how important the right amount of friction is for us to perform movements safely. The shoes you wear, the roads you drive on, and the floors, courts, tracks, and playing fields you walk, run, and jump on are all built to provide you with just the right amount of friction. Friction plays an important role in almost every movement we make, from the time we are born until we die. Biomechanists are interested in friction from both a performance and injury standpoint.

Friction has two forms: **static** (F_s) and **kinetic** (F_k). Static friction values range from 0.0N to a maximum friction force found when movement between the objects in contact is imminent. Static friction is sometimes referred to as the maximum static friction of an object, and it is the force that allows an object to initially resist moving when a motive force is applied to it. Kinetic friction is present when objects in contact slide or roll over one another.

Load vs. Friction

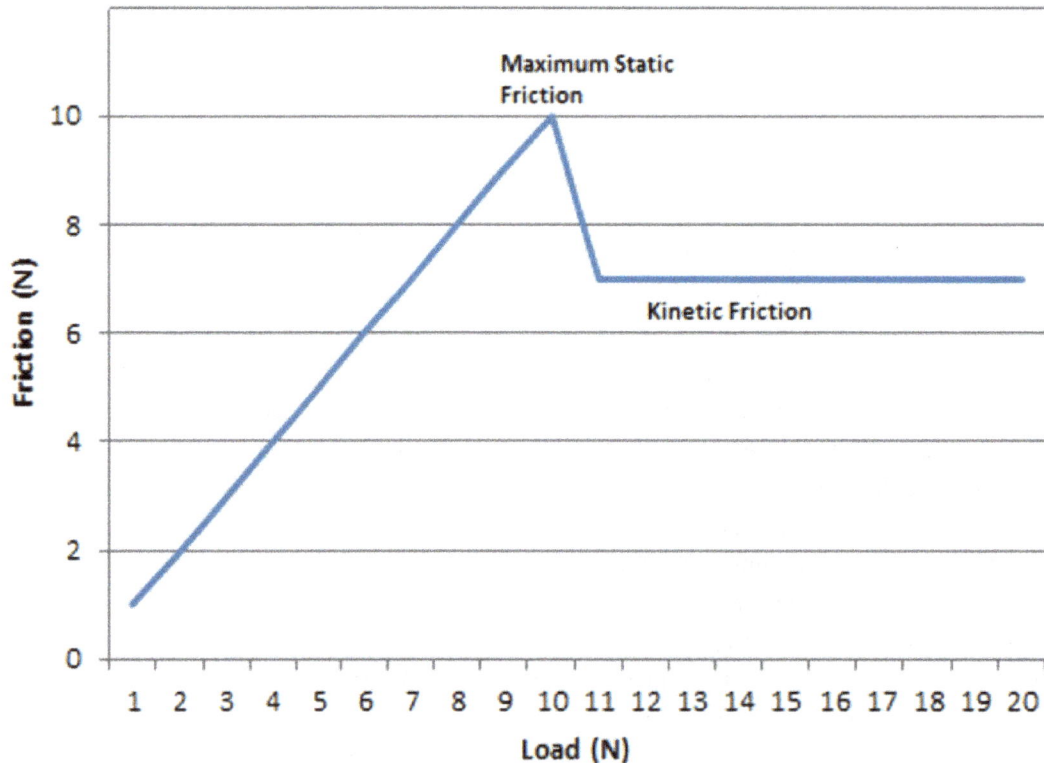

Figure 7.13   Load versus friction.

For any objects in contact with one another there are two coefficients of friction, the coefficient of static friction μ_s and the coefficient of kinetic friction, μ_k: $\mu_k \leqslant \mu_s$. Friction is present and must be handled appropriately in virtually all forms of human motion. For humans to walk, run, stand, crawl, or sit we must be able to work with friction. Friction is present whenever we move or attempt to move and are in contact with the ground or any other surface or object.

This is how it works: Let's say that there is a 10 kg box sitting on the floor and you need to slide it along the floor to a new location. If the μ_s and μ_k of the box are known to be 0.25 and 0.21, respectively, the minimum amount of horizontally directed force needed to get the box to start sliding and then to continue sliding can be easily calculated. The weight of the box would be 10kg * -9.81m/s^2 = -98.1N.

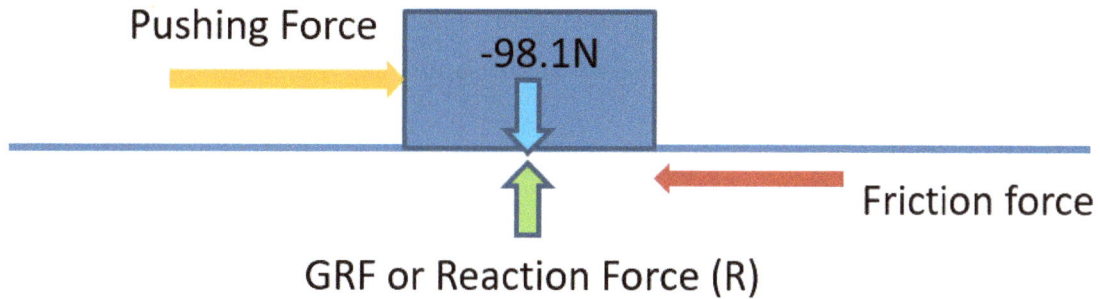

Pushing Force

-98.1N

Friction force

GRF or Reaction Force (R)

Figure 7.14   Friction diagram.

The reaction force (R) = | -98.1N | or +98.1N. The amount of friction force that must be overcome to begin sliding the box is found:

$F_s = \mu_s * R$

where F_s is the maximum static friction force of the object, μ_s is the static coefficient of friction for the object and the ground, and R is the reaction force, which is equal in magnitude but opposite in direction of the weight of the object.

$F_s = 0.25 * 98.1N$

$F_s = 24.53N$

which is the minimum amount of force needed to overcome the static friction of the box and allow it to start sliding.

Once the box starts to slide, the amount of force needed to keep it sliding is equal to F_k or the kinetic friction value of the box:

$F_k = \mu_k * R$

where F_k is the kinetic friction force of the object, μ_k is the kinetic coefficient of friction for the object and the ground, and R is the reaction force, which is equal in magnitude but opposite in direction of the weight of the object.

One or more interactive elements has been excluded from this version of the text. You can view them online here:

https://pb.cognella.com/83647-1b/?p=55#oembed-9

Please refer to the interactive ebook in Cognella Active Learning for interactive/media content.

$F_k = 0.21 * 98.1N$

$F_k = 20.6N$

What happens when the pushing force is not directed exactly along the horizontal axis of motion? In such cases the vertical and horizontal components of the pushing force must be determined and factored into the calculations for the effects of friction.

If a pushing force of 100N at 330° was applied to the box from the previous example, the static and kinetic friction values would change.

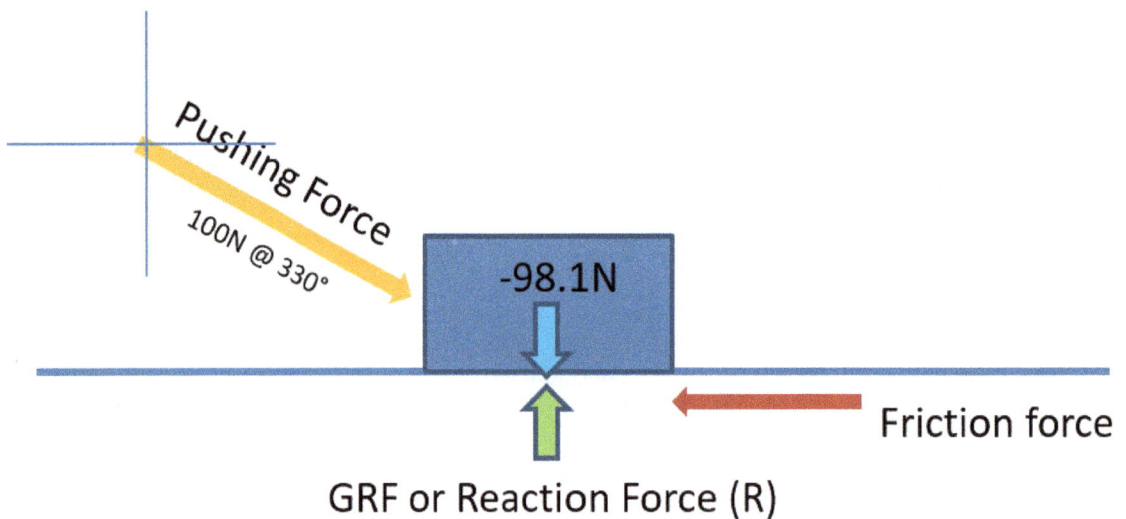

Figure 7.15   Pushing force diagram.

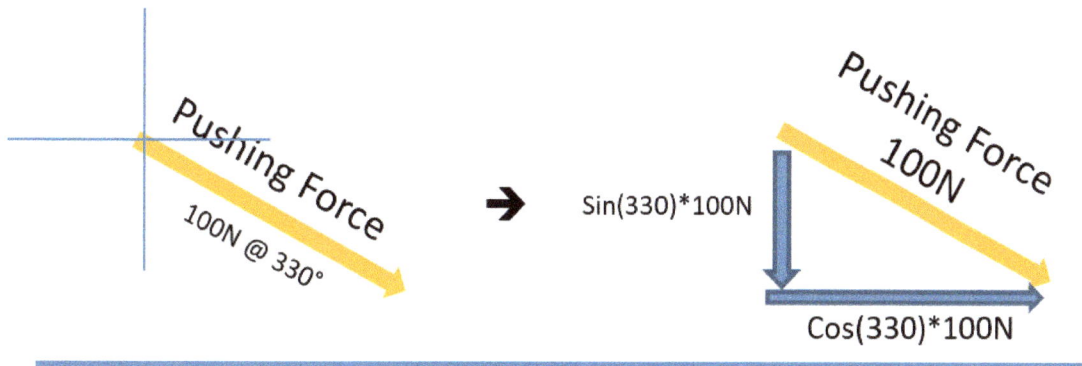

Figure 7.16   Pushing force components.

The vertical component of the pushing force is added to the weight of the box to increase the total downward vertical force that must be countered by an upward reaction force (R):

R = | -98.1N + (sin(330)*100N) |

R = | -98.1N + -50N |

R = 148.1N

Using the new reaction force value, new values for F_s and F_k can be calculated:

$F_s = \mu_s * R$ $F_k = \mu_k * R$

$F_s = 0.25 * 148.1N$ $F_k = 0.21 * 148.1N$

$F_s = 37.03N$ $F_k = 31.10N$

Any pushing force that is applied to an object in a downward direction (-vertical component 0.0N) increases the friction experienced by the object since it effectively increases the reaction force. For pushing force directed upward (+vertical component) decreases the reaction force and the friction experienced by the object during sliding.

Why don't people always move objects utilizing an upward pushing force? The answer is left up to the student.

One or more interactive elements has been excluded from this version of the text. You can view them online here:

https://pb.cognella.com/83647-1b/?p=55#oembed-10

Given the same box and friction coefficients, determine the maximum static and kinetic friction for the box if it was placed on a 30° incline.

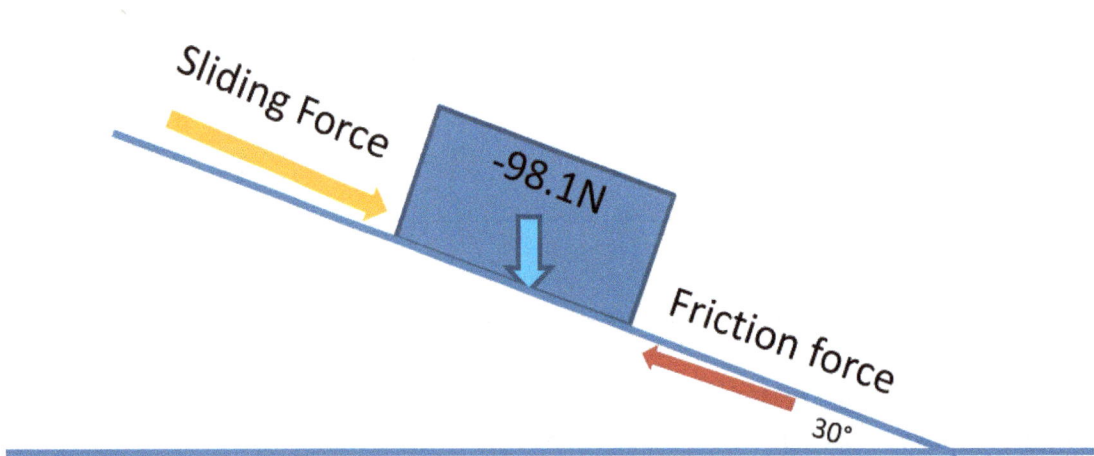

Figure 7.17   Sliding box.

Determine components of weight.

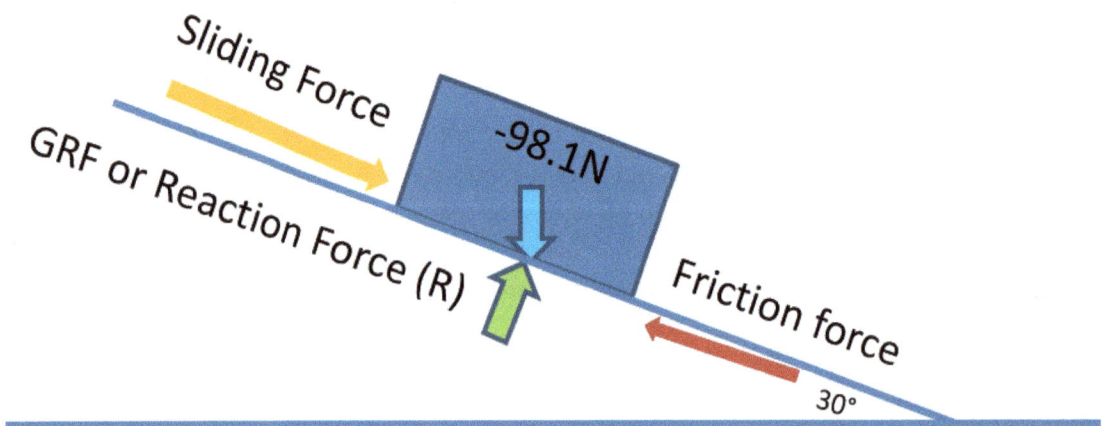

Figure 7.18   Sliding box components.

Note that the reaction force has been realigned to counter the normal component of the weight force. Graphically it can be illustrated as Figure 7.19.

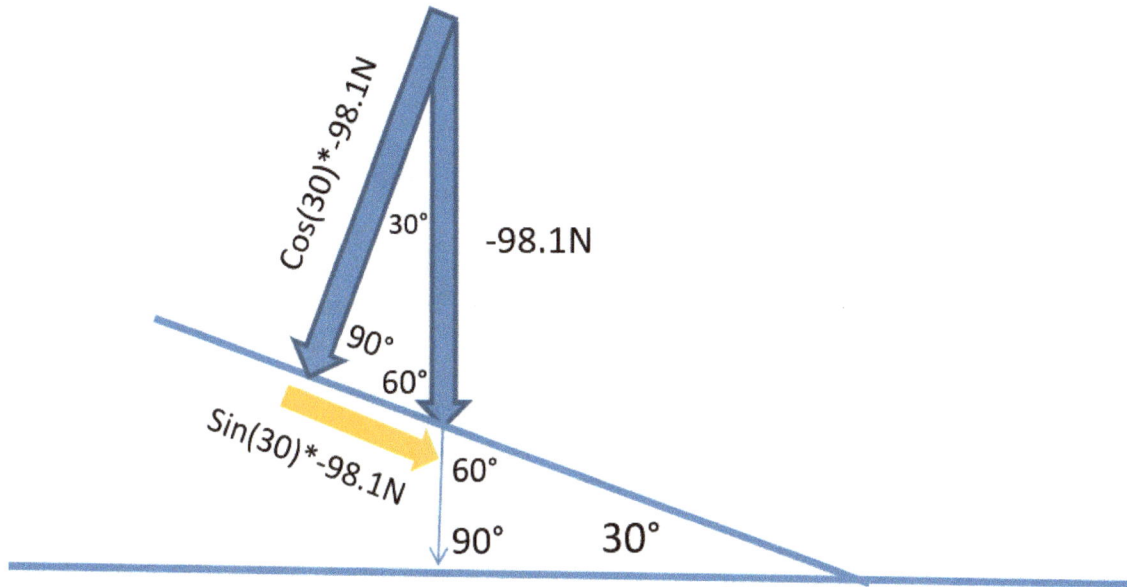

Figure 7.19   Normal force.

This shows that the normal component of the weight force is equal to cos(30)*-98.1N, or -84.96N. The reaction force (R) is equal to the absolute value of the normal weight force, so it is equal to 84.96N. The fact that the weight is on an incline means that it wants to slide down the ramp. The sliding force is determined by finding the remaining side of the weight force triangle. The sliding force, which will be opposed by the maximum static friction force (F_s) is sin(30)*-98.1N, or -49.05N:

$$F_s = \mu_s * R$$

$$F_s = 0.25 * 84.96N$$

$$F_s = 21.24N$$

which is less than the sliding force of 49.05N. Therefore, the box will start sliding down the ramp. Since $F_s > F_k$, once started the box will continue to slide down to the bottom of the ramp.

Friction is a critical component of human locomotion. Friction provides our ability to brake and push forward during walking. It is the cyclical ability to create braking and propulsive forces that allow humans to walk. A braking force is created by friction when heel strike occurs. The braking force disappears during mid stance and then is used to push us forward during the toe off phase.

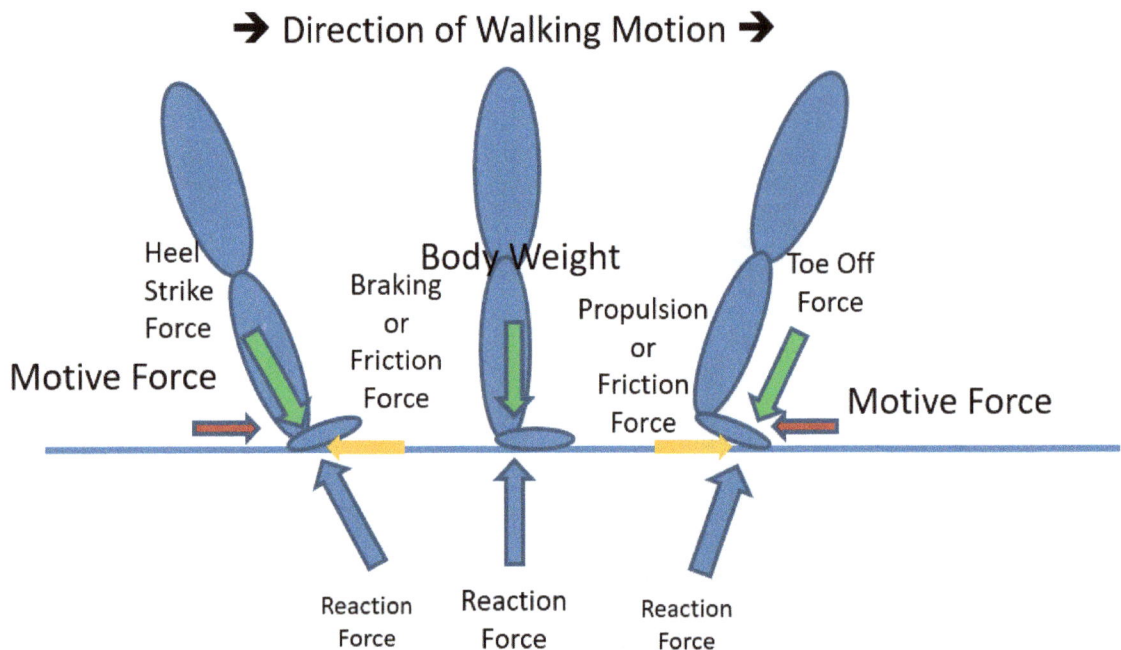

→ Direction of Walking Motion →

Heel
Strike
Force

Body Weight

Toe Off
Force

Braking
or
Friction
Force

Propulsion
or
Friction
Force

Motive Force

Motive Force

Reaction
Force

Reaction
Force

Reaction
Force

Figure 7.20   Friction during gait.

Friction is considered a retarding force since it always opposes motion. Drag is another form of retarding force and will be covered in more detail in a later chapter.

Work and Power

Whenever a force is applied against a resistance over a measurable displacement, mechanical work is done. **Mechanical work (W)** is a type of mechanical energy that is a vector expressed in units of joules (j). The equation for mechanical work is $W = F * d * \cos(\Theta)$, where W is the mechanical work done by a force (F) applied over a measurable displacement (d) of resulting motion, times the cosine of the angle between the applied force and the displacement. It is important to understand that Θ is the angle between the force and displacement and is not just the angle of force or the angle of the displacement. *That means that if both the force and displacement are in the same direction, then the difference between them is zero.*

One or more interactive elements has been excluded from this version of the text. You can view them online here: https://pb.cognella.com/83647-1b/?p=55#oembed-11

Please refer to the interactive ebook in Cognella Active Learning for interactive/media content.

For example, if a lifting force of 25N @ 90° is applied to a weight of 25N that results in the weight being lifted 30cm, the amount of mechanical work done would be

W = F * d *cos(Θ)

W = 25N * 0.3m * cos(0)

Note that the difference between the force and displacement is zero, resulting in cos(0), which equals 1 being multiplied by the product of the force = 25N and displacement =0.3m.

W = 7.5j

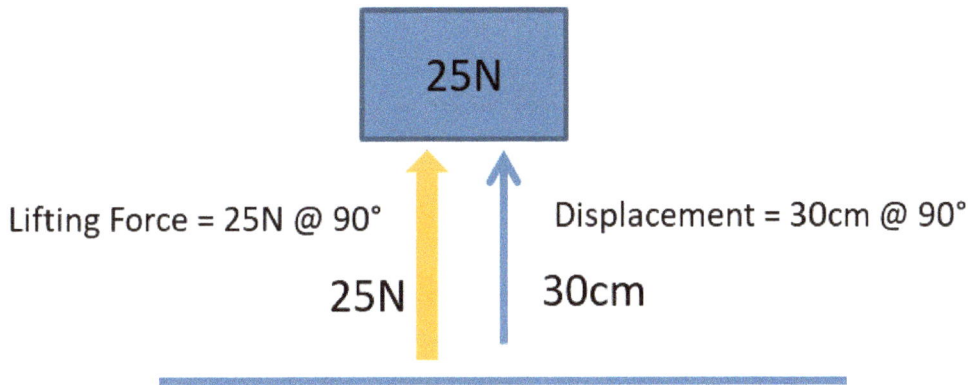

Figure 7.21   Free body diagram lift.

If the same weight was again lifted to a height of 30cm, but this time as the result of an applied force of 100N @ 45°, the resulting work would be the same, but there would have been an excess amount of force applied. The vertical (or lifting force component) of the applied force would be equal cos(45)*100N, or 70.7N @ 90°. Since only 25N @ 90° was necessary to lift the weight, there was an excess of 47.5N of vertical lifting force. The extra lifting force would cause the weight to be lifted faster but would not change the amount of mechanical work generated.

Since work is a vector, it can be either positive (+) or negative (-) in direction. By convention, work done in an upward vertical direction is considered positive, as in the previous example. But what happens when you lower the 25N weight back to the ground? Since the displacement and lifting forces are now acting at 180° to one another and the cos(180) = -1, the work done lowering the weight is -7.5j. That means that the total work accomplished lifting and lowering a weight is a net of 0j of mechanical work! So why do people go to the gym to lift weights if the total work generated is zero? Seems like they would be better served spending more time studying biomechanics!

The rate at which mechanical work is accomplished is often important in the success or failure of the physical activity. Think about what types of physical qualities make an athlete successful. You might immediately think of things such as height, weight, or muscle mass. All those factors play into the "package" of the successful athletic physique. However, for most athletes who perform at a high level in dynamic activities it is their ability to generate large amounts of mechanical work, repeatedly and whenever needed, that tends to set them apart from their competition. It is their ability to generate power that may be their most important physical skill. **Power (P)** is defined as the rate of mechanical work production: $P = W/\Delta t$. Power is a vector, which is reported in units of watts (w). There is a greater physical cost to generate mechanical work over short periods of time. For example, it is physically more difficult to sprint 100 meters than to walk 100 meters. The amount of mechanical work might be the same to move the body 100 meters against wind and frictional forces, but sprinting requires the body to produce the mechanical work much faster than walking. Sprinting requires the body to be able to convert its metabolic energy stores more quickly into muscle actions to perform mechanical work compared to walking the same distance. Sprinting is a high-power activity. Walking is a low-power activity.

Time always plays an important role in the success or failure or safety of a motion. The same is true for the role of time in work generation.

For example, if a person were to walk from field level to the top of a football stadium, they would have had to generate a specific amount of mechanical work to raise the weight of their body vertically from the beginning to end of the task. It would take some amount of time for them to walk up the steps, so they would have done mechanical work over some measurable period of time. Therefore, mechanical power could be calculated for the ascent. Neglecting all friction forces, if the 675N person had to climb 108 steps, each 20cm high, in 65 seconds to get to the top of the stadium, how much work and power did they generate?

W = F * d

W = 675N * (108 steps * (20cm/1 step))

W = 675N * 21.6m

W = 14580 j

$P = W/\Delta t$

P = 14580j / 65s

P = 224.31 w

What if the person ran up the steps in 30 seconds; did they have to work harder? Technically, the answer is no. They performed the same amount of work, 14580j, but the power required to accomplish the task increased:

$P_{Walking}$ = 224.31w

$P_{Running}$ = $W/\Delta t$

$P_{Running} = 14580j\ /30s$

$P_{Running} = 486w$

Momentum

When an object is moving, it possesses momentum. **Momentum (p)** is the product of the mass of an object times its velocity: $p = mv$, where m is the mass of the object and v is its velocity. It is a vector with units of kg m/s. Momentum can be thought of as a form of "moving inertia." The greater an object's momentum, the larger the opposing force needed to alter its movement. For example, little force is needed to change the motion of a rolling tennis ball, but a bus moving at the same velocity as the ball requires a much larger force to stop or change in its direction of motion.

Momentum is important to the biomechanist because it provides a bridge between kinematic values and kinetic values. In fact, it allows the force values to be calculated using often easily obtainable kinematic values found in complex collisions.

The **conservation of linear momentum** states that the sum of all momentum present in all colliding bodies immediately before they collide is equal to the sum of the momentum of all colliding bodies immediately after they collide. The equation for linear momentum can be found here:

$p_{prior\ to\ impact} = p_{after\ impact}$

This can be rewritten as

$m_1v_1 + m_2v_2 = v_{combined}\ ^*(m_1 + m_2)$

$m_1v_1 + m_2v_2 = v_{combined}\ ^*m_{combined}$

In this way, the velocity of the combined masses of two or more objects can be determined immediately following an impact. In situations in which the combined velocity is known, it may be possible to determine the individual contributions of each of the individual objects before the impact. Such information is especially important when re-creating accidents.

Another very useful characteristic of momentum is its relationship to impulse:

$Imp = F * t$

$Imp = \Delta p$

$F * t = p_{Final} - p_{initial}$

$F * t = m_{total}v_{final} - m_{total}v_{initial}$ assuming $v_{initial} = 0m/s$

$F * t = m_{total}v_{final}$

$F = m_{total}v_{final} / t$

This equation allows for the calculation of force present at impact between colliding bodies if the combined mass of the objects, their combined velocity, and the time of impact is known.

For example, what was the force exerted on the driver of a car that slid off an icy road into a ditch? The driver weighed 742N and was traveling at 27m/s as the car began to slip off the roadway. The car stopped 1.37s later:

$F * t = p\text{Final} - p_\text{Initial}$

$F * 1.37s = (((742N*(1kg/9.81N))*0m/s) - ((742N*(1kg/9.81N))*27m/s))$

$F * 1.37s = (75.64kg * 27m/s)$

$F = (2042.28 \text{ kg m/s}) / 1.37s$

$F = 1495.09N$

Energy

What is needed to "get the ball rolling," literally? Muscles must be tasked to contract before they generate force, but what is present that allows them to act? Where does a force large enough to hurl the object into the air come from? What is needed for the forces of motion to come into being? The answer is energy.

Energy is the ability to do work. The theory of the conservation of energy states that energy cannot be created nor destroyed. Scientists believe that all the energy of the universe was created at the time of the Big Bang and has just been changing its form to meet the needs of the universe ever since. Energy comes to us in a variety of forms, such as mechanical, potential, kinetic, strain, nuclear, electromagnetic, and chemical. In this chapter we will focus on energy in the forms of mechanical, potential, kinetic, and strain.

We have already discussed mechanical energy in the form of mechanical work. When energy is measured as the outcome of force acting against a resistance, we have mechanical work. If energy incorporates the motion of an object, we are talking about kinetic energy. Kinetic energy (KE) is the energy an object possesses as a result of it being in motion and is highly dependent on the velocity at which an object is moving. The equation for kinetic energy is $K_E = 1/2mv^2$, where m is the mass of the object, and v represents the velocity of the object at the time of observation. K_E is a vector quantity with units of joules (j). The larger the velocity of an object, the more kinetic energy it possesses, and the larger the amount of work it can accomplish when it contacts another object.

One or more interactive elements has been excluded from this version of the text. You can view them online here: https://pb.cognella.com/83647-1b/?p=55#oembed-12

Please refer to the interactive ebook in Cognella Active Learning for interactive/media content.

The location of an object relative to a reference plane determines the potential energy (PE) of the object. The greater the displacement between the object and the reference plane, the greater the potential energy of the object. The equation for potential energy is P_E = mgh, where m is the mass of the object, g is the constant of gravity, and h is the displacement of the object above the plane of reference. P_E is a vector quantity with units of joules (j). For a projectile, the sum of the potential and kinetic energy of an object remains constant throughout its flight: C_E = | P_E + K_E |, where the constant energy of an object is equal to the sum of the potential and kinetic energy of the object. This assumption of constant energy is true in situations in which air resistance is ignored. This concept will be discussed in more detail in Chapter 9.

The fourth and final type of energy that will be discussed in this chapter is that of strain energy. **Strain energy (SE)** is the energy potential that an object stores within itself when the object is deformed as the result of actions by an external force or forces. The equation for strain energy is S_E = $1/2kx^2$, where k is the spring constant of the material undergoing strain, and x is the measured displacement of the object. The spring constant k is determined through experimentation and is equal to the result of the change in applied force divided by the measured change in length of the body: k = Δforce/Δlength. S_E is a vector quantity with units of joules (j).

Exercises such as plyometrics take advantage of the ability to "teach" deformable materials such as human tendons and ligaments to capture and return strain energy to improve athletic performance. For example, a person of mass 60kg performs a plyometric jump exercise. They begin the exercise by positioning themselves at the edge of a 75cm-high box. The exercise requires the person to step off the edge of the box, landing with both feet on the ground and immediately bounding as high as possible. In this example, the person managed to jump straight back up to a height of 78 cm.

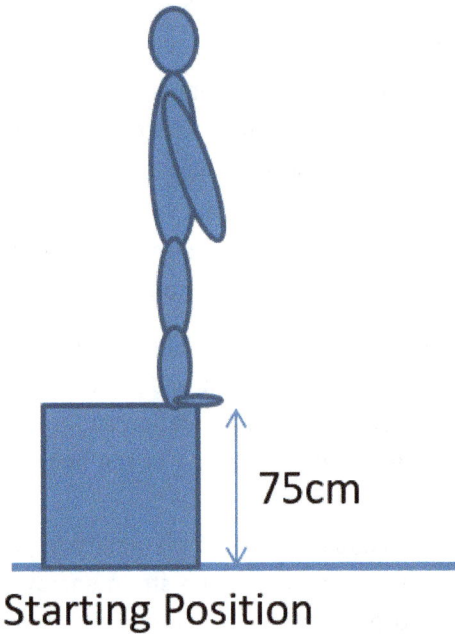

75cm

Starting Position

Figure 7.22   Standing on box.

What are the values for potential and kinetic energy of the person waiting to begin the motion?

Potential energy:

$$P_E = mgh$$

$$P_E = (60kg)*(-9.81m/s^2)*(0.75m)$$

$$P_E = -441.45j$$

Kinetic energy:

$$K_E = 1/2mv^2$$

$$K_E = \frac{1}{2}*(60kg)*(0.0m/s)^2$$

$$K_E = 0j$$

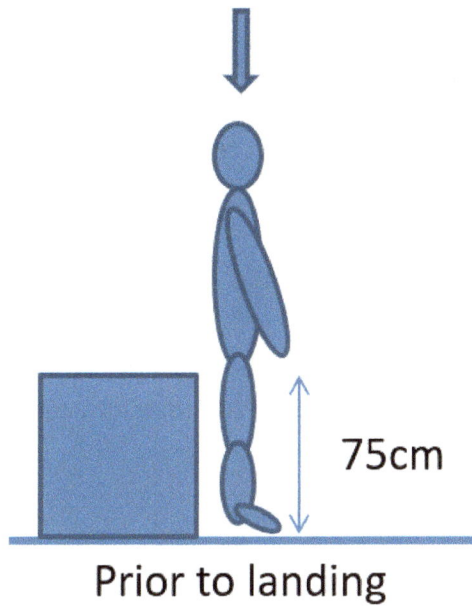

Figure 7.23   Dropping from box.

Immediately before contacting the ground, what are the potential and kinetic energies of the individual?

Potential energy:

$P_E = mgh$

$P_E = (60kg)*(-9.81m/s^2)*(0.0m)$

$P_E = 0j$

Kinetic energy:

$K_E = 1/2mv^2$

$K_E = \frac{1}{2}*(60kg)*(-3.84m/s)^2$

$K_E = -441.45j$

How did I arrive at the person's velocity of -3.84m/s? Remember that for projectiles the total energy of the system remains constant during flight. That means that $C_E = |\ P_E + K_E\ |$, and since the total energy at the beginning of the jump was 441.45j, it would also be the same just before landing. Therefore, you can solve for velocity:

$C_E = |\ P_E + K_E\ |$

$441.45j = |mgh + 1/2mv^2|$

$441.45j = 0j + 1/2mv^2$

$441.45j/(1/2*60kg) = v^2$

$\sqrt{(441.45j/(1/2*60kg))} = v$

$3.84m/s = v$

Remember that the direction of motion is down, so v = -3.84m/s

You can also check the value using the equations of constant acceleration for projectiles from Chapter 7.

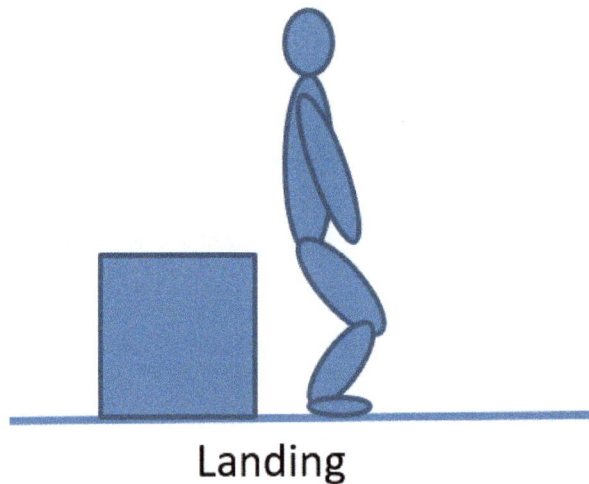

Landing

Figure 7.24   Landing.

Upon landing on the ground, the tendons of the legs stretch, which converts some of the kinetic energy of the body into strain energy. The Achilles tendons of the lower legs stretch approximately 5%, which returns about 70j of work to assist the person in their jumping motion.

If the person jumps straight up 78cm, what vertical velocity did they generate, and what was their potential energy at the apex of the jump?

Potential energy:

$P_E = mgh$

$P_E = (60kg)*(-9.81m/s^2)*(0.78m)$

P_E = -459.11j

Since the total energy of the flight is constant and equal to the absolute value of the sum of the potential and kinetic energies, we can use that information to calculate the takeoff or initial vertical velocity of the person using the kinetic energy equation:

Kinetic energy:

$$K_E = 1/2mv^2$$

$$459.11j = \frac{1}{2} \times (60kg) \times (v_{initial})^2$$

$$\sqrt{(459.11j)}/30kg = v_{initial}$$

$$3.91m/s = v_{initial}$$

Summary

Kinetics is the study of force, and force is the common factor behind all motion. Contact force is a vector that has a point of contact with the mass that it influences. Both the time of application and the area of application change the outcome of how an applied force affects a mass. To move safely and efficiently we must be able to generate, accommodate, and utilize internal and external forces. Newton's laws of motion provide us with the rules that explain the relationship between, mass, force, and interactions of forces during contact. We apply our understanding of how to generate and use muscle forces to propel and reorient our body during movement. Being able to overcome forces such as friction or air resistance are necessary for us to accomplish tasks such as walking and running. The concept of momentum provides a way to tie kinematic information to kinetic outcomes. Energy is the ability to do work, and the ease of converting from one form of energy to another makes all forms of movement possible.

List of Key Takeaways

- Kinetics is the study of force and how it effects motion. Force is a special type of vector that, in addition to having a magnitude and direction, also must have a point of application to be relevant. To gauge how a force may affect the motion state of an object, the mass of the object must be known.
- Forces occur in many forms, but all must have time to act. The combination of force times time provides a value called impulse, which is directly related to the momentum of an object. The relationship between changes in momentum allows for the calculation of force when certain kinematic values and the mass of the object are known.
- Energy is the ability to do mechanical work. Mechanical energy represents the sum of the kinetic (energy of motion) and potential (stored energy of position) energy of a body.

Table 7.1 Equations and Problems for Linear Kinetics

Variable and Equation	Units	Vector or Scalar	Comments
Force $F = ma$	N	Vector	
Weight $f_{weight} = m * a_{gravity}$	N	Vector	
Impulse $imp = F * t$	Ns	Vector	
Pressure $P = F/A$	Pascals or N/cm^2	Vector	
Stress $\sigma = F/A$	Pascals or N/cm^2	Vector	
GRF $GRF = f_{vertical} + | m_{object}a_{gavity} |$	N	Vector	$f_{vertical} = m_{object}(\Delta v/\Delta t)$
Friction $F = \mu R$	N	Vector	
Mechanical work $W = F * d * \cos(\Phi)$	joules	Vector	
Power $P = W/\Delta t$	watts	Vector	
Momentum (p) $p = mv$	kgm/s	Vector	
Conservation of linear momentum $m_1v_1 + m_2v_2 = v_{combined} *(m_1 + m_2)$	kgm/s	Vector	
Impulse and momentum $F * t = p\text{Final} - p\text{initial}$	Ns	Vector	
Potential energy $P_E = mgh$	joules	Vector	
Kinetic energy $K_E = 1/2mv^2$	joules	Vector	
Strain energy $S_E = 1/2kx^2$	joules	Vector	$k = \Delta force/\Delta length$

Image Credits

Fig. 7.9b: Copyright © by Jim Lamberson (CC BY-SA 4.0) at https://commons.wikimedia.org/wiki/File:EnPointeFoot.jpg.

Chapter 8

Angular Kinetics

Preparing to Learn: *Watch*

Angular motion results from forces asking to cause or halt rotation. By changing body position, it is possible to change the effects of rotational force. Reorienting body segments can make the body more or less likely to rotate when torque is applied. We take advantage of realigning body mass to increase or decrease body rotation for a given amount of torque.

The following videos provide visual examples of how torque and body alignment can be optimized resulting in rotational movement.

One or more interactive elements has been excluded from this version of the text. You can view them online here: https://pb.cognella.com/83647-1b/?p=56#oembed-9

Please refer to the interactive ebook in Cognella Active Learning for interactive/media content.

One or more interactive elements has been excluded from this version of the text. You can view them online here: https://pb.cognella.com/83647-1b/?p=56#oembed-10

Please refer to the interactive ebook in Cognella Active Learning for interactive/media content.

One or more interactive elements has been excluded from this version of the text. You can view them online here: https://pb.cognella.com/83647-1b/?p=56#oembed-11

Please refer to the interactive ebook in Cognella Active Learning for interactive/media content.

Preparing to Learn: *Respond*

Directions: Based on what you saw in the video, respond to the following questions:

1. Sport video: How did the orientation of the diver change from takeoff to entry, and what did repositioning his body do to the observed motion?
2. Daily life: Climbing or descending stairs is a difficult physical task that most of us take for granted. What type of angular motion is necessary to negotiate stairs, and what are the primary lower body muscles needed when climbing and descending stairs?
3. Medicine: Transitioning from one type of assistive device to another requires a strategy that does not put a person at risk of injury. Describe how body position changes assist the transition from seated in a wheelchair to standing with a walker.

Introduction to the Chapter

In this chapter we will discuss how forces applied to objects can cause the objects to rotate about their center of mass. We will also explore the importance of structures comprised of levers, axes, and forces with regard to rotational motion. Finally, we will look at how torque, occurring within the human body, or in a mechanical system, plays a central role in the many forms of rotational movement we experience each day.

Understanding how and where to most appropriately apply rotational force allows us to walk, run, sit down, stand up, lift, carry, and reposition objects. While we tend to think about motion as linear, the underlying rotational components of motion often determine the success or failure of our linear actions.

Learning Objectives

After completing this chapter, students should be able to do the following:

*   Define angular kinetics
*   List the basic components of a lever system
*   Identify simple lever systems found in the human body
*   Explain the relationship between radius of rotation and applied torque
*   Solve problems and determine torque values associated with angular motion

Angular Kinetics Concepts and Variables

In Chapter 7, the importance of forces relative to movement was introduced, and Newton's three laws of motion set the foundation for our understanding of the causes and effects of motion. In this chapter we will discuss the fundamental role that forces also play in rotational or angular motion.

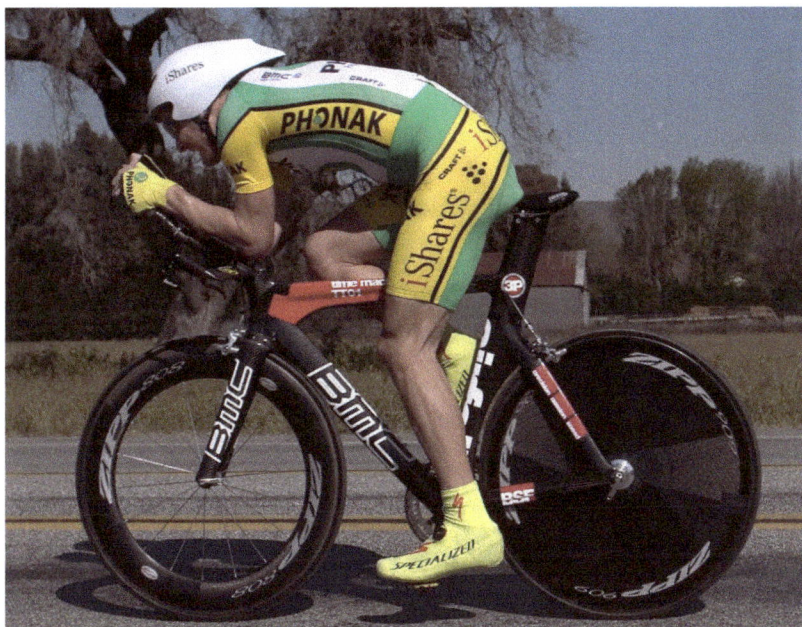

Figure 8.1   Praying mantis cyclist.

Before we go too far, we need to review some concepts about some simple machines: levers. There are three types of lever systems: first-, second-, and third-class levers. Each **lever system** is a simple machine that consists of a minimum of a lever, fulcrum, a resistance force, and motive force. A **lever** can be defined as any rigid or semi-rigid structure resting on a pivot. The **fulcrum** or pivot provides a physical location for the axis of rotation of the lever to exist. The **resistance force** is the force in opposition of the applied torque generated by the lever system, and the **motive force** is the applied force generating the torque created by the use of the lever system to overcome a resistance. All lever systems provide some form of advantage to their users. The advantage may be in balancing a resistance force, multiplying the effect of a motive force or increasing the linear velocity at the end of a lever. All three types of lever systems can be found within the human body. A value called a **mechanical advantage (MA)** can be calculated for a lever system as a ratio of the distance of the point of motive force application from the fulcrum, $L_{motive\ force}$, divided by the distance of the resistance force from the fulcrum, $L_{resistance\ force}$; $MA = L_{motive\ force} / L_{resistance\ force}$. The greater the MA the lower the amount of motive force needed to overcome the resistance.

A first-class lever system can be thought of as a balance scale in which the fulcrum is positioned between the resistance and motive forces. A teeter totter is an example of a first-class lever system. Within the human body, the balancing of the head on top of the spine is another example of a first-class lever system. The mechanical advantage of a first-class lever system can be > 1, = 1, or < 1.

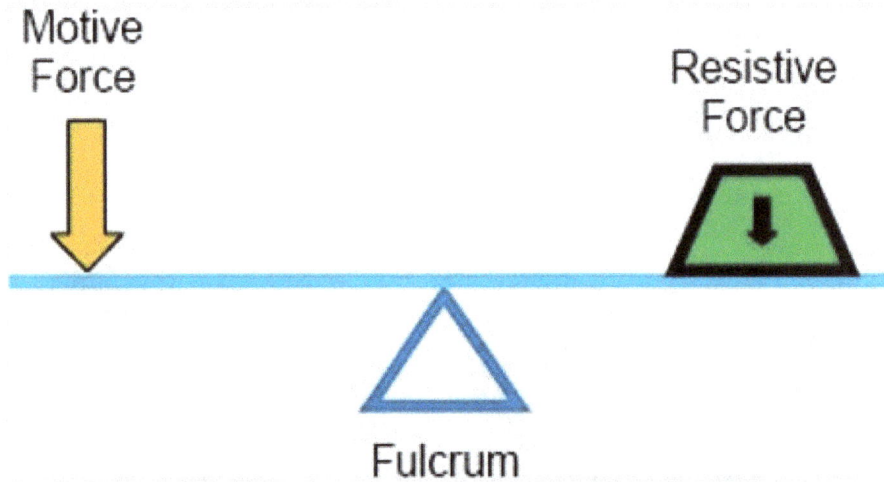

Figure 8.2   First-class lever.

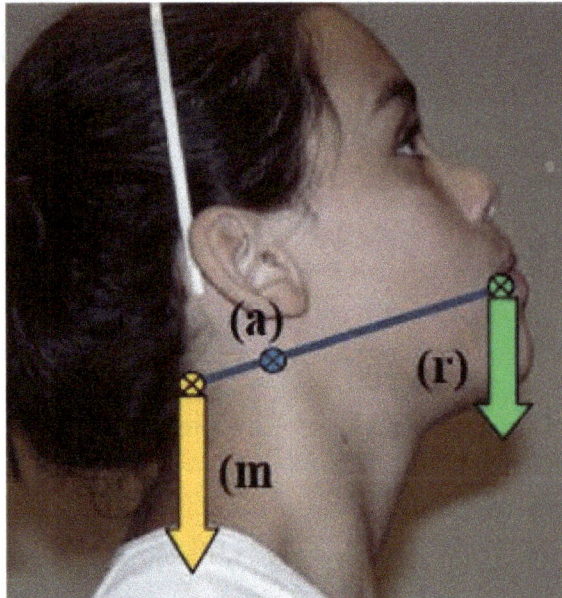

Figure 8.3   First-class lever in the human body.

A second-class lever system is the most mechanically efficient type of lever system at multiplying the effect of the motive force. It allows for a relatively small motive force to counteract the resistance force. Second-class lever systems are good for force transmission but poor for increasing distal velocity at the end of the lever. A wheelbarrow is an example of this type of lever. In the human body an example of a second-class lever system is the foot ankle complex, along with the Achilles tendon and associated lower limb musculature that allows for balancing the human body on two feet with a minimum of applied motive force. The mechanical advantage for a second-class lever system is always > 1.

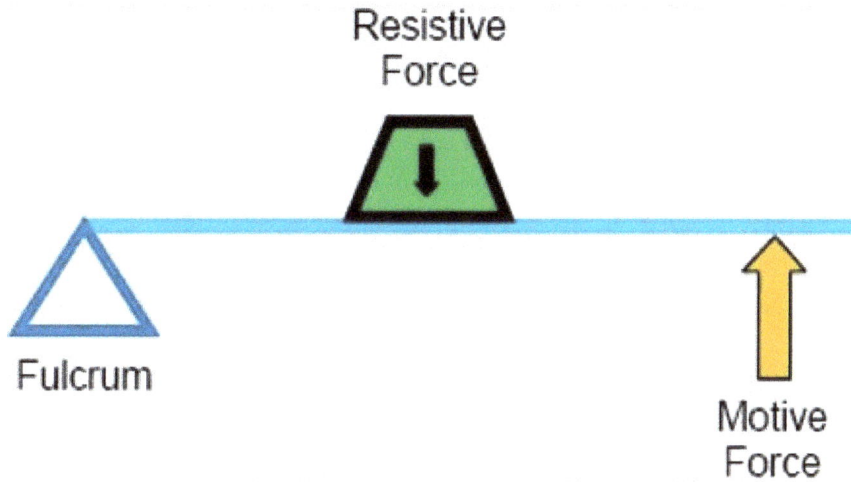

Figure 8.4   Second-class lever system.

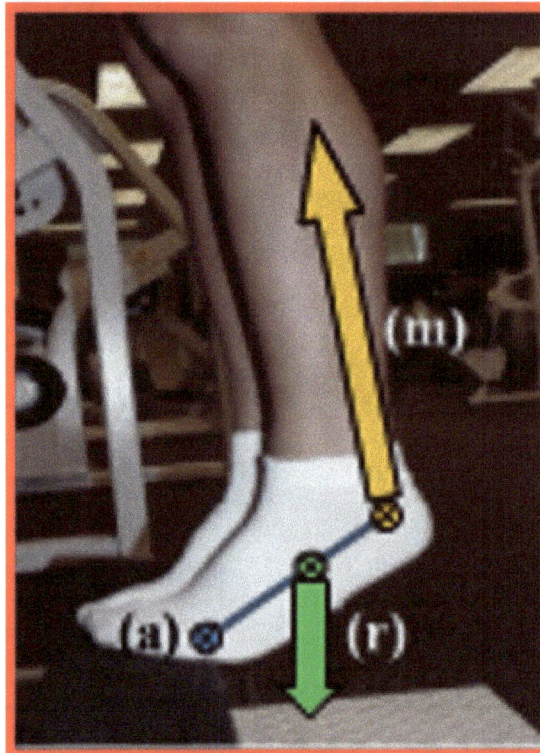

Figure 8.5   Second-class lever system found in the human body.

Third-class lever systems are most effective in creating high distal velocities at the end of the lever but require large motive forces to overcome inertia and the resistance force of the system. A catapult is a real-world example of such a lever system, as is the upper arm, elbow, and forearm of a human. A large motive force must be applied by the biceps muscle to initiate elbow flexion, but once started large distal velocities can be generated at the hand and wrist, which are ideal for throwing or striking activities. The mechanical advantage for a third-class lever system is always < 1.

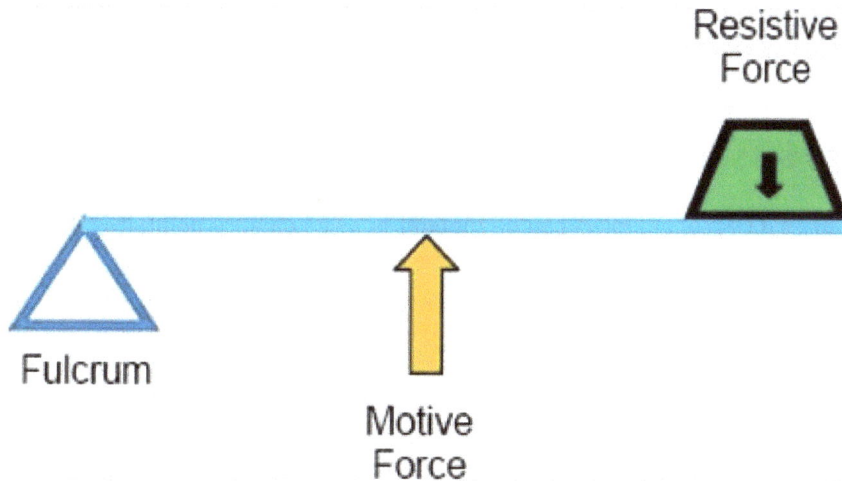

Figure 8.6   Third-class lever system.

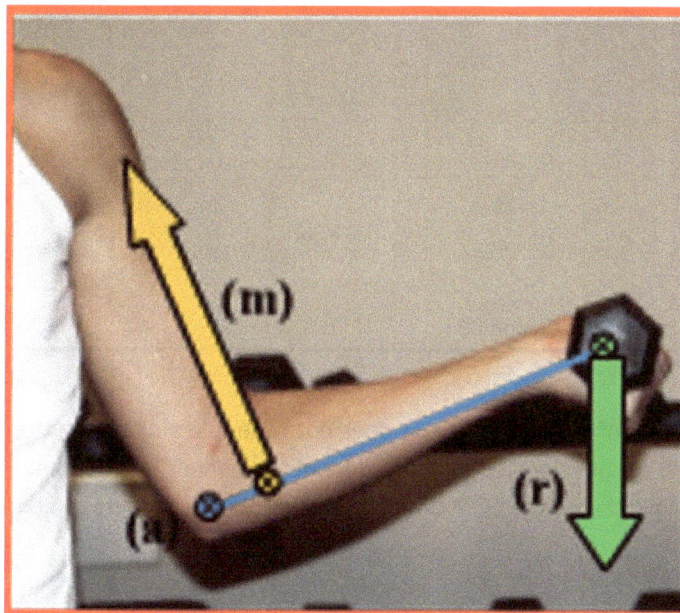

Figure 8.7   Third-class lever system in human body.

Torque (τ), which is sometimes referred to as a "moment," is the outcome of a perpendicular force applied to a lever at a greater than zero distance from the axis of rotation. The equation for torque is $\tau = \perp F * d$. Torque is a vector with units Nm. Note that torque and mechanical work are essentially equivalent terms, where $W = F * \perp d$ refers to work accomplished in a linear system and $\tau = \perp F * d$ refers to angular work performed in a rotating system. The **radius of rotation** (or moment arm) is a measure of length that represents the distance from the center of rotation along the lever arm to the point of force application.

In the calculation of torque the radius of rotation provides us with the value of distance. In lever systems, there are two radii of rotations and are equivalent to $L_{motive\ force}$ and $L_{resistance\ force}$.

Center of Mass and Center of Gravity

The **center of mass** (**COM**) of an object can be thought of as its balance point. It is the point through which the line of gravitational attraction would act if all of the mass of the object were consolidated into a single point of mass. The COM for a malleable or multisegmented body may be repositioned by shifting the distribution of mass of the object.

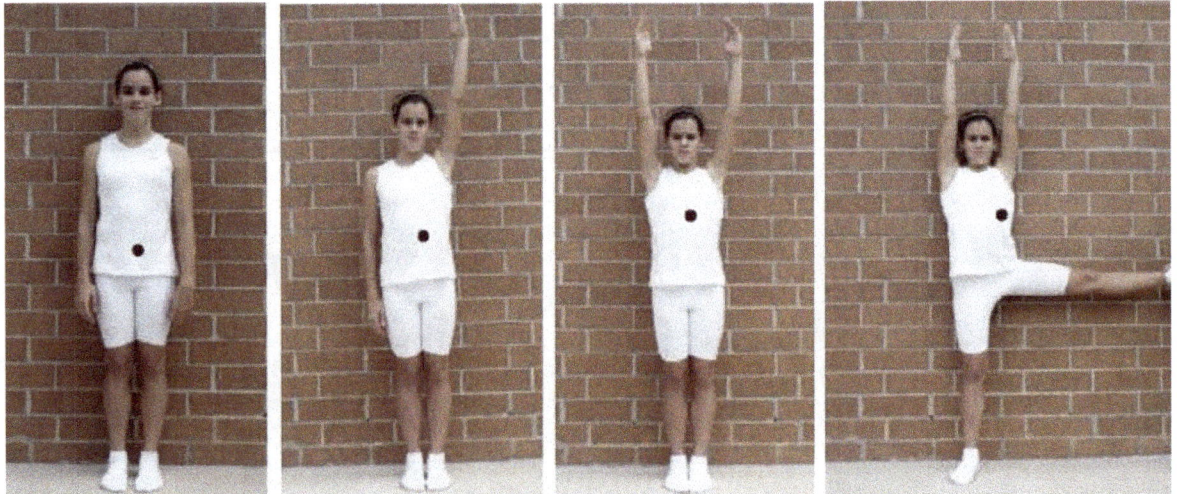

Figure 8.8   COM movement in the human body.

A fascinating property of the COM is that it does not have to reside within the physical boundaries of the object. The COM of a donut is located in the middle of the donut hole. Bending over to touch your toes with arms and legs straight causes the COM of most people to move outside the body.

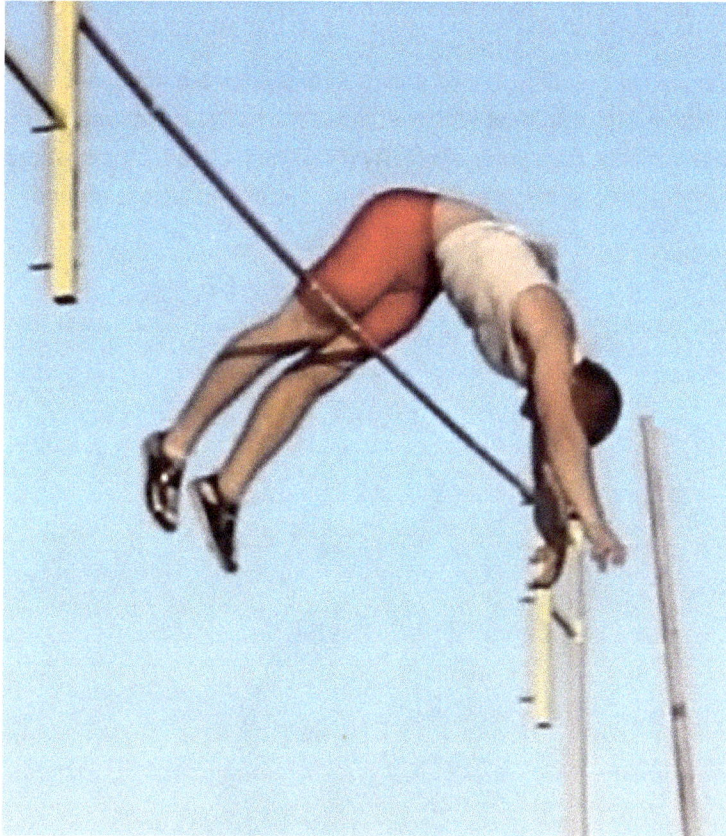

Figure 8.9   Pole vaulter COM outside of body.

The hyper extension of the back while high jumping does the same. This phenomenon allows the athlete to clear the bar while the athlete's COM may actually pass below it.

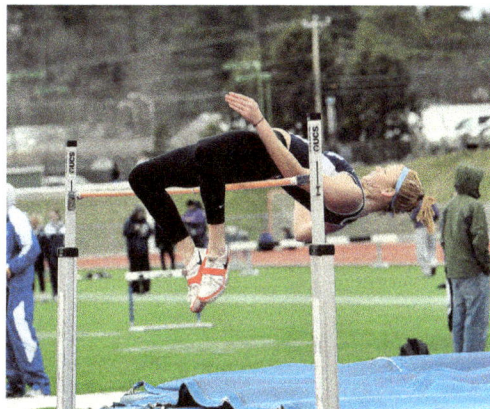

Figure 8.10   High jumper COM outside of body.

Center of Gravity

Often the terms *center of mass* and *center of gravity* are used interchangeably, but technically that is incorrect. While COM describes the point at which all mass of a body is centered and through which the line of gravitational acceleration acts, the **center of gravity (COG)** refers to a location where the line of action of the acceleration of gravity acting through the COM of an object contacts the ground.

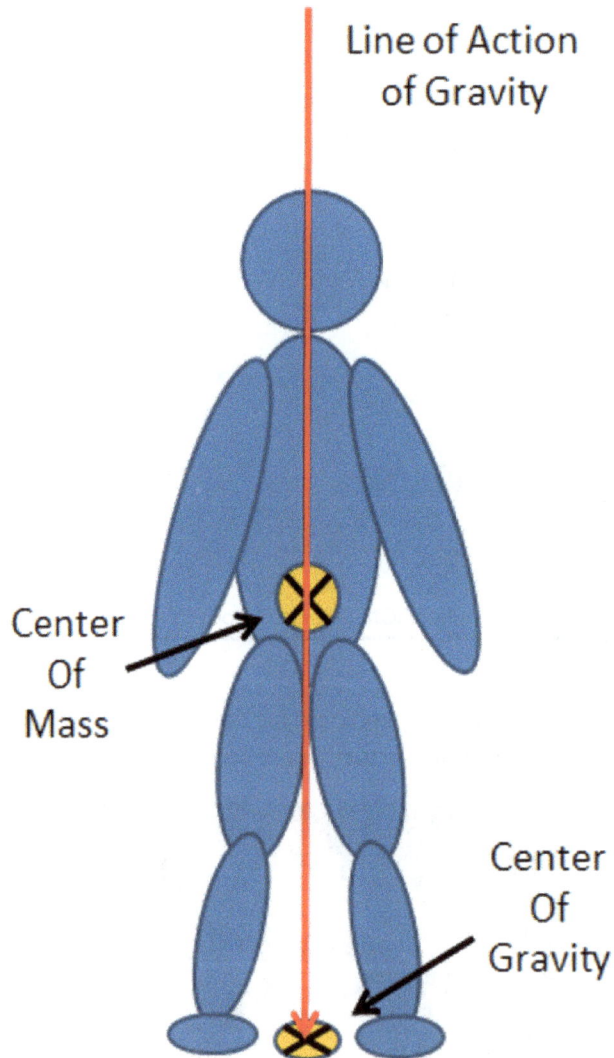

Figure 8.11   COM and COG.

The line of action of a force determines whether the outcome results in mechanical work (linear translation of the object) or torque, which is angular work (rotation of the object about an axis), or a combination of both mechanical and angular work. The location of the motive force also determines, in anatomical terms, whether the force acts to stabilize (pull or push toward the center of rotation of a joint) or dislocate (pull or push away from the center of joint rotation).

For example, two popular types of serves in volleyball are the float and topspin serves. Both require the ball to be tossed forward above the head of the server, who jumps toward the ball, striking it to propel it over the net. While there is often a difference in the amount of force used in the striking motion, with the topspin shot being struck more violently, the key difference is the location relative to the COM of the ball where the force is applied. For the float serve, the motive force is applied through the COM of the ball, which is referred to as a **centric** application of force. The outcome in movement is translation without rotation of the ball.

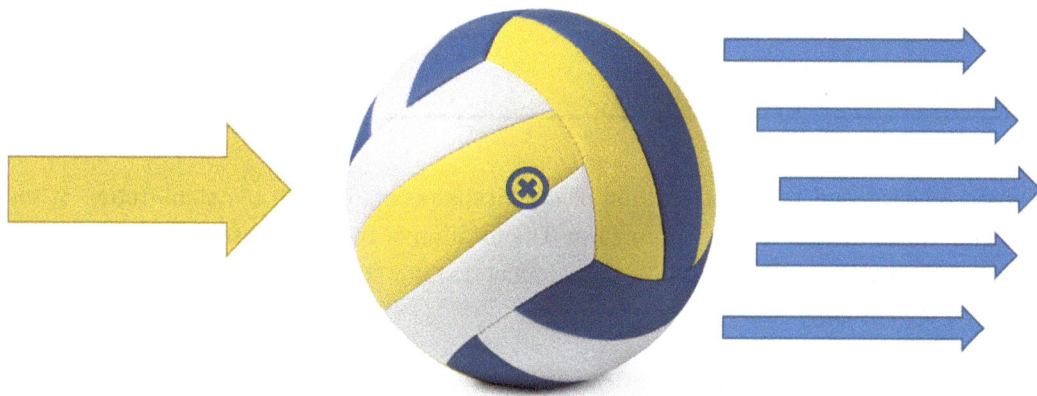

Figure 8.12   Centric force.

For the topspin serve, the outcome is a combination of translation and rotation since some of the motive force is directed at a point above the COM of the ball. A force applied to an object not through its COM is considered an **eccentric** force. The merits of both serve types from a flight and game strategy perspective will be discussed in more detail in Chapter 9.

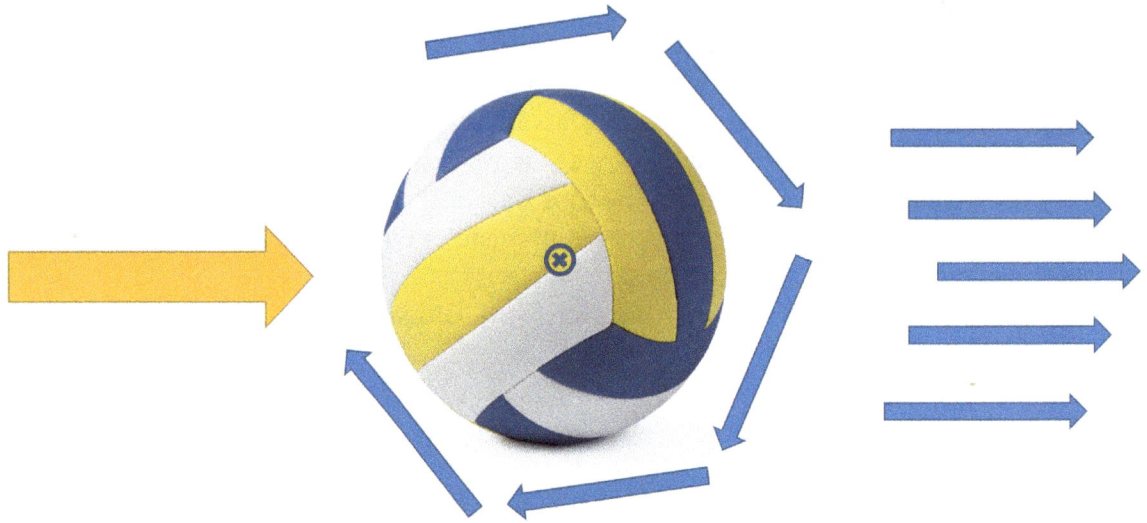

Figure 8.13   Eccentric force.

During a biceps curl the muscle action of the biceps results in both the stabilization of the elbow and flexion between the upper arm and forearm. The location of the distal insertion of the biceps tendon into the proximal end of the ulna results in this combined elbow stabilization and flexion outcome when a biceps pulling force is generated.

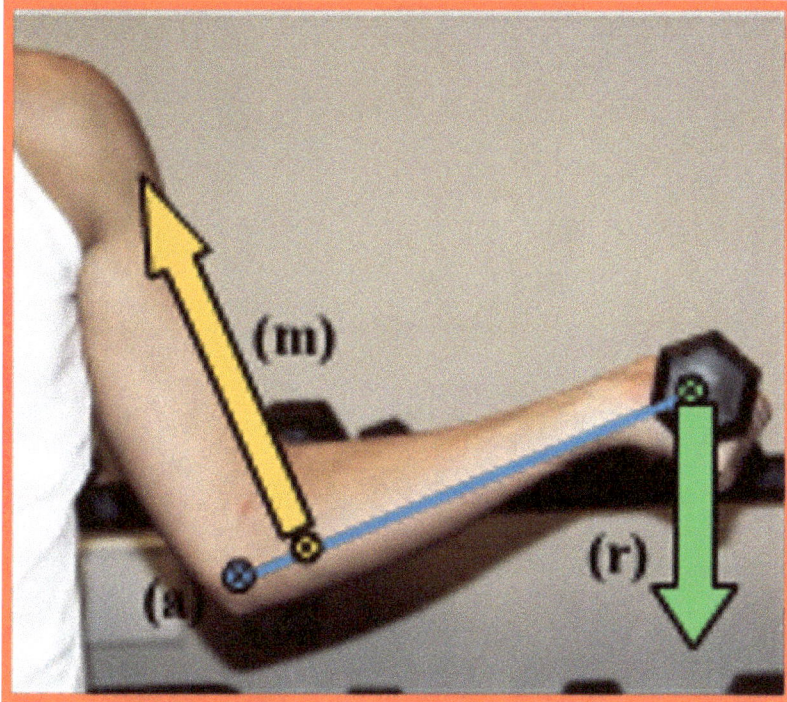

Figure 8.14   Biceps curl.

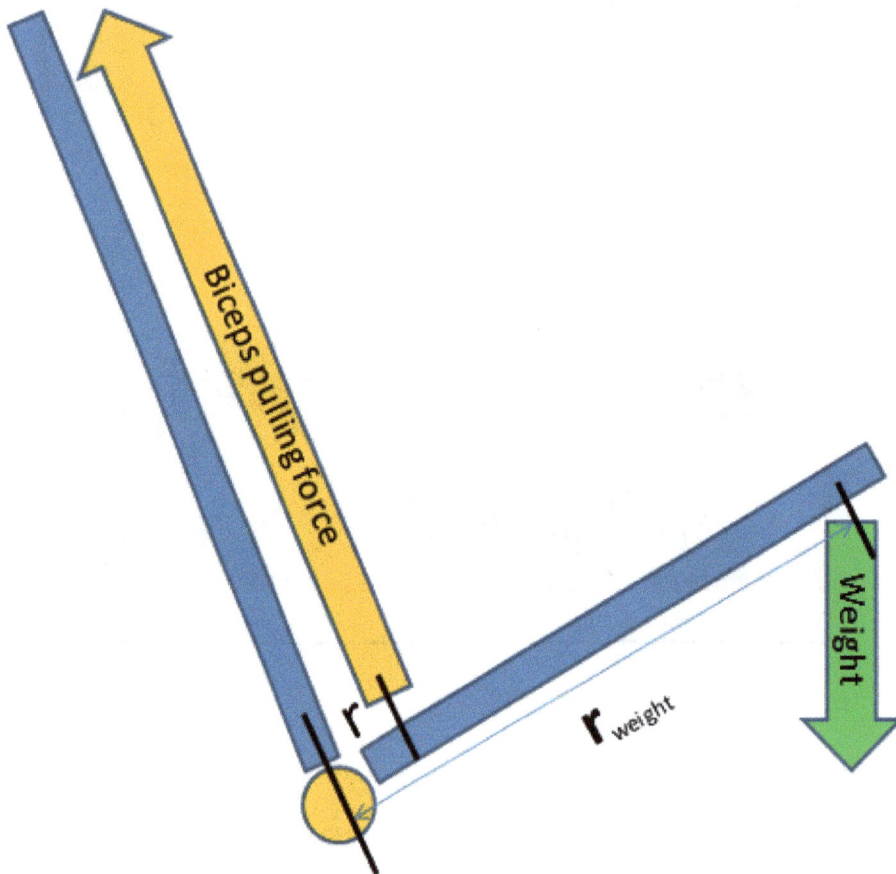

Figure 8.15   Free body diagram biceps curl.

The **radius of rotation** (r) seen in Figure 8.15 represents the $\perp$ distance away from the elbow joint center that allows some of the pulling force of the biceps to create a flexion torque. The remaining pulling force stabilizes the elbow. The distal insertion point for the biceps is located about 3cm from the axis of rotation of the elbow for adults, so a good estimate for "r" for most of us is 3cm. Therefore, if the r_{weight} value in our example was 25.5cm and the weight 22.4N, then the biceps force required to keep the upper and lower arms in equilibrium would be

$\tau_{biceps} = \tau_{weight}$

$F_{biceps} * r_{biceps} = F_{weight} * r_{weight}$

$F_{biceps} * 0.03m = 22.4N * .255m$

$F_{biceps} = (22.4N * .255m)/0.03m$

$F_{biceps} = 190.4N$

Note that because of the mechanical disadvantage inherent in a third-class lever systems such as the upper arm, elbow, and forearm, a biceps force of 850% of the resistance weight force is needed to keep the segments motionless! Why would you ever build a machine like us if we require such large internal forces to deal with relatively small external forces? What advantages do human third-class lever systems have related to motion?

Most of us had heard of Newton's three laws of motion prior to reading this text; however, many probably didn't realize that there are also three corresponding laws of angular motion that are the analogs of Newton's original set of laws. Angular motion conforms to essentially the same laws of motion as linear motion; it's just now we have to account for a "twist."

Newton's First Law of Angular Motion

Newton's first law of angular motion (inertia) states that any rotating system will continue its rotation about an axis at a constant rate and direction unless the system is acted upon by an external torque. The inertia that is battled by torque is defined as the moment of inertia of a body.

Moment of Inertia

The **moment of inertia (I)** is the resistance to change in angular acceleration demonstrated by a body due to the distribution of its mass relative to an axis of rotation. When representing a body as a two-dimensional object, $I = \Sigma mr^2$, where m represents individual point masses that make up a body and r is the radius of rotation of their associated radius of rotation values. The farther mass is located from the axis of rotation, the larger the moment of inertia. A human's moment of inertia relative to rotation about their center of mass is greatest when standing upright with arms extended overhead; it is smaller when in a piked position and at a minimum when the person is tucked tightly into a ball.

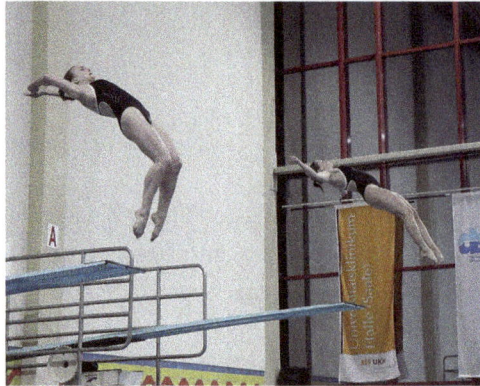

Figure 8.16   Diver large I.

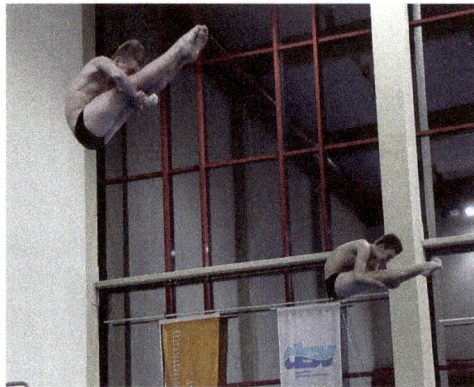

Figure 8.17   Diver smaller I.

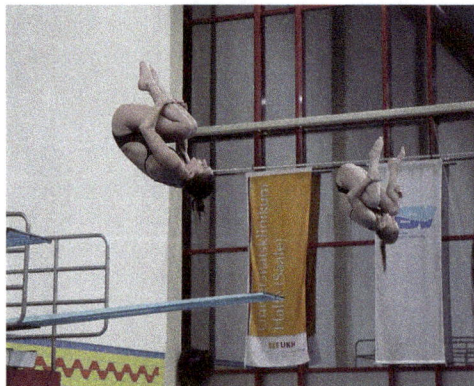

Figure 8.18   Diver smallest I.

The rapid relocation of the moment of inertia allows an athlete to complete a complex gymnastics trick.

One or more interactive elements has been excluded from this version of the text. You can view them online here: https://pb.cognella.com/83647-1b/?p=56#oembed-1

Please refer to the interactive ebook in Cognella Active Learning for interactive/media content.

For example, given the diagram (Figure 8.19) of the mass and radii of gyration values of a man, determine the moment of inertia of his whole right leg.

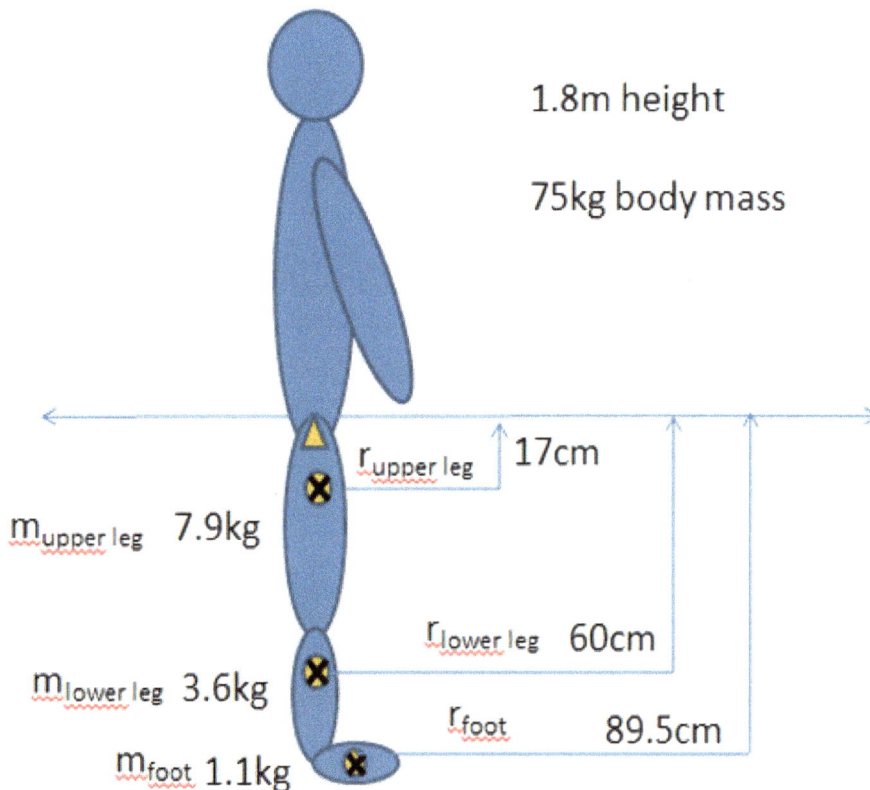

1.8m height

75kg body mass

$r_{upper\ leg}$ 17cm

$m_{upper\ leg}$ 7.9kg

$r_{lower\ leg}$ 60cm

$m_{lower\ leg}$ 3.6kg

r_{foot} 89.5cm

m_{foot} 1.1kg

Figure 8.19   COM location for lower body segments.

$I = \Sigma\ mr^2$

$I = (m_{upper\ leg} * r_{upper\ leg}^2) + (m_{lower\ leg} * r_{lower\ leg}^2) + (m_{foot} * r_{foot}^2)$

$$I = (7.9\text{kg} * (0.17\text{m})^2) + (3.6\text{kg} * (0.6\text{m})^2) + (1.1\text{kg} * (0.89\text{m})^2)$$

$$I = 1.62 \text{ kg m}^2$$

Note that even though the upper leg is the most massive of the segments because its radius of rotation is by far the smallest, it contributes less to the moment of inertia of the whole leg than the shank. The relatively small moment of inertia of the leg results in significant muscular force savings when performing hip flexion and extension movements such as walking or running.

I is a function of the total mass of the body, or selected body segments, and is identified as a location where the lumped mass of the body acts to resist angular change. The location of the moment of inertia can be found for a combination of segments simultaneously by determining where the combined mass of the segments would be located to produce the same result as the combined value derived by summing the individual contributions of each segment. Human body segments tend to have their COM located closer to the proximal end of the segment, reducing the segment moment of inertia, facilitating our ability to rotate them through muscle-generated torques about the joints to which they are connected.

Finding the true moments of inertia of an object as complex and variable, as the human body provides ongoing difficulty for biomechanists. People come in too many shapes and sizes to formulate a general but accurate value of I for everyone. It is currently impossible to develop a working model that can accurately determine the exact inertial characteristics of all humans. It is not for lack of trying; there have been many attempts to develop databases and equations to estimate I for all people. Work by Dempster (1967), Zatsiorsky (2003), and Jensen (1993), to name a few, have greatly contributed to our knowledge and understanding of the human moment of inertia, but none have been able to solve the problem. So, work will continue, but for us to be able to begin to understand the mathematics behind moment of inertia calculations we will use the tables created by Dempster and his team.

Torque

Torque (τ) is also equivalent to the product of the moment of inertia multiplied by the angular acceleration of an object: $\tau = I\alpha$. The angular acceleration of an object is directly proportional to the applied torque, causing the acceleration inversely proportional to the moment of inertia of the object, which resists the effect of the applied torque.

At first glance it might be hard to recognize how that relationship for torque is equivalent to the more familiar mechanical work value of F * ⊥d. The easiest way to mathematically verify that they are indeed equal is to check to see if their units match:

$\tau = I\alpha$ and $\tau = F\perp d$

$I\alpha = F\perp d$

Table 8.1 pairs the parameters of the torque and mechanical work with their correct units.

Table 8.1. Parameters and Units

Parameter	Units

Table 8.1. Parameters and Units

I	kg m^2
α	rad/s^2
F	kg m/s^2
d	m

If we substitute a value of 1 for each of the parameters of the equation,

$I\omega = F\bot d$

$1\text{kg m}^2 * 1\text{ rad/s}^2 = 1\text{ kg m/s}^2 * 1\text{ m}$

$1\text{kg m}^2/\text{s}^2 = 1\text{kg m}^2/\text{s}^2$ ✓

They are equivalent!

The relationship $\tau = I\alpha$ demonstrates how torque, moment of inertia, and angular acceleration are related to one another. The net torque applied to a body is directly proportional to the angular acceleration it experiences and the rotational inertia (moment of inertia) exhibited by the body.

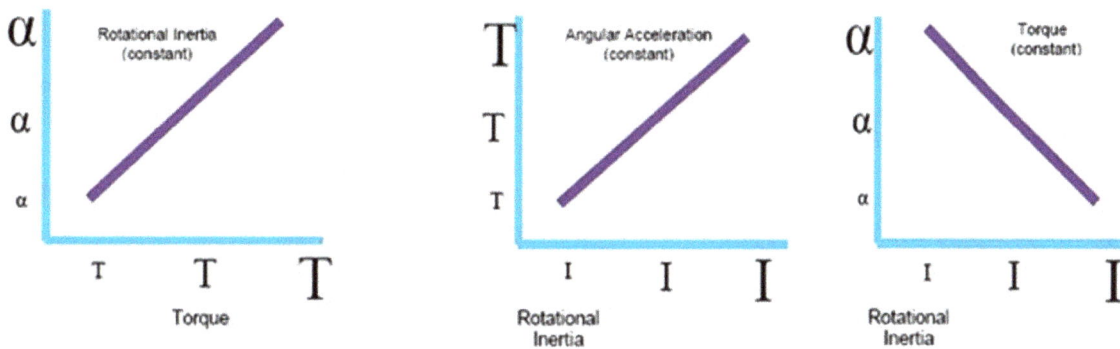

Figure 8.20   Torque acceleration moment of inertia.

This relationship is important because it allows the easy calculation of the moment of inertia of any object if the applied torque and angular acceleration are known. As demonstrated previously, many assumptions and calculations must be made to determine the moment of inertia of human body. This relationship among torque, moment of inertia, and angular acceleration provides a much simpler way to accurately determine the moment of inertia.

In many complex movements a person is required to coordinate the application of torques from multiple muscles activating in rapid succession. At the same time, angular acceleration and changing moments of inertia must be properly accounted for to generate a successful motion outcome such as during a tennis serve or performing an Olympic style lift.

One or more interactive elements has been excluded from this version of the text. You can view them online here: https://pb.cognella.com/83647-1b/?p=56#oembed-2

Please refer to the interactive ebook in Cognella Active Learning for interactive/media content.

One or more interactive elements has been excluded from this version of the text. You can view them online here: https://pb.cognella.com/83647-1b/?p=56#oembed-3

Please refer to the interactive ebook in Cognella Active Learning for interactive/media content.

For example, what is the moment of inertia of a parkour runner as he completes a somersault following a jump from the roof of a small house? If angular acceleration of the runner's body was 13.2rad/s^2 and the torque applied to his body as he tucked and pushed off the ground was 18.2Nm, what was the moment of inertia of his body during the somersault?

$\tau = I\alpha$

$18.2\text{Nm} = I * 13.2\text{rad/s}^2$

$I = (13.2\text{rad/s}^2) / 18.2\text{Nm}$

$I = 7.3 \text{ kgm}^2$

To arrive at the proper units for I, remember that the placeholder "rad" may be discarded if not needed, as in this case, and that the units of "s^2" for the angular acceleration term cancels with the "s^2" of the base units of "N" for the torque value.

Newton's Second Law of Angular Motion

Newton's Second Law of Angular Motion *(angular acceleration)* states that "the angular acceleration of a rotating body is directly proportional to and acts in the same direction as the applied torque but is inversely proportional to the moment of inertia of the body." Therefore, if a torque of sufficient magnitude is applied to a body such that it causes an angular acceleration of the body, it will accelerate in the direction of the applied torque. That means a body with a large moment of inertia requires a large torque to generate a small angular acceleration. It also means a body with a small moment of inertia will experience a large angular acceleration if a large torque is applied.

Angular Power

Angular power (P_{ang}) is generated by torque being multiplied by the angular velocity of a rotating object: $P_{ang}\ \tau = {}^* \omega$, where τ is applied torque and ω the angular velocity represented in units of rad/s, and the units for P_{ang} are watts.

For example, as a person pushes down on the pedal of bicycle, she is generating angular power, which will be transformed into mechanical energy to propel the bike forward at a pedaling cadence of 60rpm. If she pushes on the pedal attached to a 170mm long shaft oriented at 40° with 100N @ 338°, how much torque is she creating on the crank? Remember that torque is the product of the ⊥ component of the applied force and the radius of rotation. If the torque value found in this problem represents the average torque applied to pedals during her ride, what is her average power output?

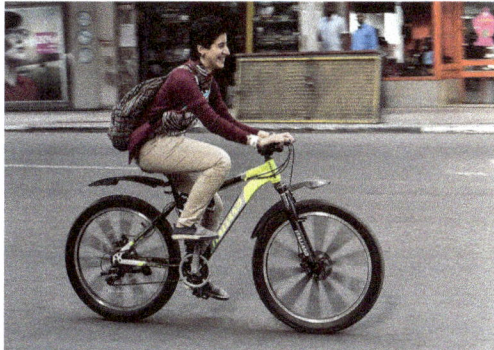

Figure 8.21   Cyclist pushing down on pedal.

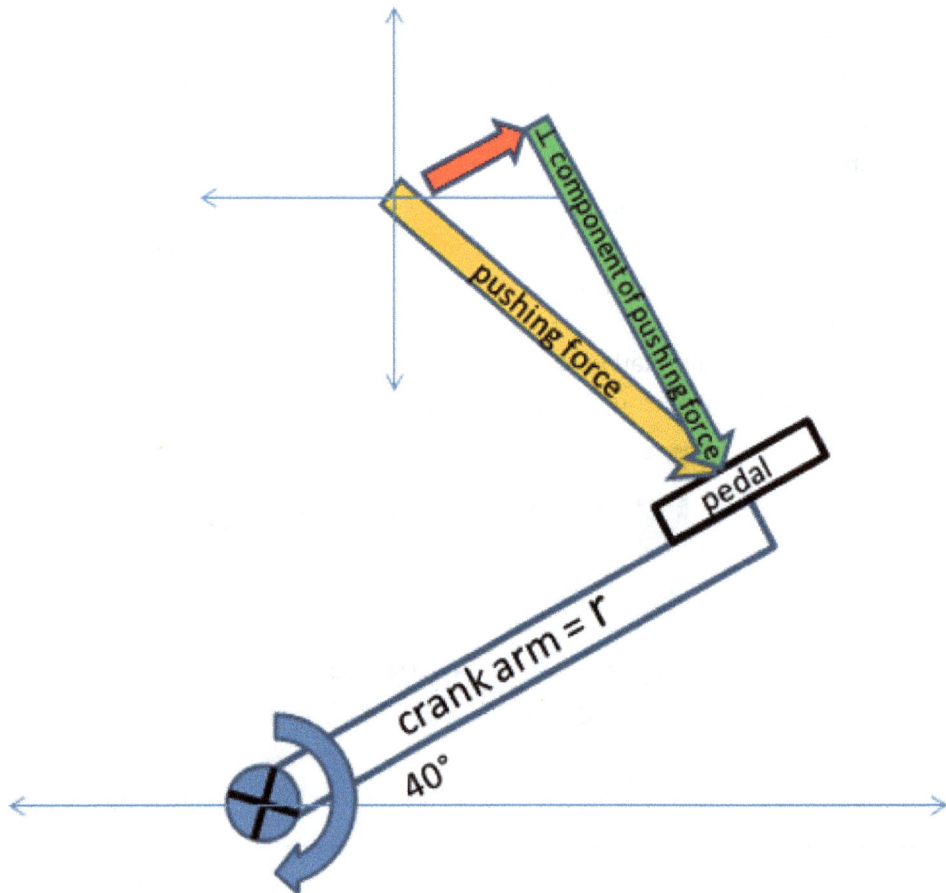

Figure 8.22   Forces pushing down on pedal.

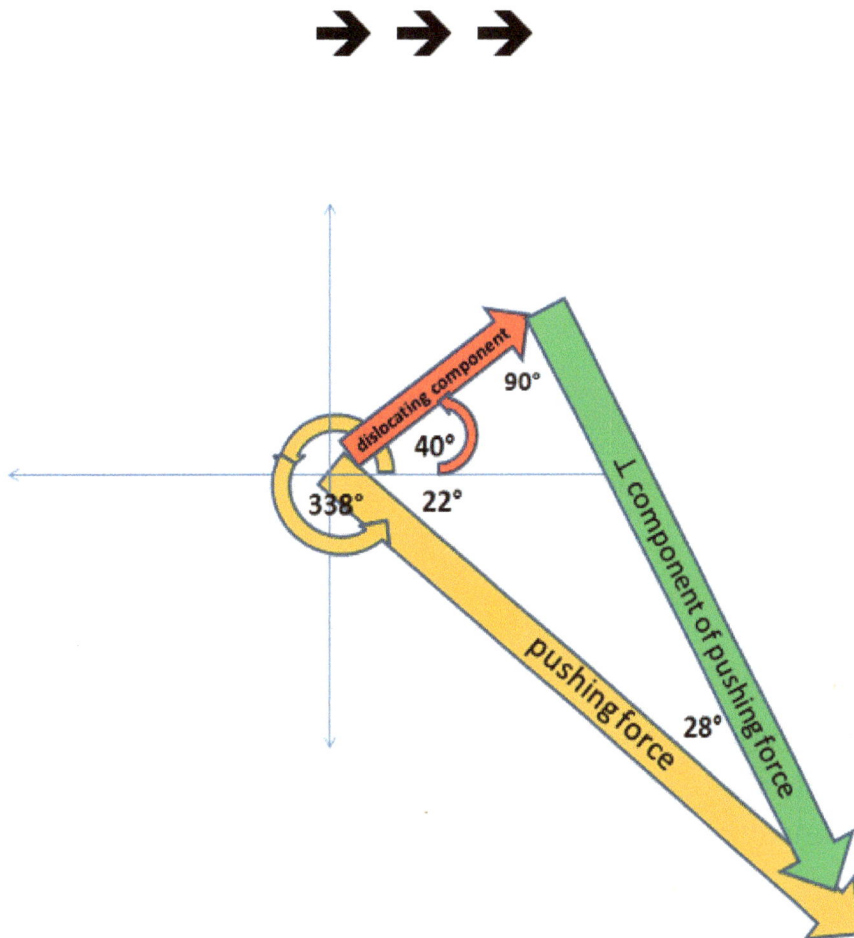

Figure 8.23   Force components acting on pedal.

Since we know that the crank arm is at 40°, the dislocating component of the pushing force must be parallel. So, related to the Cartesian coordinate axis located at the origin of the pushing force, the dislocating force must also be directed at 40°. To reduce the pushing force into its right-angle components, the force applied to the pedal that will generate torque, that is, the ⊥ component of the pushing force, must be oriented at 90° to the dislocating component of the pushing force. That knowledge allows us to determine the interior angles of the pushing force right triangle into angles of 62° = 40° + (360° - 338°) between the pushing force and the dislocating pushing force component and 28° = 180° - 90° -

62° between the pushing force and the ⊥ component of the pushing force that will generate torque when applied to the pedal.

The instantaneous torque generated can now be calculated as

$\tau = F * \perp d$

$\tau = (\perp$ component of the pushing force$) *$ crank length

$\tau = (\sin (62) *100N) * 0.17m$

$\tau = 88.29N *0.17m$

$\tau = 15.01Nm$

The average angular power is

$P_{ang} = \tau * \omega$

$P_{ang} = 15.01Nm * \omega$

$\omega = 60rpm \Rightarrow 60$ rev/min $\Rightarrow (60rev * 360°/1rev)/ (1min *(60s*/1min)) \Rightarrow 360°/s$

$\omega = 360°/s * (6.28rad/360°) \Rightarrow 6.28rad/s$

$P_{ang} = 15.01Nm * 6.28rad/s$

$P_{ang} = 94.26$ w

Force needs to be applied in a downward direction onto the pedal during the phase when maximum force can be generated.

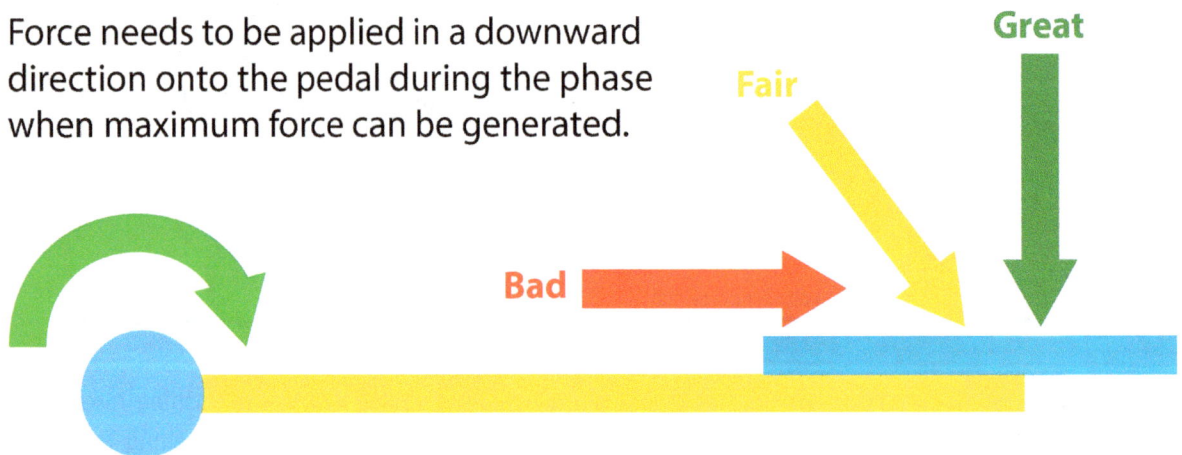

Figure 8.24   Various force application angles on pedal.

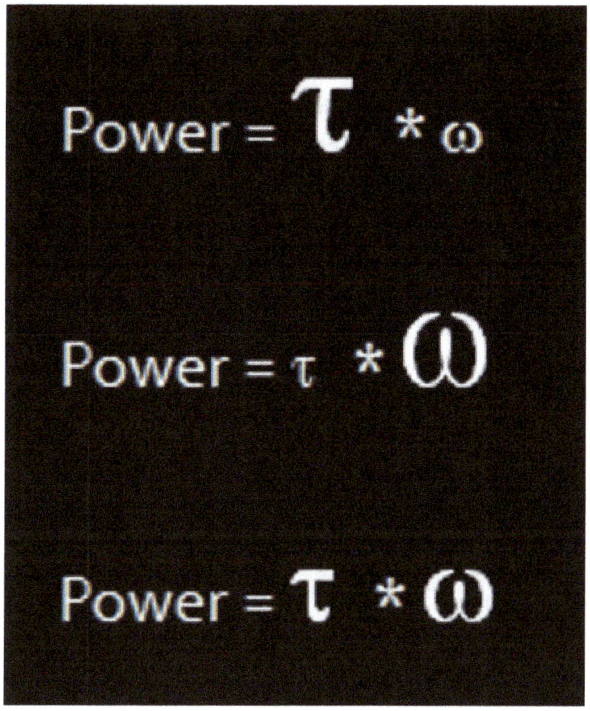

$$Power = \tau * \omega$$

$$Power = \tau * \omega$$

$$Power = \tau * \omega$$

Figure 8.25   Power, torque, angular velocity.

We humans take advantage of this second law of angular motion in many of the complex movements that allow us to run, jump, throw, and strike objects. Elite sprinters generate over four steps per second as they blaze down the track. To accomplish such a feat, they take advantage of the segmented architecture of the human body. By flexing at the hip, they pull the mass of the upper leg, lower leg, and foot closer to the center of rotation of hip, reducing the moment of inertia of the whole lower extremity. The decrease in the moment of inertia of the leg reduces the amount of torque that must be generated by the hip flexors to pull the leg mass forward and up against the acceleration of gravity. Then, as they extend the hip, knee, and plantar flex, the foot preparing for their next foot contact, they move the leg mass away from the hip, which increases the moment of inertia, slowing the rotation of the leg as it comes down to the ground. Even though the moment of inertia is increased, it doesn't take more effort from the hip extensors since they are now being aided by gravity, which helps drive the leg downward.

One or more interactive elements has been excluded from this version of the text. You can view them online here: https://pb.cognella.com/83647-1b/?p=56#oembed-4

Please refer to the interactive ebook in Cognella Active Learning for interactive/media content.

Newton's Third law of Angular Motion

Newton's Third Law of Angular Motion *(action–reaction)* states that "when one body exerts a torque on another body, the second body will respond by exerting a torque of equal magnitude but opposite direction on the first body." Human balance is a wonderful example of Newton's third law in action. We learn at a very early age if we begin to fall in one direction to immediately throw out a limb in the opposite direction to help regain our balance. That balancing act is our kinesthetic response to a torque, which will lead us to topple over unless a counter active torque is quickly generated.

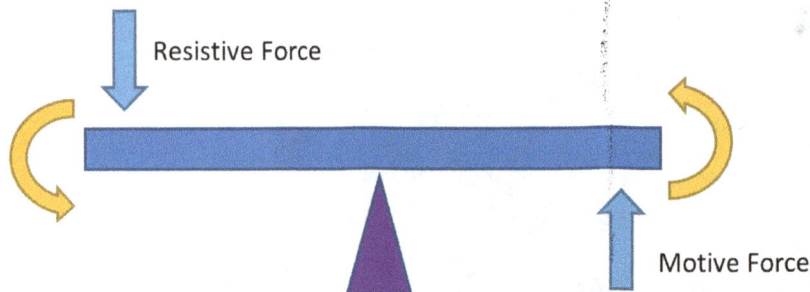

Resistive Force

Motive Force

Figure 8.26   Diagram showing a torque couple.

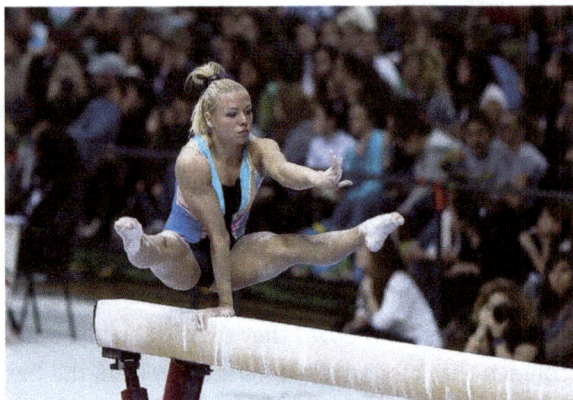

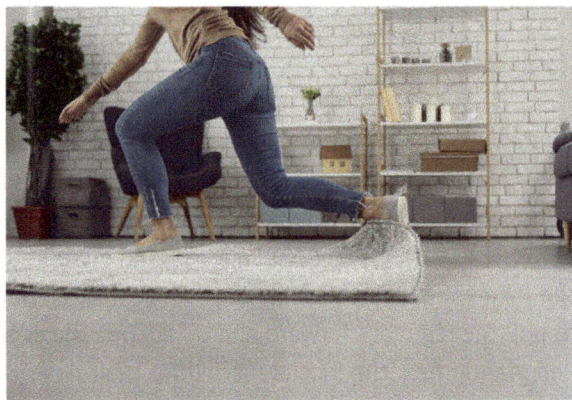

Figure 8.27   Regaining balance.

We use a variety of different strategies to maintain balance and allow us to safely propel ourselves from one place to another. Sometimes adjusting the orientation of our limbs provides that balance and stability; other times it may require a brace or other gait assistive device.

One or more interactive elements has been excluded from this version of the text. You can view them online here: https://pb.cognella.com/83647-1b/?p=56#oembed-5

Please refer to the interactive ebook in Cognella Active Learning for interactive/media content.

📱 *One or more interactive elements has been excluded from this version of the text. You can view them online here:*
https://pb.cognella.com/83647-1b/?p=56#oembed-6

Please refer to the interactive ebook in Cognella Active Learning for interactive/media content.

📱 *One or more interactive elements has been excluded from this version of the text. You can view them online here:*
https://pb.cognella.com/83647-1b/?p=56#oembed-7

Please refer to the interactive ebook in Cognella Active Learning for interactive/media content.

Angular Momentum

Angular momentum (**L**) is a measure of an object's tendency to maintain its rotational motion. **Angular momentum** is the product of the moment of inertia of the object (*I*) and its angular velocity (ω) reported in units of rad/s. The units of **L** are kg m^2/s. For example, rotating at the same angular velocity it is much easier to stop a spinning tennis ball than a bowling ball due to their differences in angular momentum.

Angular momentum is utilized by humans in all forms of motion since almost all human motion is the product of angular changes occurring around joint centers. Any time a mass of a body changes its angular position over time, the body possesses angular momentum. In humans, angular momentum is most often the result of internal muscle forces that, with practice, optimize changes in *I* and ω in such a way as to allow the motions to be executed with a minimum of muscle force.

Conservation of Angular Momentum

The **conservation of angular momentum** states that the angular momentum of a body will remain constant unless the moment of inertia or the angular velocity of the body is changed by the application of a net external torque greater than zero. That means that while a gymnast may start a trick in a layout position, change to a twisting tucked position, and end with a forward roll, the angular momentum measured at any point during the sequence would be the same. *Airborne angular momentum is generated during takeoff and cannot be increased or decreased by the performer during their flight.* This is an important fact for athletes to understand: All of the angular momentum you will have to work with during your flight is generated at takeoff. For the extreme athlete to successfully complete the multiple flip trick on their bike, they must take off with the right amount of angular momentum or the attempt is doomed to fail regardless of their mid-air attempt to salvage the trick.

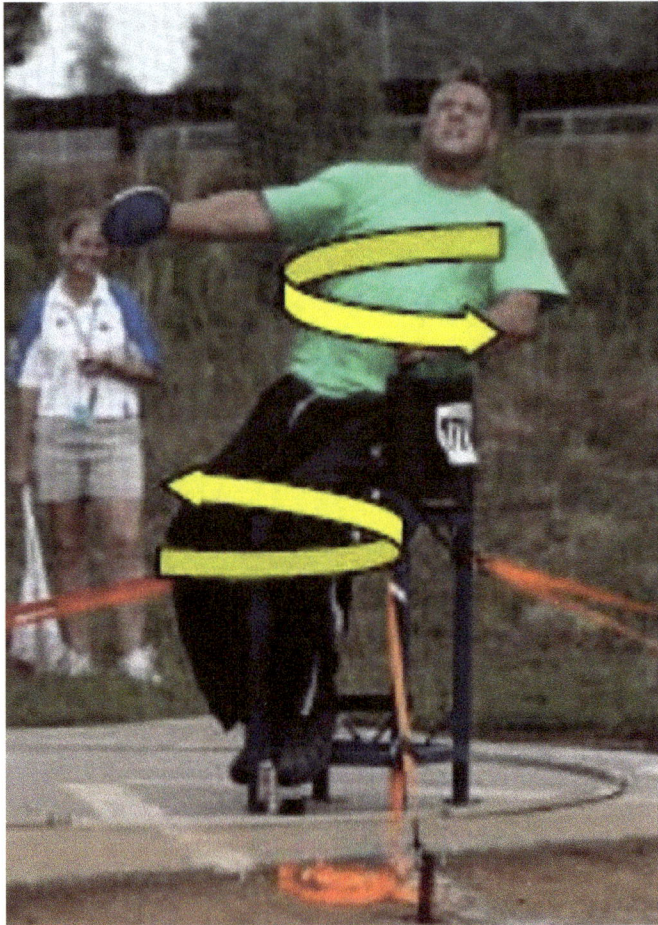

Figure 8.28   Seated athlete angular rotation.

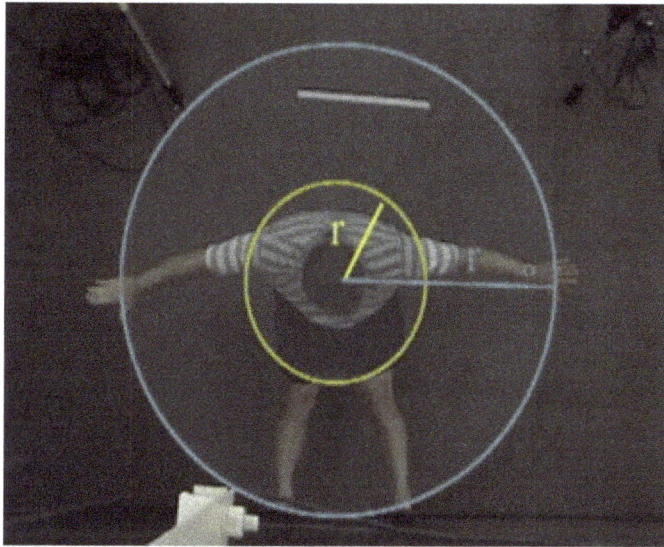

Figure 8.29   Seated with large moment arm.

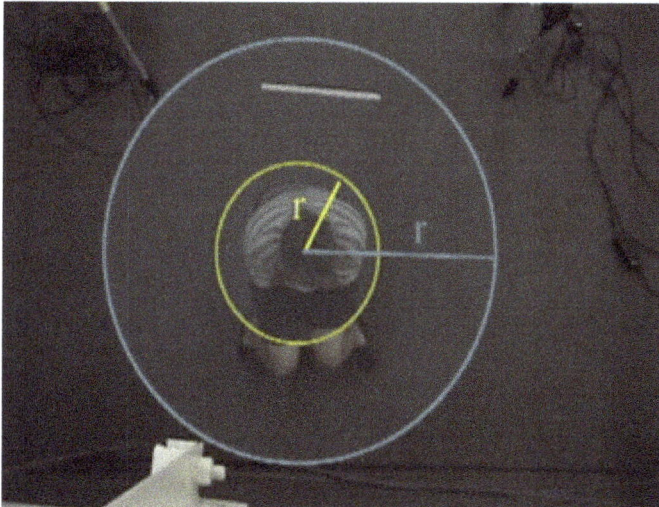

Figure 8.30   Seated with small moment arm.

Note the example of the diver in Figure 8.31 as she performs her dive. By assuming a pike position (bending at the waist and wrapping your arms around your legs while they are kept fully extended), she decreases her moment of inertia, greatly increasing her angular velocity. She exits the pike position by extending her arms and legs, maximizing her moment of inertia, which slows her angular velocity to a minimum just prior to entry into the water.

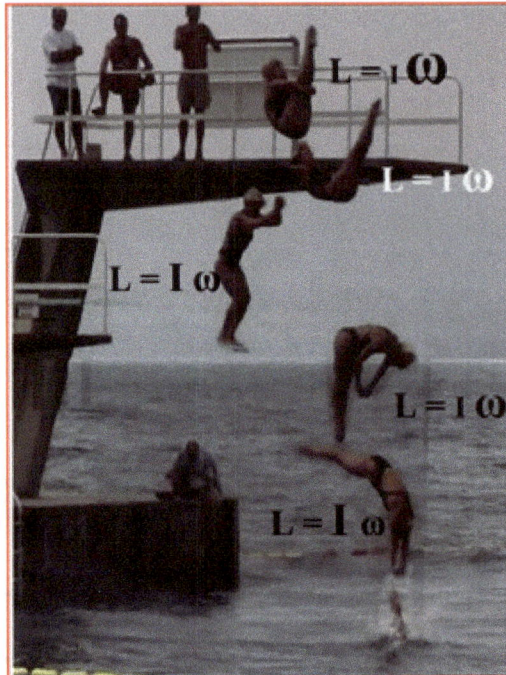

Figure 8.31   Diving example relationship between moment of inertia and angular velocity.

The same concepts are illustrated in the following video in which a student demonstrates a back flip.

One or more interactive elements has been excluded from this version of the text. You can view them online here: https://pb.cognella.com/83647-1b/?p=56#oembed-8

Please refer to the interactive ebook in Cognella Active Learning for interactive/media content.

Transfer of Angular Momentum

The total amount of angular momentum in a projectile remains constant, but that does not mean that through various changes of segment orientations that some parts of a multisegmented body cannot increase or decrease their angular momentum during flight. In fact, thoughtful shifting of angular momentum allows for many of the complex aerial movements accomplished by gymnasts, divers, extreme motocross, and other athletes that thrill us with their skills.

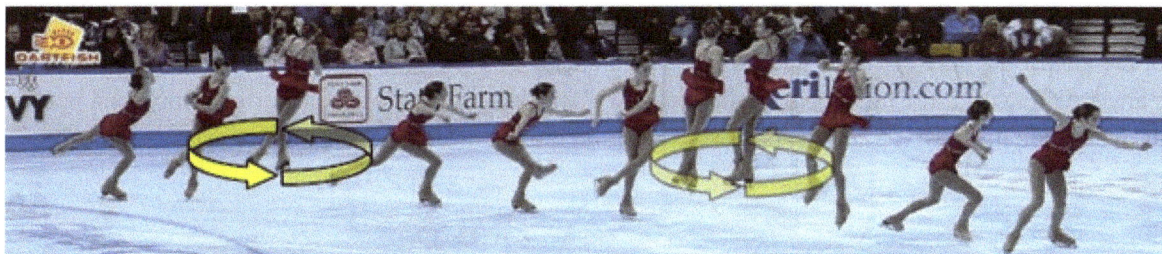

Figure 8.32   Skater stromotion angular momentum.

Total angular momentum is a vector with its own direction and magnitude that remains constant through the aerial portion of a movement. However, the angular velocity vector, which is a component of total angular momentum, does not have to align with the total angular momentum vector during the execution of a complex aerial movement. That means that during a movement that includes both twisting and somersaulting, some of the total angular momentum of the body can be transferred from twisting to somersaulting or somersaulting to twisting without changing the total angular momentum of the body.

When a body is in contact with a support surface, such as the ground (or other massive object), it is possible for momentum that is generated in the segment(s) in contact with the ground to transfer that momentum to the rest of the body. Such transfer occurs when a tennis player hits a serve or groundstroke, or a softball player swings at a pitch. When a body is not in contact with the ground, however, say during an aerial movement, it is very difficult to transfer any significant amount of momentum from a body segment to the rest of the body.

It may seem counterintuitive, but for a person to perform a somersault or a twist in the air, the momentum transfer that results in the movement must be initiated while still in contact with the ground, vaulting horse, diving board, ramp, motorcycle, and so on. Once airborne, individual segments can be reoriented, but they produce very little whole-body movement changes unless there was angular momentum already present (from takeoff) that could be redirected.

Some athletes appear to defy the laws of physics by generating twists and turns while in mid-air, but upon closer inspection, trick jumping cyclists use the motorcycle or bicycle as their support surface, pushing or pulling on their bike to initiate the movements.

One or more interactive elements has been excluded from this version of the text. You can view them online here: https://pb.cognella.com/83647-1b/?p=56#oembed-12

Please refer to the interactive ebook in Cognella Active Learning for interactive/media content.

Angular Impulse

Angular impulse (ΔL) is a value that represents the result of a torque applied to an object over a short time period. Angular impulse is a vector found using the equation ΔL = τ * Δt, where τ represents the applied torque and Δt the time of torque application. The units for ΔL are Nms. An example of an angular impulse is any striking event in which the outcome imparts a torque on the object being struck, such as a pop-up hit in baseball in which the contact point of the bat on the ball is below the center of mass of the ball.

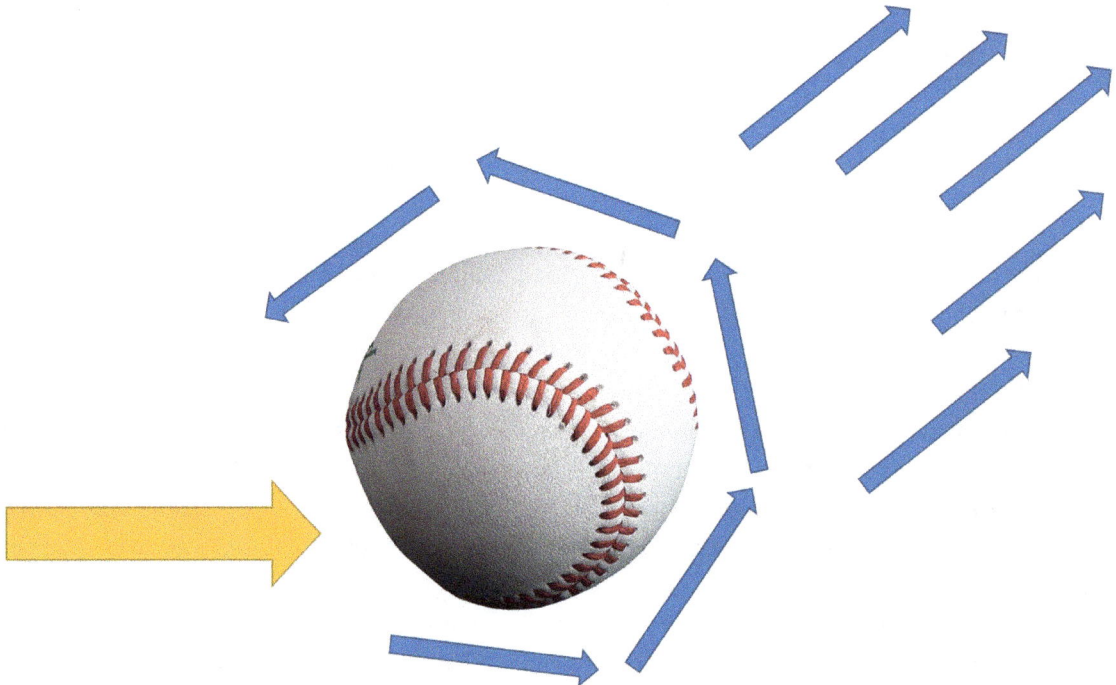

Figure 8.33   Baseball angular impulse.

Angular impulse is often expressed as a change in angular momentum: τΔt = Δ(Iω).

Oscillations

In many movements, it is common for all or part of the moving body to oscillate back and forth as it waits or moves from one location to another. A person "standing still" is actually constantly moving forward and backward, right and left. If their instantaneous center of gravity location were recorded as they stood still, the graph would appear to be a jumbled line radiating in all directions about a point located between their feet. This type of constant adjustment is common and necessary for a system as complex as a human to maintain upright balance.

The side-to-side oscillations of a cyclist as they pedal a bike are easier to see and help maintain balance as bike and rider moves forward. Every time a movement occurs, there is some shifting of mass, and Newton's third law must be satisfied with the body required to make a compensatory adjustment to deal with the new demands of alignment to achieve equilibrium. Too much or too little adjustment and balance cannot be maintained. Excessive oscillating movements can result in greater and greater swings of the COM, eventually resulting in total loss of balance. Most of us at an early age learn and remember through practice how to make the necessary small adjustments that allow us to walk or ride a bike while maintaining our balance. This is demonstrated in the extreme with the elite cyclist shown in Video 8.13 during a sprint.

🖳 *One or more interactive elements has been excluded from this version of the text. You can view them online here: https://pb.cognella.com/83647-1b/?p=56#oembed-13*

Please refer to the interactive ebook in Cognella Active Learning for interactive/media content.

Basic motor skills related to balance become ingrained and automatic at a relatively young age. Because of this, we don't have to spend time or effort later in life focusing our attention on constantly solving the very complicated biomechanical problem of balance. Occasionally we are reminded how important simple movement skills are in our daily lives. When conditions change unexpectedly, either due to injury, illness, or mechanical alterations, we may be quickly reminded that our motor skill set is not up to the task, as seen in Video 8.14.

🖳 *One or more interactive elements has been excluded from this version of the text. You can view them online here: https://pb.cognella.com/83647-1b/?p=56#oembed-14*

Please refer to the interactive ebook in Cognella Active Learning for interactive/media content.

An excellent example of how linear and angular motion come together in a sport can be seen in pole vaulting. An athlete uses horizontal linear velocity to generate momentum that is transferred into the pole, causing it to bend, which is then transferred back to the individual as they transition from a runner to a projectile. Watch the Chapter 8: Interactive video and try to identify all of the linear and angular components of the complex pole-vaulting motion.

Table 8.2 lists the relationships between angular kinetic variables, how they are calculated, their units, and vector or scalar status.

Table 8.2 Angular Kinetics Equations, Units, and Parameters

Variable and Equation	Units	Vector or Scalar	Comments

Table 8.2 Angular Kinetics Equations, Units, and Parameters

			First-class lever system can be =, < 1
Mechanical advantage $MA = L_{motive\ force} / L_{resistance\ force}$	unitless	Scalar	First-class lever system can be =, < 1 Second-class lever system, 1 Third-class lever system, < 1
Torque or moment $\tau = \perp F * d$	Nm	Vector	
Moment of inertia $I = \Sigma\ mr^2$	kgm^2	Vector	
Torque and moment of inertia $\tau = I\alpha$	Nm	Vector	
Angular power $P_{ang}\ \tau = * \omega$	watts	Vector	
Angular momentum $L = I * \omega$	$kg\ m^2/s$	Vector	
Angular impulse $\Delta L = \tau * \Delta t$ or $\tau\Delta t = \Delta(I\omega)$	Nms	Vector	

Think of It This Way

One or more interactive elements has been excluded from this version of the text. You can view them online here: https://pb.cognella.com/83647-1b/?p=56#oembed-15

Please refer to the interactive ebook in Cognella Active Learning for interactive/media content.

How do gears work, and why they are so useful? Are there examples in the human body where a gear-like structure helps with force transfer?

Mechanical gears allow for the transfer of energy from one rotating axis, either through direct contact of the gears or by a connecting chain, strap, or band. Connecting gears of different diameters change the effective force output at the different gears. For example, a fast-rotating smaller diameter gear interfaced with a larger diameter gear results in a slower rotation speed of the larger gear, but with a greater force output from the larger gear. When an equivalent amount of force is transferred to two different diameter gears, the outcome results in the faster rotation of the smaller gear that generates a lower output force, compared to a larger gear, which rotates slower but outputs more force. The images of force output given the same applied pedal force of a bicycle are illustrated in Figure 8.34. This ability to change the output force through the use of gears demonstrates how changing the mechanical advantage as needed can allow a rider to vary speed and deal with changes in track elevation without varying applied pedal force.

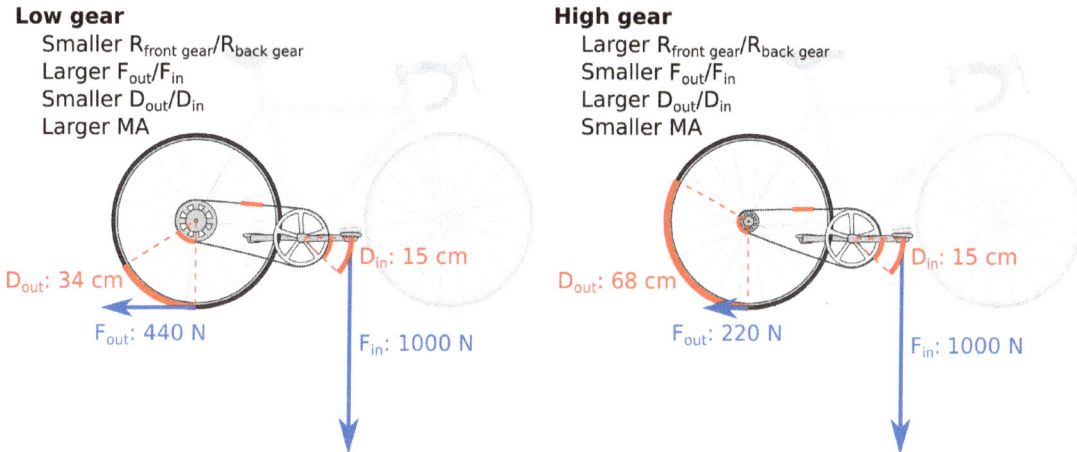

Low gear
  Smaller $R_{front\ gear}/R_{back\ gear}$
  Larger F_{out}/F_{in}
  Smaller D_{out}/D_{in}
  Larger MA

High gear
  Larger $R_{front\ gear}/R_{back\ gear}$
  Smaller F_{out}/F_{in}
  Larger D_{out}/D_{in}
  Smaller MA

D_{in}: 15 cm
D_{out}: 34 cm
F_{out}: 440 N
F_{in}: 1000 N

D_{in}: 15 cm
D_{out}: 68 cm
F_{out}: 220 N
F_{in}: 1000 N

Figure 8.34   Bicycle gear diagram.

The patella of the human knee also demonstrates how a change in the radius of rotation, or moment arm, of a force transferred from one location to another around an axis of rotation can provide a movement advantage. The average thickness of an adult patella is ~4mm, but that small distance is enough to provide a significant increase of the torque acting across the knee when the quadriceps actively attempt to cause knee extension. With the patella extending the radius of rotation by 4mm an 8000N, quadriceps force increases the torque by 32Nm.

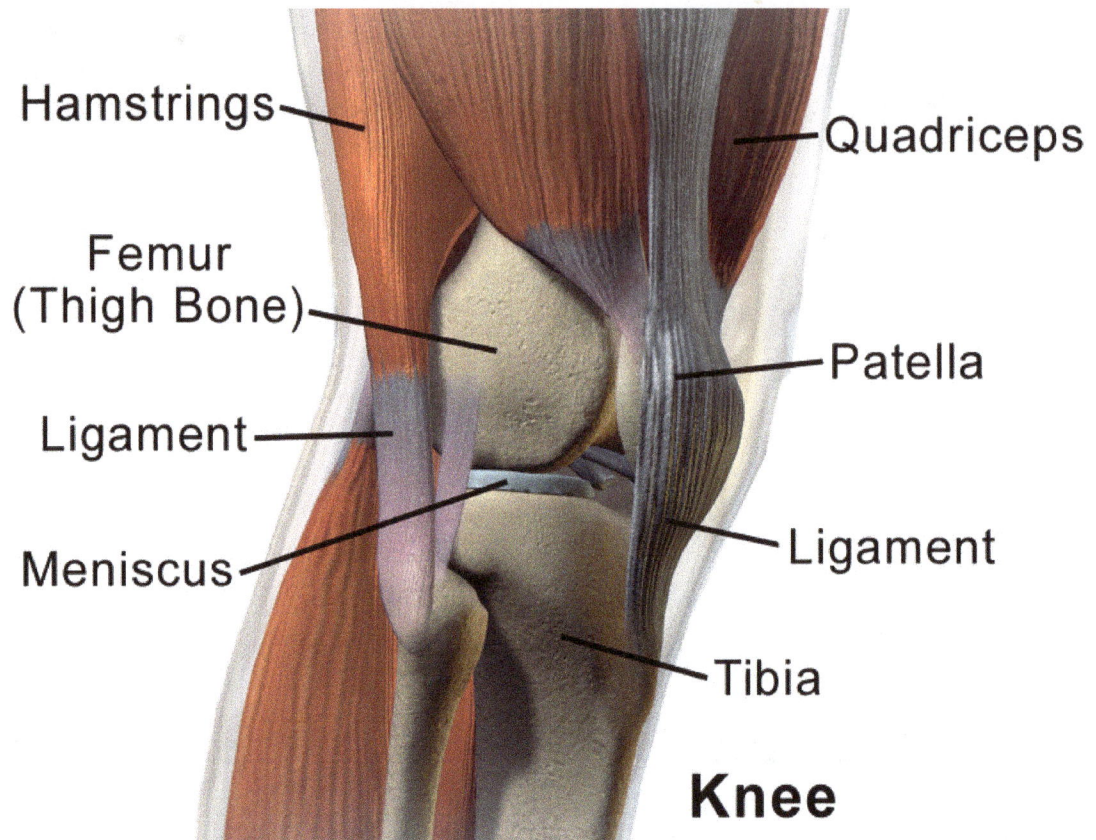

Figure 8.35   Human knee diagram.

What if the patella thickness could be adjusted as needed, similar to switching gears on a bicycle? How thick would the patella need to be to create the same 32Nm of toque with 5500N of quadriceps extension force?

Summary

In this chapter we talked about how force may cause a change in angular motion when applied to a body. Angular motion is a key component of most forms of human motion. Newton's three laws of angular motion provide us with basic rules governing the rotational motion we commonly experience. Lever systems found throughout the body help us utilize our muscles to generate a wide variety of movement outcomes. Changes in the location of the COM result in changes in the moment of inertia of the body. When a force is applied, causing a rotation, it is referred to as torque. Various equations relating mass, its location, and how its rotational state can be changed by the application of torque were explained and examples presented.

Equations for torque, angular momentum, angular impulse, moment of inertia, and others provide the tools necessary to appreciate how angular motion can be created or modified.

List of Key Takeaways

- Angular kinetics is the study of how forces effect rotational motion.
- Simple machines found throughout the body use angular kinetics to assist in simple and complex movements.
- The moment of inertia of a body can be altered by reorientation of body segments, making a given torque more or less likely to result in rotation.
- Newton's laws of angular motion describe how torques effect a body.
- Torque is a measure of angular work.
- Angular power represents the rotational work accomplished by torque.
- Angular momentum is directly related to moment of inertia.
- Angular impulse allows for the calculation of torque for a given moment of inertia and rotational velocity.

References

Dempster, W. T., and Gaughran, R. L. (1967) Properties of body segments based on size and weight. *American Journal of Anatomy*, 120(1), p 33-54.

Jensen, M.D., Kanaley, J.A, Roust, L.R., O'Brien, P, C., Braun, J.S., Dunn, W. L, and Wahner, H.W. (1993). Assessment of Body Composition with use of Dual-Energy X-ray Absorptiometry: Evaluation and Comparion with other Methods. *May Clinic Proceedings*, 68(9), p 867-873.

Zatiorsky, V. M., (2003). Measuring body segment parameters: X-ray versus gamma scanning. *Journal of biomechanics*. 36(9), p 1405-1406.

Image Credits

Fig. 8.1: Copyright © by Michael David Murphy (CC BY-SA 2.0) at https://commons.wikimedia.org/wiki/File:Floyd-landis-toctt.jpg.

Fig. 8.10: Copyright © by Scott Ray (CC BY 2.0) at https://commons.wikimedia.org/wiki/File:Womens_high_jump_5.jpg.

Fig. 8.12: Copyright © 2019 Depositphotos/gresey.

Fig. 8.13: Copyright © 2019 Depositphotos/gresey.

Fig. 8.16: Copyright © by Martin Rulsch (CC BY-SA 4.0) at https://commons.wikimedia.org/wiki/File:2020-01-25_47._Hallorenpokal_Synchronized_diving_Women_(Martin_Rulsch)_135.jpg.

Fig. 8.17: Copyright © by Martin Rulsch (CC BY-SA 4.0) at https://commons.wikimedia.org/wiki/File:2020-01-25_47._Hallorenpokal_Synchronized_diving_Men_(Martin_Rulsch)_113.jpg.

Fig. 8.18: Copyright © by Martin Rulsch (CC BY-SA 4.0) at https://commons.wikimedia.org/wiki/File:2020-01-25_47._Hallorenpokal_Synchronized_diving_Women_(Martin_Rulsch)_155.jpg.

Fig. 8.21: Copyright © by Haleem Elshaarani (CC BY 2.0) at https://commons.wikimedia.org/wiki/File:Sarah_Hegazy_riding_a_bicycle.jpg.

Fig. 8.27a: Copyright © by Alby.1412 (CC BY 2.0) at https://commons.wikimedia.org/wiki/File:Dorina_B%C3%B6cz%C3%B6g%C5%91%2C_balance_beam%2C_2013.jpg.

Fig. 8.27b: Copyright © 2021 Depositphotos/lacheev.

Fig. 8.33: Copyright © by Tage Olsin (CC BY-SA 2.0) at https://commons.wikimedia.org/wiki/File:Baseball_(crop).jpg.

Fig. 8.34: Copyright © by Becarlson (CC BY-SA 3.0) at https://commons.wikimedia.org/wiki/File:Bicycle_mechanical_advantage.svg.

Fig. 8.35: Copyright © by BruceBlaus (CC BY 3.0) at https://commons.wikimedia.org/wiki/File:Blausen_0597_KneeAnatomy_Side.png.

Chapter 9

Fluid Dynamics

Preparing to Learn: *Watch*

Swimmers must deal with moving through two fluids while participating in their sport: air and water. Water is the fluid that provides the most concern since the viscosity of water slows and resists the movement of the athletes. The study of movement in and through water is called hydrodynamics.

Improving the aerodynamics of a car can greatly improve its fuel efficiency. Other aspects of how air passes around a car's exterior when understood and appropriately modified provide improvements in the ride quality and safety.

One or more interactive elements has been excluded from this version of the text. You can view them online here: https://pb.cognella.com/83647-1b/?p=57#oembed-4

Please refer to the interactive ebook in Cognella Active Learning for interactive/media content.

Medical practitioners realize the value of exercising in water. In the following video a series of exercises designed to treat low back issues are shown.

One or more interactive elements has been excluded from this version of the text. You can view them online here: https://pb.cognella.com/83647-1b/?p=57#oembed-5

Please refer to the interactive ebook in Cognella Active Learning for interactive/media content.

Preparing to Learn: *Respond*

Directions: Based on what you saw in the video, respond to the following questions:

1. Have you ever noticed the vortex generators found on most cars? Did you have any idea of their purpose? How would you explain to someone what a vortex generator does to improve the ride quality and safety in modern cars?
2. Did you realize that medical personnel needed to understand the effects of fluid dynamics to best serve their patients? What other types of rehab do you think would be effective in a water environment?

Introduction to the Chapter

We live in a world of fluid. The air that surrounds us and the water that we swim in are examples of fluids that we must negotiate every day. We are so accustomed to dealing with air pressure, wind, and air resistance that they are mostly ignored. We do appreciate a cool evening breeze on a hot summer day or realize we are working harder to overcome a head wind when biking, but unless we are placed in a situation that requires us to focus on our interaction with air it is "just the way it is," and we get on with our lives.

However, if you are interested in almost any form of motion, knowing how fluids work and how to best interact with them is essential. One of the first things you realize working with fluids is that that the faster you try to move through them, the more they resist our efforts (Newton's third law). This can be very frustrating when the goal is to move through the fluid with the least amount of effort. Optimizing movement through fluid has been, and continues to be, the source of much research for athletes such as cyclists who must come up with strategies to limit how air resistance effects them at high speeds.

More and more the effects of fluid drag and buoyance are being used to our benefit in rehab and exercise settings. The same properties of fluids that are often the nemesis of athletes are being used for whole-body or targeted programs for strength, flexibility, and rehab purposes.

Learning Objectives

After completing this chapter, students should be able to do the following:

- Define fluids and list their properties
- List different types of fluids, their similarities and their differences
- Explain the difference between lift and drag
- List key parameters related to fluid dynamics and know how to solve for their values

Fluid Dynamics values and concepts

We all owe our lives to fluid mechanics, and yet when the topic shows up in a classroom setting many of us are less than thrilled. It's a shame really, since without the "magic" of fluid dynamics the blood filled with oxygen and nutrients that our bodies rely on would not be able to get around to all the places it's needed and our chance for survival would be nil. We will not cover the internal applications of fluid mechanics in the human body in this text, but for those who are interested there are many good sources such as "Fluid hydraulics in human physiology" Royder (1997) and "Biofluid Dynamics of Human Body Systems" Goyal (2013). Unless you are an astronaut working in the vacuum of space, every movement that you will make in your life will be affected to some degree by the properties of fluid dynamics. Walking, running, jumping, cycling, swimming, hitting a golf ball, and so forth involve aerodynamics, hydrodynamics, or a combination of both. All fall under the umbrella term of fluid dynamics.

Viscosity

Fluids have no fixed shape. Their shapes are usually easily modified when forces act upon them. They can be liquids or gases. Fluids have thickness, or viscosity, which is a measure of how easily the fluid will flow or change shape when a force is applied to it. Fluid viscosity is the result of the density (mass per given volume) and specific weight (weight per given volume) of the matter constituting the fluid. The viscosity of a fluid is influenced by the environmental properties of temperature, atmospheric pressure, and humidity.

The more viscous a fluid, the less likely and slower it is to flow and change its shape. Honey, a viscous fluid, flows much slower than water, another liquid fluid, which has a much lower viscosity.

The molecules within a liquid are more ordered and have greater intermolecular attraction than those of gases, even though both liquids and gases are fluids. Differences in the molecular properties between liquids and gases make liquid fluids more resistant to shear forces than gas fluids. That means that liquid fluids will generate more resistance to an object attempting to push through it compared to a gas fluid. For example, air is a gas fluid, while water is a liquid fluid. Air has lower viscosity than water for a given volume, which is why it is easier to walk through air than water.

Fluid Structure

Fluids can take either the form of gases or liquids, but both can be thought of as built-in layers or strings of molecules. That layered structure of fluids requires that an object must slide through and/or push against those layers as it moves through a fluid.

If you think of air as a series of horizontal layers of molecules forming a blanket on the surface of the earth, then as a person moves horizontally with or against the air they must push their way through these layers that act to resist their movement. Even calm or nonflowing fluids resist motion based on Newton's third law of action-reaction. When an object attempts to force its way through fluid, the molecules of the leading edge of the object will push against the molecules of the fluid, resulting in a reaction that resists the object's intended movement path.

For most everyday human movements through calm air, because the density of our bodies is so much greater than air, it is easy for us to win the battle and force our way through the air molecules that attempt to resist our movement. From a practical standpoint, the air resistance we encounter is negligible compared to other resistive forces to our movement, such as ground contact friction. However, when a person moves quickly through calm air, such as is the case with elite cyclists, air resistance quickly becomes a significant factor. It is estimated up to 90% of the muscular energy generated by a cyclist is used to overcome air resistance (Kyle and Burke (1984)!

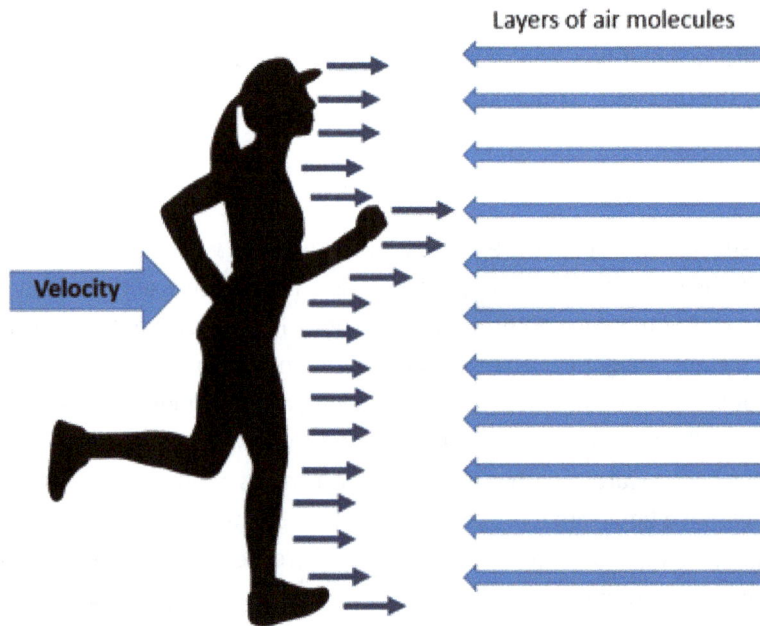

Figure 9.1   Running through layered air.

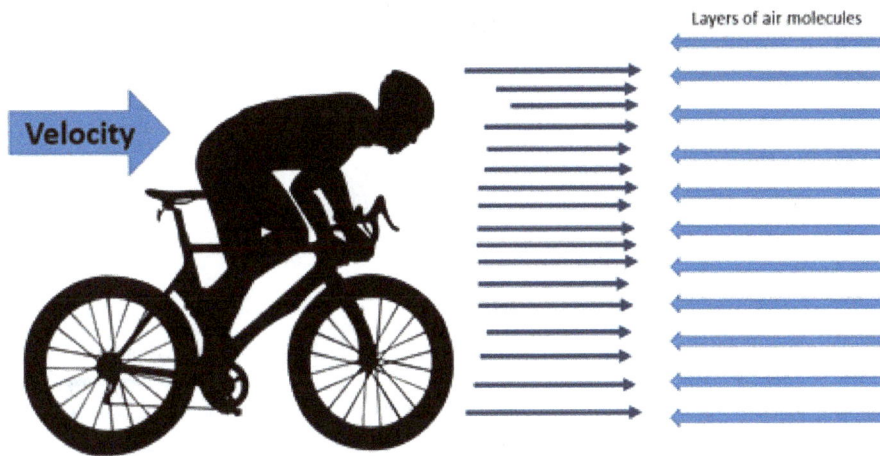

Figure 9.2   Cycling through layered air.

For example, if the velocity of a cyclist, v_c, is 20m/s, and the wind velocity, v_w, is 0m/s, then the relative velocity of the cyclist to the air is:

$v_{c \text{ to } w} = v_c - v_w$

$v_{c \text{ to } w} = 20\text{m/s} - 0\text{m/s}$

$v_{c \text{ to } w} = 20\text{m/s}$

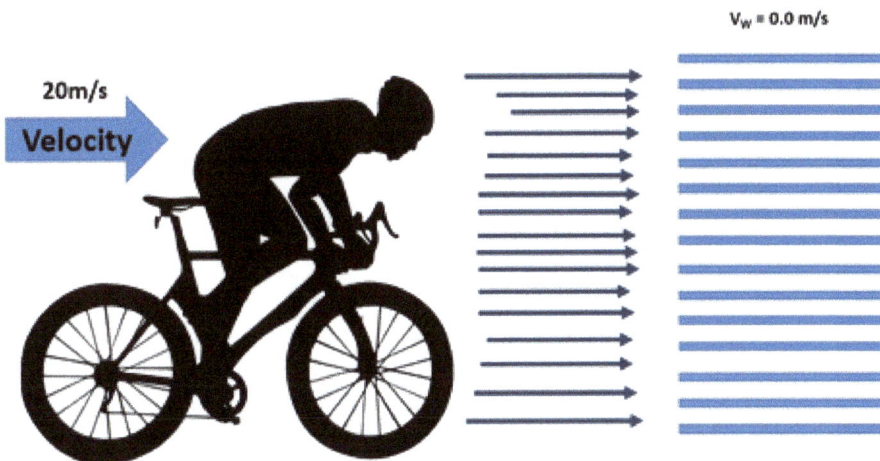

Figure 9.3   Cycling through layered air problem 1.

If conditions change such that the cyclist still proceeds with a velocity of 20m/s and runs into a head wind of -4.5 m/s, then the velocity of the cyclist becomes

$v_{c\ to\ w} = v_c - v_w$

$v_{c\ to\ w} = 20m/s - (-4.5m/s)$

$v_{c\ to\ w} = 20m/s + 4.5m/s$

$v_{c\ to\ w} = 24.5m/s$

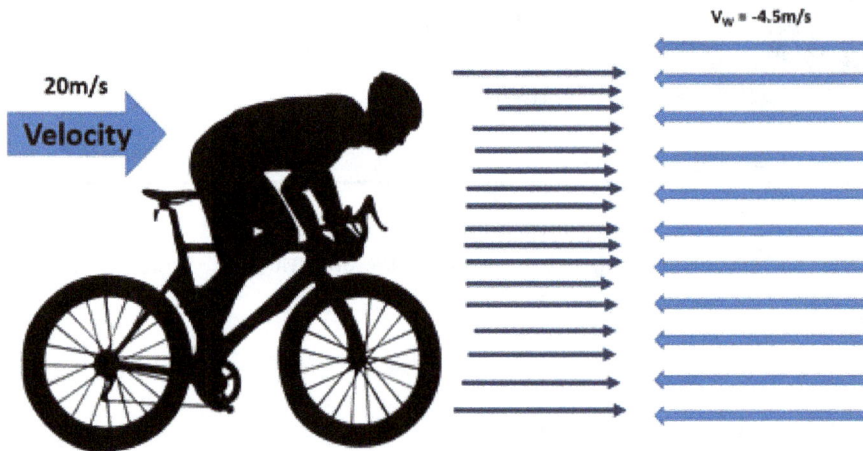

$v_w = -4.5m/s$

20m/s

Velocity

Figure 9.4   Cycling through layered air problem 2.

If later in the ride while still traveling at 20m/s he picks up a tail wind of 6.2m/s, his relative velocity becomes

$v_{c\ to\ w} = v_c - v_w$

$v_{c\ to\ w} = 20m/s - (6.2m/s)$

$v_{c\ to\ w} = 13.8m/s$

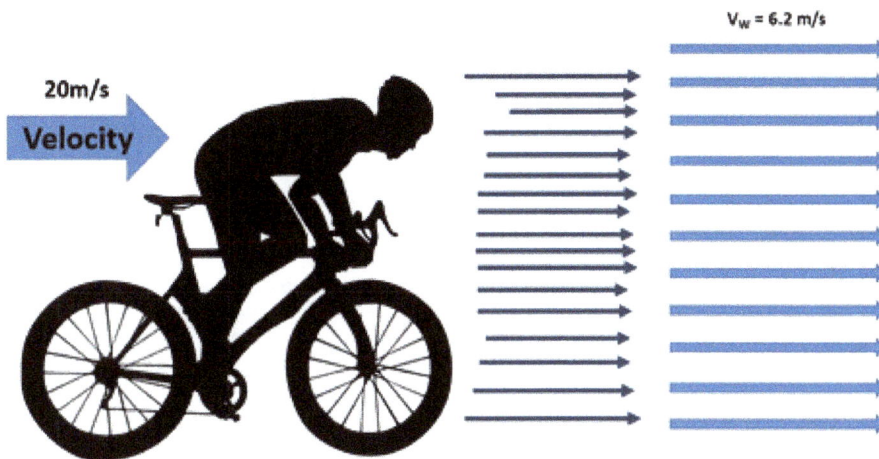

Figure 9.5   Cycling through layered air problem 3.

Turbulence and Drag

Whenever an object moves through a fluid, it disturbs the state of the fluid. If the object slices through the fluid, parting it with minimal interference to the alignment of fluid molecules and the fluid immediately returns to its previous condition, the object's movement is considered nonturbulent motion. Should the object's movement cause the layers of the fluid to mix before realigning, the movement is turbulent in nature.

Drag

When any two objects in contact with each other slide across one another, mechanical friction is present. As an object slides through a fluid, friction is also generated. The friction, or resistance to movement through the fluid, has several components. **Skin friction drag** is the friction that occurs at the surface of an object as it slides through a fluid.

Drag is dependent on the shape of the object and is called the **form drag** of the object. Form drag greatly determines how easy it is for the object to move through a fluid. If the form drag is very low, such as for a javelin, it will experience only a small amount of friction as it moves through the air.

An object such as a cardboard box has a high form drag and will experience a large amount of air resistance. Objects such as the human body have variable form drag based on how the body segments are aligned. A skater in an upright position will present a body with a large form drag as opposed to the recumbent position taken by a luge athlete during competition.

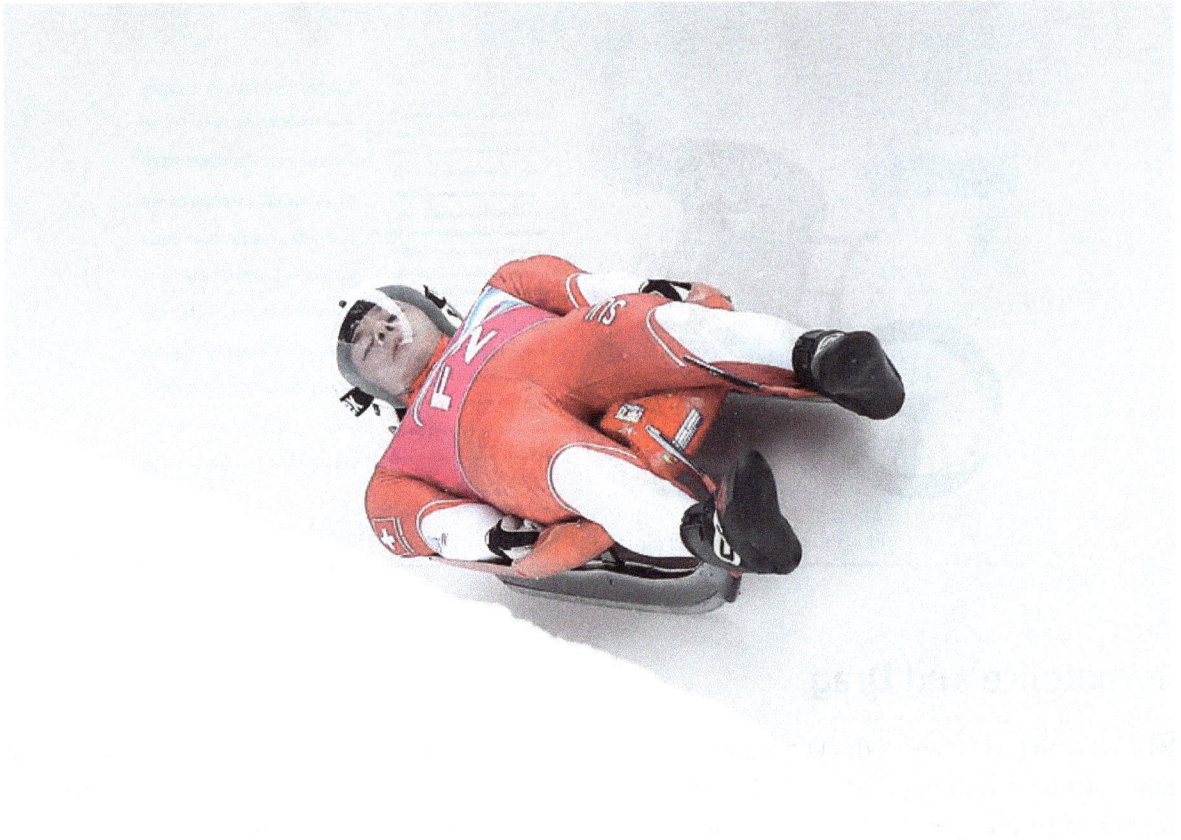

Figure 9.6   Luge.

Yet another type of drag occurs when an object or part of the object crosses between two adjacent fluids such as air and water. This type of drag is called **wave drag** and is of great concern for swimmers or any other object that may have to cross and recross the boundaries between two fluids.

The general equation for drag is $F_{drag} = 1/2C_d* \rho*A_{contact}*v^2$, where F_{drag} is drag friction; C_d is the coefficient of drag for the fluid, which is usually determined through experimentation and takes in all the complexity of the object shape and fluid it passes through; $A_{contact}$ is the contact area of the object with the fluid; ρ is the density of the fluid; and v is the relative velocity of the object moving though the fluid.

There are multiple unique considerations that go into determining the specific coefficient of drag of an object. (For a more detailed explanation of how coefficients of drag are found please see this.)

Is drag always a bad thing, and do you always want to reduce drag? Are there any other properties of drag that might need to be considered besides how it slows objects down when they attempt to move quickly through a fluid? (Remember that drag is a form of friction and as such generates heat. A little, no big deal; a lot and you burst into flame!)

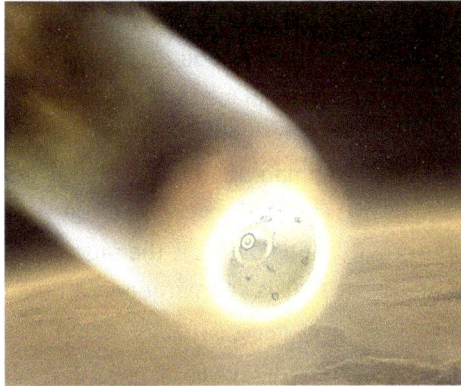

Figure 9.7   Capsule reentry.

Sometimes there is not enough drag to meet our movement needs. This occurs when we rely on drag to allow for the controlled decent of a spacecraft on an alien world. For example, the low atmospheric drag found on Mars poses significant technical problems for engineers trying to land spacecraft safely on the planet.

Viscosity describes the resistance to flow of a fluid based on the internal friction present in the fluid. **Density** is the quantity of mass present in a given volume of a fluid. The greater the density, the greater the internal friction generated by any object moving through it.

Terminal Velocity

Terminal velocity is the highest velocity an object can obtain while moving through a given fluid. It is directly related to the surface area of the object in contact with the fluid and the viscosity of the fluid. Terminal velocity will vary by object and is determined based on the drag and buoyancy of the object in the fluid. Terminal velocity is a state of zero acceleration for a projectile as the effect of gravity is no longer able to increase the velocity of the falling object. The minimum terminal velocity for a person through air during freefall in a "spread eagle" position is approximately 56m/s and can approach a maximum of ~89m/s when tucked into a tight ball configuration.

Buoyancy

As Newton correctly predicted with his third law of motion, whenever a force is applied to an object, an equal and opposite reaction force is created. Whenever a force is generated against a fluid, it follows the third law and creates a reaction force. One such type of reaction force created by fluid is buoyancy. **Buoyancy** is the upward vertical reactive force generated by a fluid when an object is placed on the surface of the fluid. Buoyancy is the force that makes an object float.

Archimedes was a Greek mathematician and scientist who first explained the physics of buoyancy. He determined that any object either partially or fully submerged in a liquid would experience a buoyancy force equal to the weight of the liquid displaced by the object: Buoyancy force = weight of the object in air – weight of the object in liquid. Archimedes also understood that the volume of an object of any shape could be determined by the amount of liquid water it displaced when submerged. That relationship with volume and displaced water also holds for partially submerged objects. In that way, it is possible to determine the volume of a complex structure such as the human hand by dipping it in water and measuring how much water it displaces.

The relative density, or specific gravity, of an object is the ratio of its density compared to the density of water. Based on the volume of an object that is submerged in a liquid and the specific gravity of that liquid, the buoyancy force may be calculated as $F_{buoyancy} = V\gamma$, where V is the volume of body submerged in the fluid and γ is the specific gravity of the fluid, or $F_{buoyancy} = PA$, where P is pressure and A the area affected by the pressure, or $F_{buoyancy} = \rho ghA$, where ρ is the density of the fluid, g is gravity, V is the volume of the body submerged in the fluid, h is the height of the submerged part of the body, and A is the area of body. The denser the liquid, the greater its specific gravity and the greater buoyancy force it will generate. Since salt water has a greater density than fresh water, a person or object will experience greater buoyancy in salt water than in fresh water. It is easier for a person to float in salt water than fresh water and boats or other watercraft will ride higher in the water in salt water than fresh water McKelvey and Grotch (1978).

How and why is it possible for a human to float in water? If the buoyancy force resulting from the product of the volume of a person submerged in water times the specific gravity of the water is greater than the weight of the person, they float! Why are there some body orientations that are better for floating than others? Because unless the body is oriented such that the net buoyancy force is aligned with the person's net body weight, a torque will be generated, which will cause the body to rotate in the water. If the body rotates, the angular momentum of the body may cause the body to dip downward at a sufficient rate to overcome the buoyancy force, and the person sinks.

For example, if a 55kg person is in an optimal floating position and has $0.056m^3$ of their volume submerged into pool water with a specific gravity of $9875N/m^3$, will they be able to float?

$F_{buoyancy} = V_{submerged\ object} * \gamma_{specific\ gravity}$

$F_{buoyancy} = 0.056m^3 * 9875N/m^3$

$F_{buoyancy} = 553N$

Body weight

$BW = m_{body} * a_{gravity}$

$BW = 55kg * -9.81m/s^2$

$BW = -539.55N$

Since the buoyancy force is greater than the body weight force, the person will float. The optimal floating orientation of the body will look like Figure 9.8.

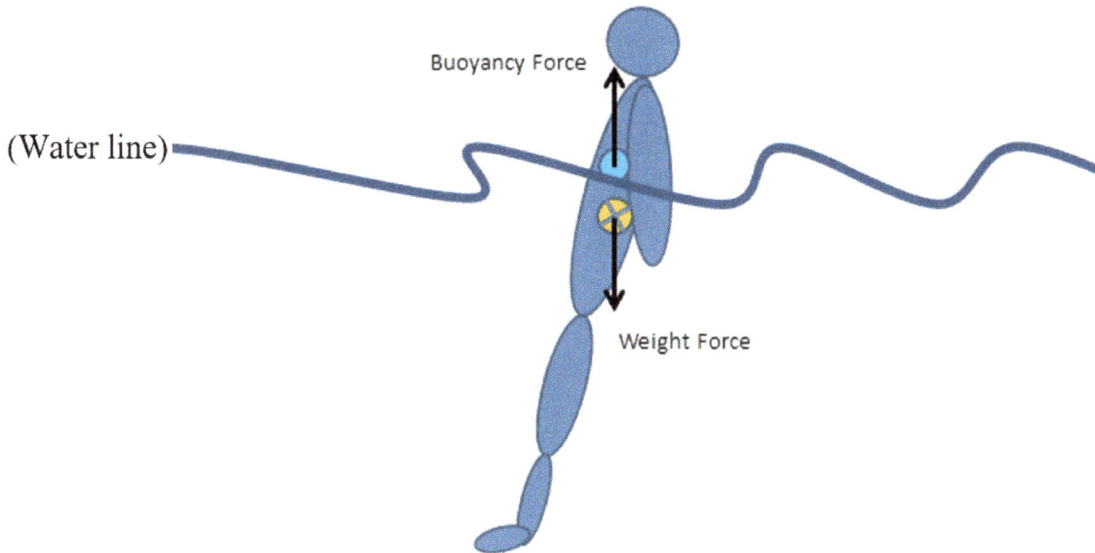

Figure 9.8   Floating 1.

If the person tried to float laying horizontally, their body would automatically rotate to try to find the optimal floating position.

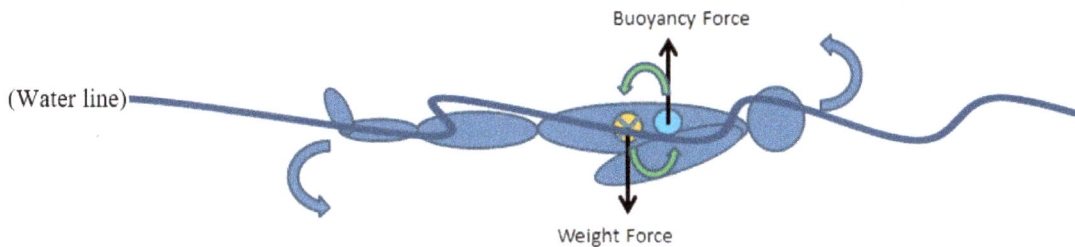

Figure 9.9   Floating 2.

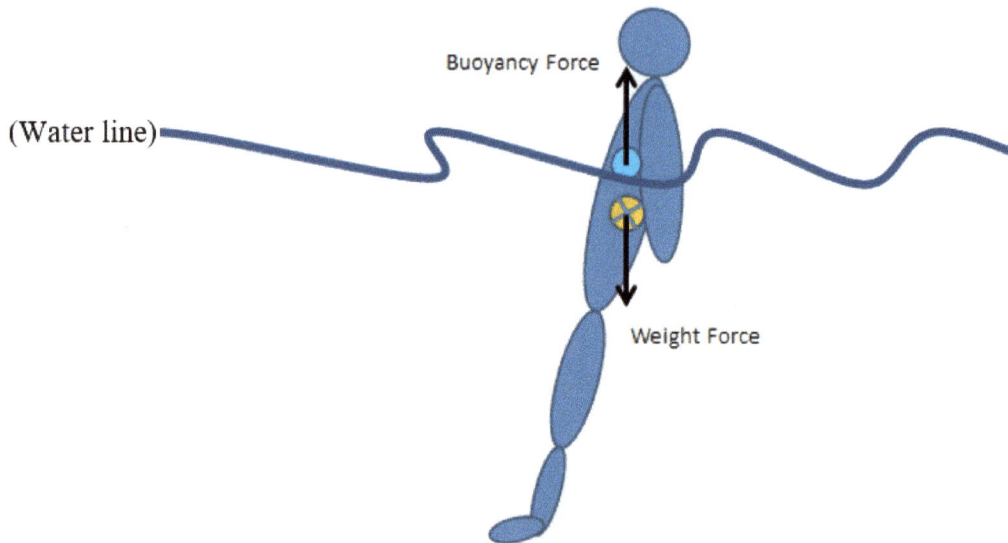

Figure 9.10   Floating 3.

Laminar Flow

When dealing with fluids, engineers typically model them as layers of material, similar to a multilayered cake. The fluid layers stack onto one another, and when the fluid flows, all molecules of the fluid layers move at similar rate and in the same direction; this is called laminar flow. This description of a fluid represents a laminar flow model of the fluid.

Laminar Fluid Flow

Figure 9.11   Laminar flow.

When an object is introduced into a laminar flow in such a way that the object's motion plane is parallel to the layers of the fluid, the layers of the fluid part, and the object may slide between them in a nonturbulent fashion. To maintain the same overall flow rate of all the layers, the fluid molecules of those closest to the object may need to speed up and for a time compress some adjacent layers.

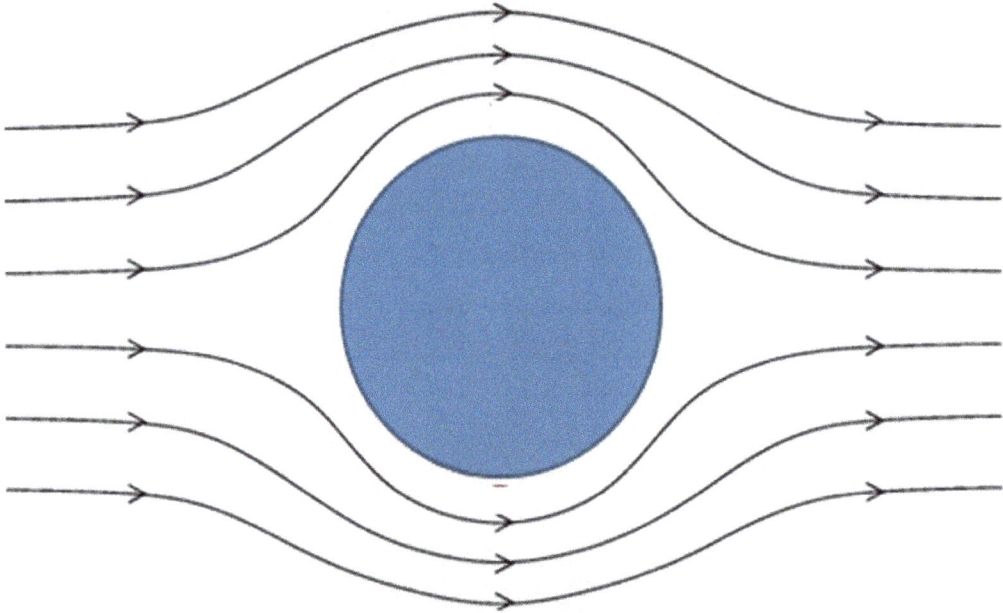

Figure 9.12   Boundary layer.

The layers of fluid closest to an object that are disrupted by its movement through a fluid represent the boundary layer of fluid. It is within the boundary layer that the smooth laminar flow is altered and where a variety of important fluid-to-object interactions occur.

Turbulence is the result of an object moving through a fluid in so disruptive a manner that the fluid layers overlap and mix. Laminar and turbulent fluid flows are two distinct conditions that result in their own set of fluid forces acting on objects in the fluid. Often, objects experience a combination of both laminar and turbulent flow simultaneously. Swimmers experience this combined laminar and turbulent flow situation whenever they are in water.

The more mass of a fluid that is supported above a given point, the greater the pressure. That means that air pressure is greatest at the surface of the earth, and water pressure is greatest at bottom of the ocean.

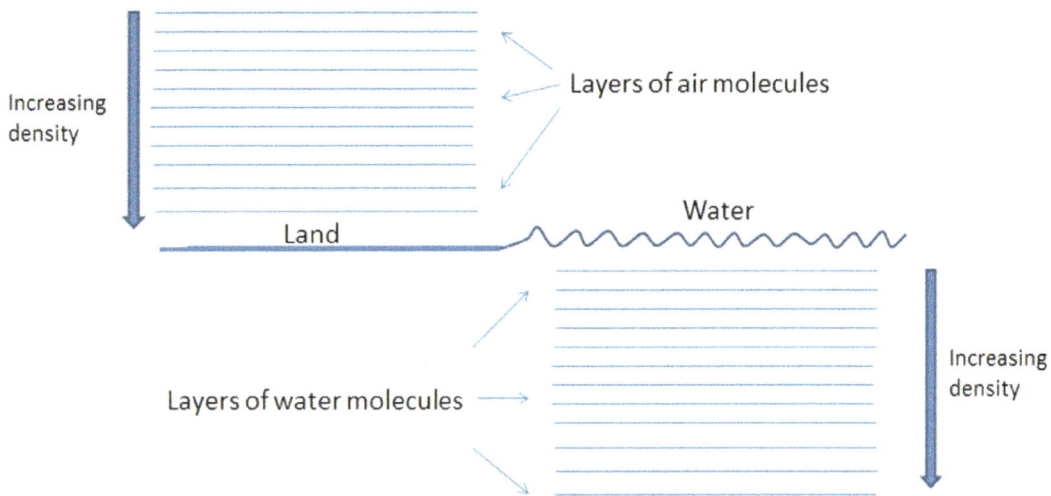

Figure 9.13   Air and water layers.

Lift

An extremely important property of objects as they move through a fluid is their ability to generate lift based on their speed and shape. Lift is the result of pressure variations between layers of a fluid when an object is moving through it. Lift is dependent on the shape of the object and the speed it is moving. The lift force is expressed as $F_{Lift} = 1/2\rho C_{Lift}A_{Lifting\ Surface}v^2$, where lift force F_{Lift} is the product of the fluid density ρ; C_{Lift} the coefficient of lift, which represents the body's ability to generate lift; the surface of the object on which the lifting force acts is $A_{Lifting\ Surface}$; and relative velocity of the object relative to the fluid squared is v^2 (https://www.grc.nasa.gov/www/k-12/rocket/lifteq.html).

For example, what is the lifting force acting on the wing of a small plane traveling at 75m/s at an altitude of 3,000m? The wing has an "active" (the area effected by lift force) surface area of $10m^2$. The air temperature is 10C with humidity of 25%. The coefficient of lift for the wing is 1.47. Air density was $0.859kg/m^3$, as determined using the air density calculator found here:

$$F_{Lift} = 1/2\rho C_{Lift}A_{Lifting\ Surface}v^2$$

$$F_{Lift} = ½(0.859kg/m^3)*(1.47)*(10m^2)*(75m/s)^2$$

$$F_{Lift} = 3551.43N \text{ of lift per wing}$$

Certain shapes are ideally suited for generating lift as they move through fluids. The best lift producing shape is called a foil. A foil is a shape with a bulbous leading edge that tapers to a smooth pointed tail.

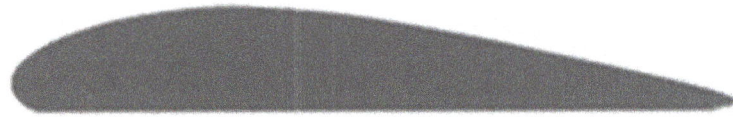

Flat Bottomed Foil

Symmetrical Foil

Semi-Symmetrical Foil

Figure 9.14   Air foils.

Bernoulli's Equation

The unique shape of a foil takes advantage of the fact that layers of fluid encountered by the front end of a foil will speed up or slow down so as to reach the end of the foil at the same time as other molecules aligned vertically with the leading edge of the foil. This property increases the speed of fluid moving over the top side of the foil relative to fluid moving along the underside of the foil. The difference in fluid speeds on the top and bottom of the foil results in lower pressure on the top surface and higher pressure on the bottom surface. This phenomenon was first explained by 18th-century Swiss mathematician Daniel Bernoulli and was expressed in his equation $p_{\text{fluid pressure}} + 1/2\rho_{\text{fluid density}}V_{\text{relative velocity}}^2 + \rho_{\text{fluid density}}a_{\text{gravity}}h_{\text{height}} = \text{constant}$,where p is the pressure, ρ is the density, V is velocity, g is the acceleration of gravity, and h is the height of the object above ground (http://hyperphysics.phy-astr.gsu.edu/hbase/pber.html)

Bernoulli's equation helps us to understand the relationship between pressure, velocity, and elevation for an object moving through a fluid. Bernoulli understood that the concept of conservation of energy could be applied to objects moving through a fluid. His equation shows that to maintain the constant energy of a system at a given height, an increase in fluid velocity corresponds directly to a decrease in the pressure exerted by the fluid.

His equation proves that by increasing the velocity of a fluid you reduce the pressure generated by the fluid over a given surface contact area. That means the pressure on the top surface of a moving foil, where fluid moves more rapidly than on the underside of the foil, is less than on the bottom surface, resulting in an upward push on the foil by the slower moving fluid below it. This difference in fluid velocity and pressure between the upper and lower surface of the foil generates lift to the foil.

The Bernoulli equation helps explain why an aircraft's velocity must increase to maintain lift at greater altitudes and why the wings of an aircraft can generate sufficient lift at lower speeds during takeoff and landing. This property holds true for objects moving in any fluid and is central to the lift-generating properties of airfoils used for air flight and hydrofoils used on many marine vehicles.

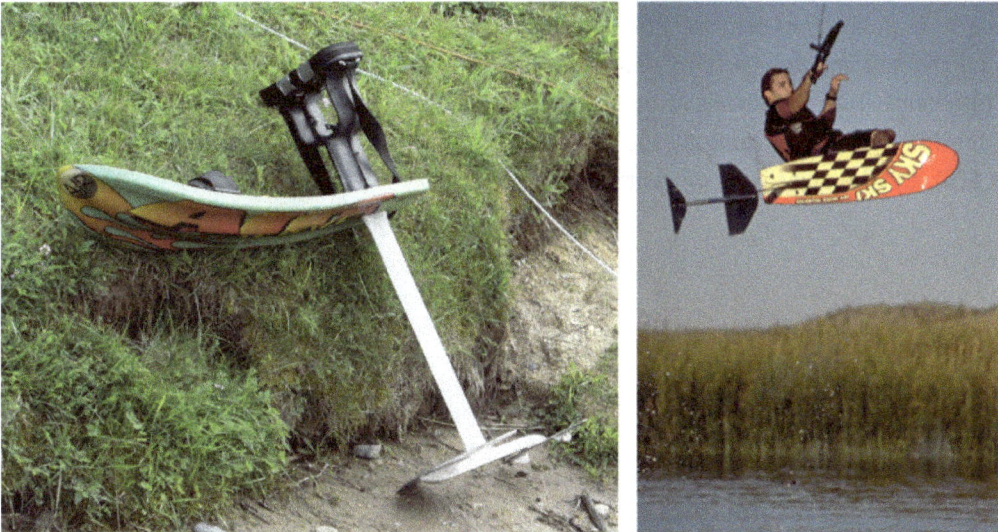

Figure 9.15   Hydro skis.

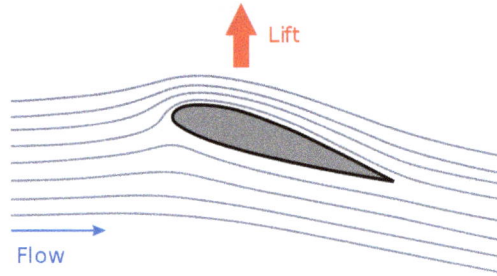

Figure 9.16   Air foil lift.

(To see this in action, see https://commons.wikimedia.org/wiki/File:Magnus-anim-canette.gif).

Angle of Attack

The angle at which an object presents its leading surface area to a fluid is called its angle of attack and changes the instantaneous lift and drag characteristics of the object. If an air or hydrofoil is oriented parallel to the layers of a fluid, it will result in both lift and drag on the foil in a state of minimum turbulence or a situation of laminar flow. By increasing the angle of attack slightly, the lift force will increase on the foil, and laminar flow will be maintained. If the angle of attack continues to increase, a state of turbulence with significant increase in drag will occur (Figure 9.17a), until eventually the lifting force on the foil will be overcome by the drag and the foil will "stall" or lose its ability to generate lift (Figure 9.17b), and the object will sink within the fluid.

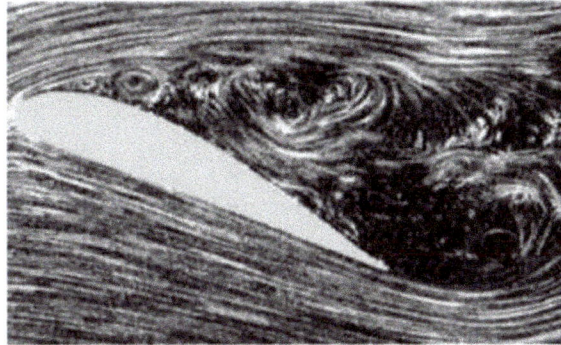

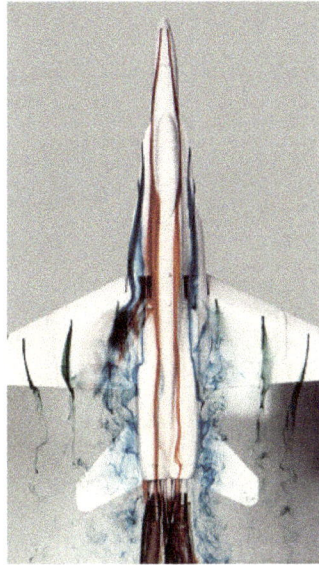

Figure 9.17   Airfoil turbulence and jet turbulence.

It is important to note that an object does not need to have a foil shape to generate lift while moving through a fluid, just that the foil is the most efficient shape for lift generation. Almost anything has some lift potential, from a frisbee to a human being. Humans take advantage of our ability to reorient our body segments to optimize movement in both air and water. The position a swimmer assumes when performing a backstroke is ideal for maximizing bouyancy and lift while decreasing drag; this allows the person to move their body effectively through the water. Cyclists and skiers often assume tucked positions, thereby reducing drag as they pedal along a road or race down a mountain.

In this chapter we have discussed what causes an object to speed up, slow down, float, rise, or sink in fluids. Thus far, we have talked about objects moving linearly through fluids, but what happens when the object moving through a fluid spins? Not only is the object affected by lift and drag, but another phenomenon called the Magnus effect also affects its motion. The Magnus effect was named for Heinrich

Gustav Magnus (1802–1870), an experimental scientist, the first person to explain why a rotating object swerves as it moves through a fluid.

Magnus Effect

The Magnus effect or Magnus force tends to cause rotating objects moving through a fluid to curve from their initial path. The Magnus effect is the result of frictional drag in the form of turbulence and pressure differentials, as explained by the Bernoulli principle, generating forces on a rotating object, causing it to swerve or veer from its straight-line path. This is not the same path change that is elicited by gravity causing an arc in the path of a projectile but additional direction changes caused by the rotational and drag properties of the object.

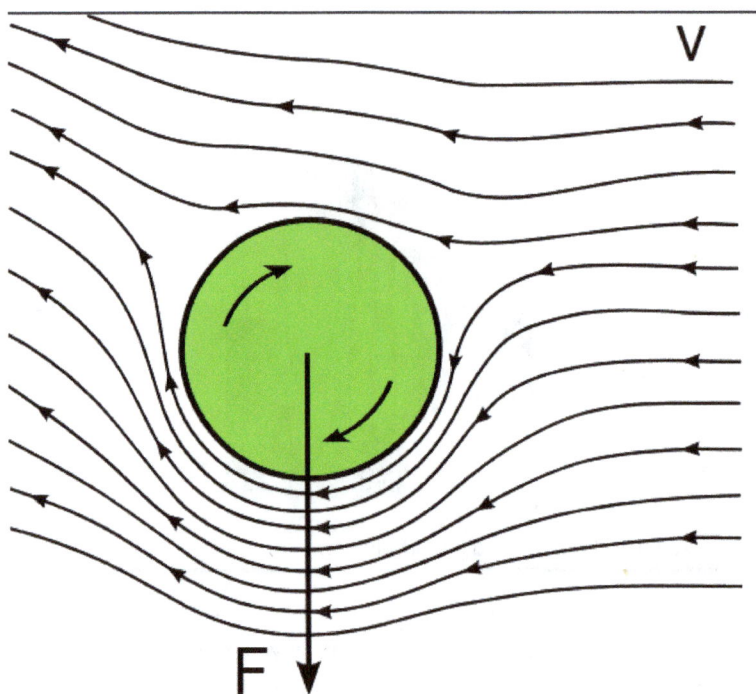

Figure 9.18   Magnus effect.

The most common examples of the Magnus effect in action occur when a ball is thrown or struck such that it has a high rate of rotation that leads to a curving of the ball's flight. The manufacture of certain types of game balls, such as a baseball, provides the ball with nonuniform surfaces that will increase the Magnus effect when the ball is thrown or struck.

The Magnus effect results when the rotation of the object causes layers of fluid on either the top (for underspin) or on the bottom (for topspin) to decrease the pressure, resulting in upward or downward lift. In addition, the rapid spinning results in significant turbulence immediately behind the object, which increases its drag. Topspin generates a Magnus force that pushes the ball downward, and underspin a Magnus force pushing it upward. Athletes in different sports use such spins to their advantage. A tennis player uses topspin, allowing them to strike the ball harder, with less chance of the ball sailing out of the court, and a golfer imparts underspin on their shot to maximize flight distance.

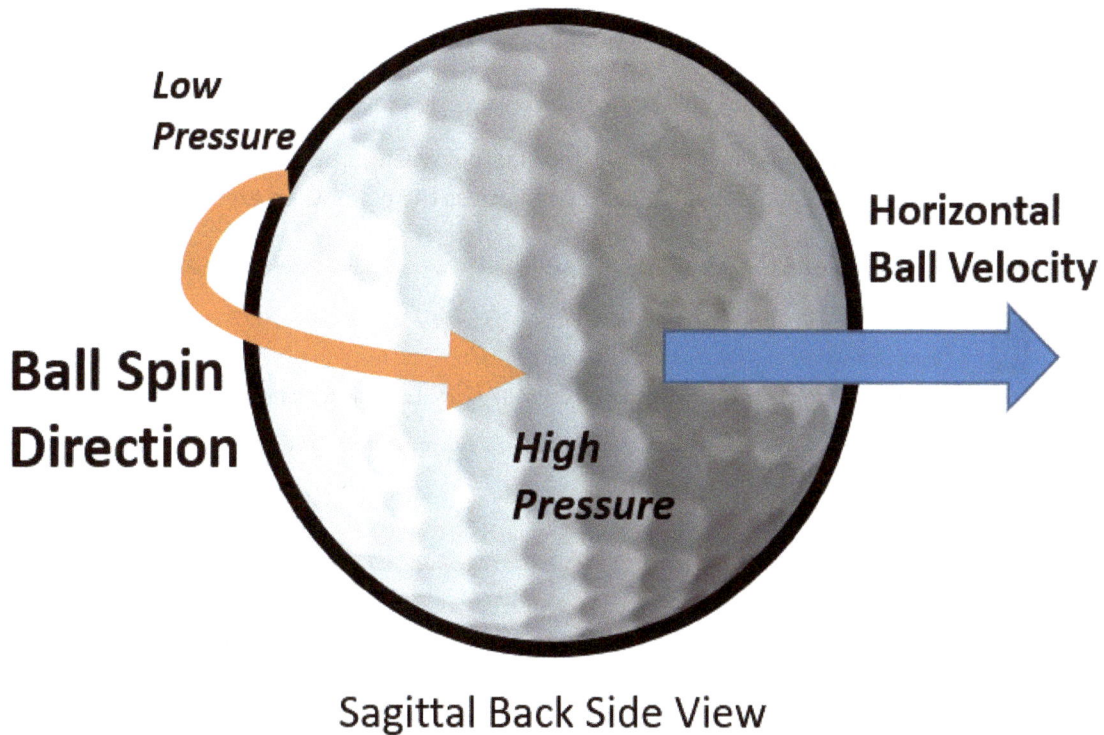

Figure 9.19   Magnus effect on a golf ball.

One or more interactive elements has been excluded from this version of the text. You can view them online here:
https://pb.cognella.com/83647-1b/?p=57#oembed-1

Please refer to the interactive ebook in Cognella Active Learning for interactive/media content.

One or more interactive elements has been excluded from this version of the text. You can view them online here: https://pb.cognella.com/83647-1b/?p=57#oembed-2

Please refer to the interactive ebook in Cognella Active Learning for interactive/media content.

One or more interactive elements has been excluded from this version of the text. You can view them online here: https://pb.cognella.com/83647-1b/?p=57#oembed-3

Please refer to the interactive ebook in Cognella Active Learning for interactive/media content.

A baseball pitcher uses a combination of topspin and sidespin when throwing a curve ball. The combined Magnus effect results in the ball dropping and swerving across the plate when executed correctly.

One or more interactive elements has been excluded from this version of the text. You can view them online here: https://pb.cognella.com/83647-1b/?p=57#oembed-6

Please refer to the interactive ebook in Cognella Active Learning for interactive/media content.

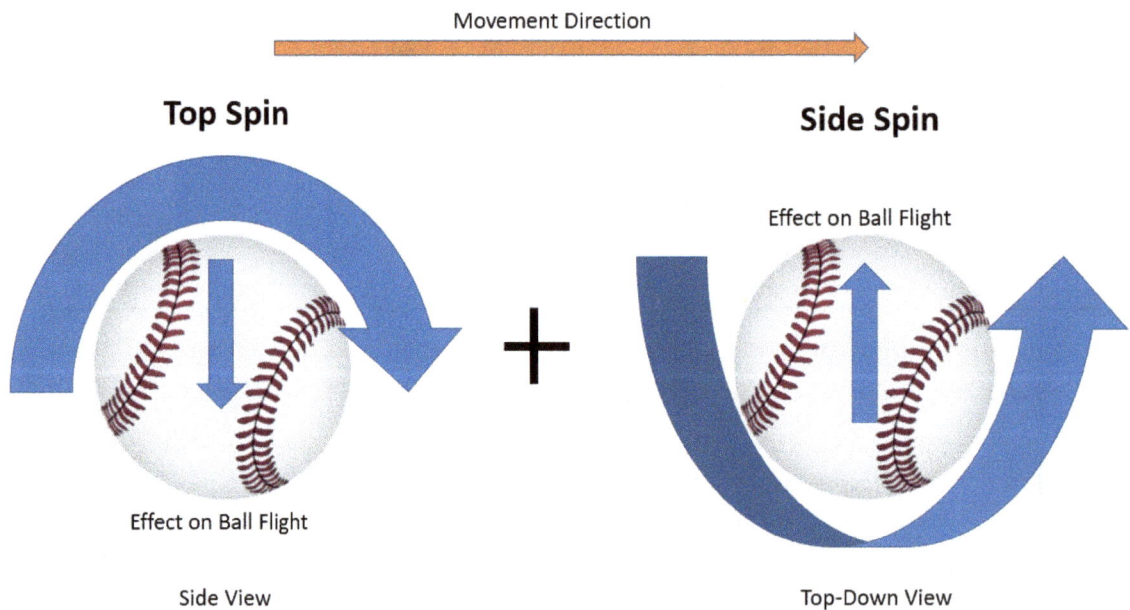

Figure 9.20   Right-hand curve ball.

How This All Works

There is a longstanding myth of a "rising" fastball in baseball and softball resulting from underspin being adding to a pitched ball. In reality, there is no "rising" fastball, but it is possible to blunt the effect of gravity using the Magnus effect. When executed properly, the pitched ball will not fall as rapidly, giving the impression that the ball rises on its way to the home plate. The "rising" fastball is an optical illusion but is still a very effective pitch for those players who can throw it.

The force of the Magnus effect can be calculated with the following equation:

$Fm = Cd (ω × v)$ Note: The "x" represents the cross product of the angular and linear velocities

where

Fm = the Magnus force

ω = angular velocity vector of the object

v=velocity of the fluid (or velocity of object, depends on perspective)

Cd = drag coefficient (or air resistance coefficient) across the surface of the object

Each object has its own unique drag coefficient based on its unique physical topography. Table 9.1 lists a variety of objects and their drag coefficient values.

Table 9.1 Drag Coefficients of Various Objects

Object	Cd	Object	Cd
Human (upright position)	- 1.3	Penguin	0.0044
Human running	0.5	Falcon	0.24
Racing cyclist	0.4	Aircraft	0.02 – 0.09
Ski jumper	1.2 – 1.3	Smooth sphere	0.1 – 0.5
Skier	1.0 – 1.1	Golf ball	0.25 – 0.3
Parachutist	1.0 – 1.4	Car	0.35 – 0.5
Human swimming	0.035	Sports car	0.3 – 0.4
Trout	0.015	Motorcycle	0.5 – 1.00
Dolphin	0.0036	Truck	0.6 – 1.00
Seal	0.004	Tractor-trailer	0.6 – 1.20

Note: From "Applied Biomechanics Concepts and Connections," by John McLester and Peter St. Pierre, Thomson Wadsworth, p. 257. Copyright 2008 by Thomson Wadsworth, a part of the Thomson Wadsworth Corporation.

For example, the dimples on a golf ball are designed to help golfers hit the ball father and with more control. Given linear and angular velocities of 35m/s and 14.5rad/s, respectively, for a golf ball and a round ball in similar size and weight, what would be the minimum and maximum drag (or lift, since the equations are the same) of the two balls?

$\rho = 1.225kg/m^3$

$v = 35m/s$

radius = .21m

$\omega = 14.5rad/s$

C_d golf ball = 0.25 – 0.30

C_d sphere = 0.1 – 0.5

$F_{drag} = 1/2\rho C_{drag}A_{Contact\ Surface}v^2$

$A_{Contact\ Surface} = \pi r^2$

$A_{Contact\ Surface} = 3.1416*(2.1cm)^2$

$A_{Contact\ Surface} = 0.1385m^2$

$F_{drag\ golf\ ball} = 1/2\rho C_{drag}A_{Contact\ Surface}v^2$ $F_{drag\ sphere} = 1/2\rho C_{drag}A_{Contact\ Surface}v^2$

Minimum drag of the golf ball Minimum drag of the sphere

$F_{drag\ golf\ ball} = 0.5*1.225kg/m^3*0.25*0.1385m^2 * 35m/s$ $F_{drag\ sphere} = 0.5*1.225kg/m^3*0.1*0.1385m^2 * 35m/s$

$F_{drag\ golf\ ball} = 0.74N$ $F_{drag\ sphere} = 0.30N$

Maximum drag of the golf ball Maximum drag of the sphere

$F_{drag\ golf\ ball} = 0.5*1.225kg/m^3*0.3*0.1385m^2 * 35m/s$ $F_{drag\ sphere} = 0.5*1.225kg/m^3*0.5*0.1385m^2 * 35m/s$

$F_{drag\ golf\ ball} = 0.89N$ $F_{drag\ sphere} = 1.48N$

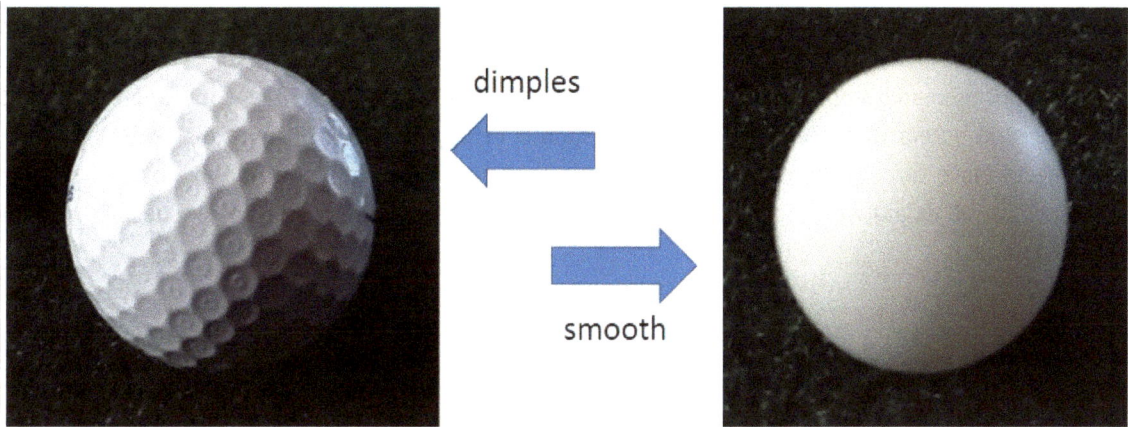

Figure 9.21   Dimpled and smooth golf balls. Dimpled golf balls increase the Magnus effect of spins and reduce aerodynamic drag during flight.

Table 9.2. Equations and Units for Fluid Dynamics

Variable and Equation	Units	Vector or Scalar	Comments
Drag force $F_{drag} = .5 \, \rho \, C_d * A_{contact} \, v^2$	N	Vector	
Buoyancy force $F_{buoyancy} = V\gamma$ $F_{buoyancy} = PA$ $F_{buoyancy} = \rho g h A$	N	Vector	
Lift force $F_{Lift} = 1/2 \rho C_{Lift} A_{Lifting \, Surface} v^2$	N	Vector	
Bernoulli's equation $P_{fluid \, pressure} + 1/2 \rho_{fluid \, density} v^2_{relative \, velocity} + \rho_{fluid \, density} a_{gravity} h_{height} = constant$	N/cm^2	Vector	
Magnus force $Fm = C_d \, (\omega \times v)$	N	Vector	

Summary

We live on a planet on which 70% of its surface is water and all of it is wrapped in a gaseous atmosphere. We learn to move in a fluid-filled sack before we are born. Our entire lives require us to negotiate various fluid-filled environments. Understanding the basics of fluid dynamics will help you appreciate how you and other objects move in our fluid-filled world.

The concepts and applications related to drag, lift, buoyancy, laminar flow, angle of attack, turbulence, and others discussed in this chapter should help you appreciate what is really happening when objects move through fluids. That knowledge can help us navigate and improve our efficiency of movement, as well as aid with the creation of machines designed to take advantage of special properties of fluid dynamics.

List of Key Takeaways

- Fluid dynamics describes and explains how objects move through fluids.
- Almost all movement occurs while interacting with some form of fluid, whether gas or liquid.
- Understanding the effects of turbulence, drag, lift, and buoyancy provides us with the basic knowledge of the physics of movement through a fluid.

References

Goyal, M.R. (2013). Biofluid Dynamics of Human Body Systems, CRC Press.
Kyle, C.R. and Burke, E.R., (1984). Improving the racing bicycle. Mech Eng 106(9):34–45.
McKelvey, J.P. and Grotch, H. (1978). "Physics for Science and Engineering", ISBN 0-06-044376-6, pg. 352).
McLester, J. and St. Pierre, P. (2008). Applied Biomechanics Concepts and Connections. Thomson Wadsworth.
Royder, J. O. (1997). Fluid hydraulics in human physiology, AAO Journal (Summer) pg 11-16.

Image Credits

Fig. 9.1: Copyright © 2018 by mohamed_hassan. Reprinted with permission.
Fig. 9.2: Copyright © 2018 by mohamed_hassan. Reprinted with permission.
Fig. 9.3: Copyright © 2018 by mohamed_hassan. Reprinted with permission.
Fig. 9.4 : Copyright © 2018 by mohamed_hassan. Reprinted with permission.
Fig. 9.5: Copyright © 2018 by mohamed_hassan. Reprinted with permission.
Fig. 9.6: Copyright © by Sandro Halank (CC BY-SA 4.0) at https://commons.wikimedia.org/wiki/File:2020-01-18_1st_run_Luge_Women%27s_Double_(2020_Winter_Youth_Olympics)_by_Sandro_Halank%E2%80%93003.jpg.
Fig. 9.7: Source: https://commons.wikimedia.org/wiki/File:Entry.jpg.
Fig. 9.15a: Copyright © by Deana Hunter (CC BY 2.0) at https://commons.wikimedia.org/wiki/File:Air_Chair_01.jpg.
Fig. 9.15b: Copyright © by WaterHound (CC BY-SA 3.0) at https://commons.wikimedia.org/wiki/File:Sky_Skier_performs_jump,_1998.jpg.
Fig. 9.16: Copyright © by Michael Paetzold (CC BY-SA 3.0 DE) at https://commons.wikimedia.org/wiki/File:DeflectionAndLift_W3C.svg.
Fig. 9.17a: Copyright © by Jaganath (CC BY-SA 3.0) at https://commons.wikimedia.org/wiki/File:Flow_separation.jpg.
Fig. 9.17b: Source: https://commons.wikimedia.org/wiki/File:110444main_fvf_165.jpg.
Fig. 9.18: Copyright © by Gang65 (CC BY-SA 3.0) at https://commons.wikimedia.org/wiki/File:Magnus_effect.svg.
Fig. 9.19: Copyright © by Urbanuntillll (CC BY-SA 3.0) at https://commons.wikimedia.org/wiki/File:Golf.png.
Fig. 9.20: Source: https://commons.wikimedia.org/wiki/File:Baseball.svg.

Chapter 10

Advances and the Future of Biomechanics

Preparing to Learn: *Watch*

As we move into the future, biomechanics will be there to continue its quest of reducing injury while improving/maintaining human movement possibilities. With advances in technology come new opportunities for biomechanists to apply their understanding of physics, anatomy, and instrumentation in new and exciting ways. Science fiction will continue to become science fact, with solutions found to previously unsolvable problems. People will be able to move closer to reaching or even surpassing the physical limitations of the human machine!

Enjoy watching the following videos that show how biomechanically inspired advances change what we know about human movement.

One or more interactive elements has been excluded from this version of the text. You can view them online here: https://pb.cognella.com/83647-1b/?p=58#oembed-1

Please refer to the interactive ebook in Cognella Active Learning for interactive/media content.

One or more interactive elements has been excluded from this version of the text. You can view them online here: https://pb.cognella.com/83647-1b/?p=58#oembed-2

Please refer to the interactive ebook in Cognella Active Learning for interactive/media content.

Preparing to Learn: *Respond*

Directions: Based on what you saw in the videos, respond to the following questions:

1. In the video "When Sports Meets Science," what was the most surprising relationship between sports and science to you and why?
2. Video 10.3 describes some of the future ties between medicine and biomechanics. What are the three measures done on bone and implants to determine their appropriateness for patient use? Why is a knowledge of biomechanics critical to the optimization of implant development and use?

Introduction to the Chapter

Biomechanics is a continually changing field of study. As we learn more about ourselves and continue to push our physical limits, biomechanics will be there to help improve our movement capabilities while trying to keep us from injury. Human anatomy is slow to radically change its form and function, but the technology that humans use from advances in sport equipment to "smart apparel", to intelligent joint replacements, means that biomechanists must continually monitor and evaluate the human condition.

Every day, science fiction is becoming science fact. If the new science fact is to provide real benefits related to movement from birth to death, then it must be understood how these advances affect people. Biomechanics provides the perfect bridge between technological advances and our human movement goals.

Learning Objectives

After completing this chapter, students should be able to do the following:

- List examples of technology designed to be used by people to improve their movement ability and/or reduce their likelihood of injury in sport, daily life, and clinical settings
- List possible advances in sport performance linked to applied biomechanics
- List three or more examples of future improvements in the daily lives of people due to advances in biomechanically inspired devices
- Discuss how joint replacement innovations may improve performance beyond "normal human" limits and what that may mean for future athletic competition

Possible Future of Sport Biomechanics

The study and understanding of human and animal movement continues to evolve. From the early observations of our distant ancestors to the sophisticated analyses possible today, people have and will continue to be fascinated with all of the many forms of movement. Today we have the science of biomechanics, which links musculoskeletal anatomy with mechanics and specialized instrumentation to understand our world of movement better than ever before.

But what about the future? How will biomechanics change? What will be the big biomechanical questions of tomorrow? The three primary areas of biomechanical research, sports, daily life, and medicine, continue to provide new challenges for the researcher and applied biomechanist. We are gathering new and interesting data on how the musculoskeletal system works and remodels when under stress. While mechanical physics and its associated mathematics has not changed significantly over the past centuries, the ability to link them directly to real-time data has. What once took years of painstaking manual calculations can now be performed in fractions of seconds based on data from wearable technologies.

Advances in Sport

Sport biomechanics often acts as a testing ground for innovation and the advancement of human movement study. Throughout the text and certainly during this chapter there are noticeable overlays of the types of problems, attempted solutions, and advances in technology seen across the areas of sport, daily life, and medicine. People are people, and they move between the three areas of biomechanical research often on a daily basis, so it makes sense that biomechanists will MacGyver solutions based on the proven results from another area.

New designs in athletic footwear have reduced the energy cost of wearing shoes while still maintaining the basic form and function necessary to enhance performance and safety. An example is the Vapor Fly Next 2% Running Shoe Tech from Nike. Shoe companies, just like every other company, want to impress customers with their use of technology. They like to tease their audience with just enough familiar terms to make the consumer believe the technology is state-of-the-art and then throw in some special jargon and maybe an acronym or two to make their product special. With the Nike Vapor Fly, Nike uses all of those tricks and more, from mentioning a carbon fiber midsole plate (carbon fiber is always a good thing related to high performance, right?) which they say "creates a propulsive sensation to help you push the pace" to dropping the name of a famous athlete like Eliud Kipchoge, the first person to run a sub 2-hour marathon (someone we might have heard of but will never be able to personally match his performance), to adding their special secret ingredient, the ZoomX foam, that is too important to actually explain but we are assured it is patented. The business of selling athletic equipment often is more art than science. However, at the core of every good piece of equipment is the correct tool to help the athlete perform at their best. With the Nike Vapor Fly, the lightweight, lower energy cost shoe that they have developed provides one of the best athletic tools for those serious about running.

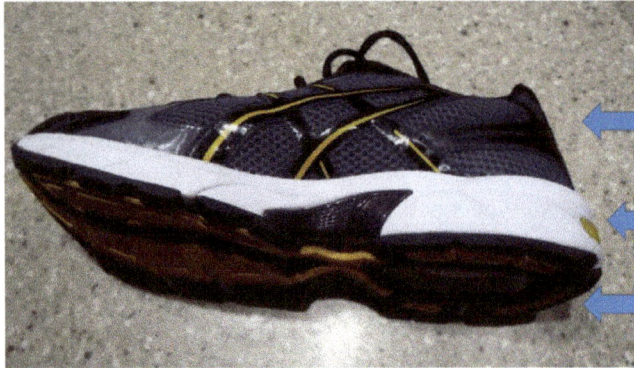

Top layer: "Upper" is a slipper with nothing on the bottom

Middle layer: "Midsole" the cushion the plantar surface of the foot rests in when wearing the shoe

Bottom layer: "Outsole" the part of the shoe that contacts the ground.

Figure 10.1   Basic anatomy of every running shoe .

Wearable Tech: Smartphones, Watches, Sleep Bands, and Sport Apparel

Athletes and their coaches are always trying to gather more data, looking for an edge. Many are now looking at measurements recorded directly from sensors worn on the body of the athlete. Whether it's a GPS-type app on a smartphone that records times, distances, and other information to be analyzed during each workout, or specialty devices that focus on our coping with fatigue and evaluating sleep efficiency, there is an app or gadget for just about any measure thought useful related to sport performance, injury prevention, or rehab efficiency.

There is even a strong push to develop active sports apparel that will measure, record, and analyze everything from heart rate to sweat response, to force production and muscle activity levels—essentially a wearable biomechanics laboratory woven into the clothes that you wear!

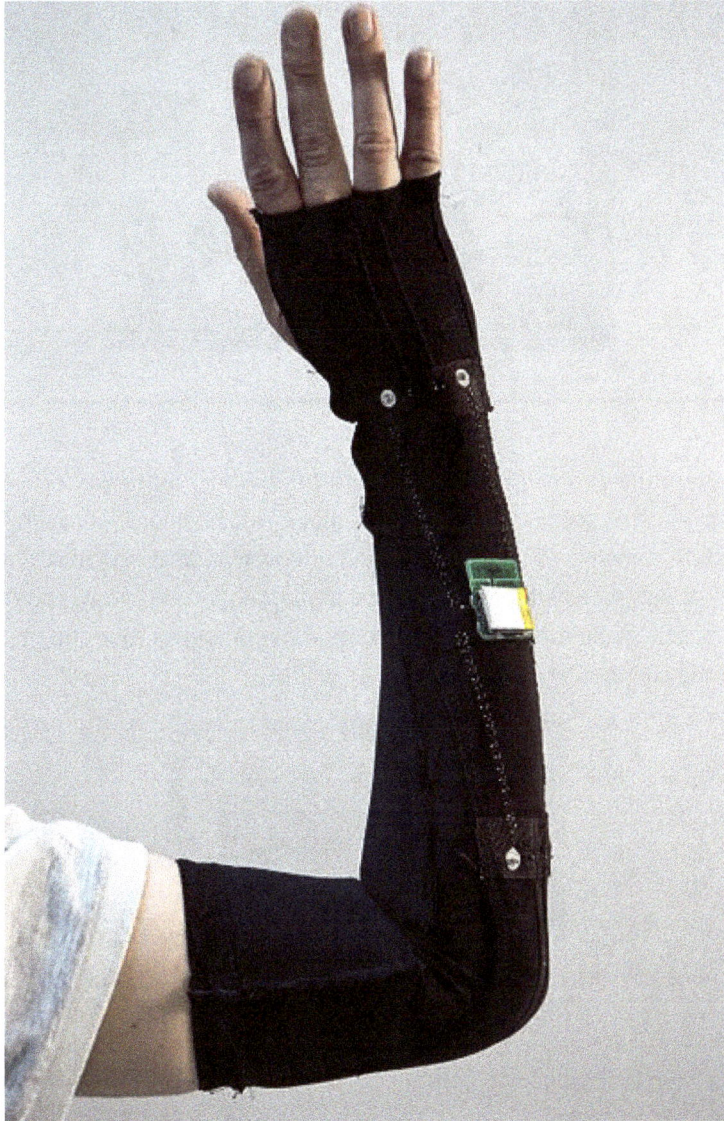

Figure 10.2   Apparel tech.

Cyborgs!

A cyborg is a person whose physical abilities have been enhanced beyond what is normally possible as the result of mechanical systems being embedded in their bodies. Sound like science fiction? What about someone with a pacemaker? Over 1 million are implanted worldwide each year (Hbaita and El-Chami, 2018) or cochlear implants with about ¾ million worldwide (National Institute on Deafness and Other Communication Disorders, 2016)? Technically, they are cyborgs. What about someone with artificial legs? Yep, cyborg.

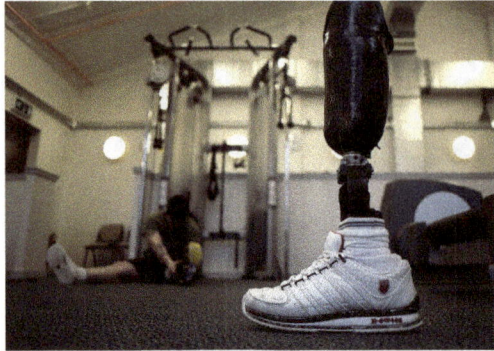
Figure 10.3   Leg prosthetic.

Science fiction literature and comic books used to be the only place you could read about cyborgs and their superhuman feats of strength, speed, and agility. Not anymore. Through the advancement of technology and the understanding of how the human body works, creating real-life cyborgs is no longer just in the realm of sci-fi. Advancements in prosthetics, implantable technology, and the miniaturization of electronic components now make it possible for cyborgs walk among us. But don't worry, unlike the plots of many sci-fi novels, they are not here to take over the world!

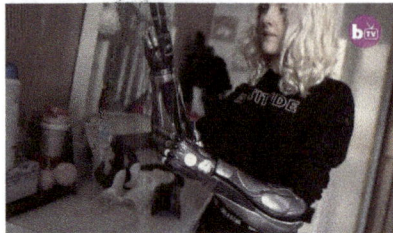
Figure 10.4   Real-life female cyborg image.

What happens in sport when an enhanced human, a cyborg, wishes to compete against nonmechanically enhanced humans? It is much the same debate that has been raging for decades related to the use of performance-enhancing drugs.

This is a question that used to be just a philosophical one but now is an actual issue that should be addressed by today's sports scientists. If someone gains a perceived advantage due to some form of technological enhancement, who needs to determine if the advantage is real or not? Biomechanics, along with other sport scientists, need to be involved in determining if the advantage is real. They should also assist with ensuring that enhancements don't produce unexpected or unwanted side effects that could lead to injury. In that way, they can help ensure that sports competitions are safe and fair for everyone.

Advances in Daily Life

The world of Biomechanics is increasingly becoming the world of everyday life. Applications that used to only happen in laboratories, or with specialized teams working with very specific populations are now becoming commonplace, and we all benefiting!

Possible Future of Daily Life Biomechanics

As mentioned earlier, advances in sport biomechanics often migrate into the other areas of biomechanical interest such as daily life and medicine. Highly functional prosthetics, pioneered with athletes and injured military personnel, have yielded options for the general population that would likely not have been available nearly as soon. Robust wearable tech has made it into the daily lives of millions who rely on smartwatches or phone apps to track and analyze their movements or a host of physiological responses. From the very youngest to the oldest among us, biomechanically inspired technology has become part of our lives.

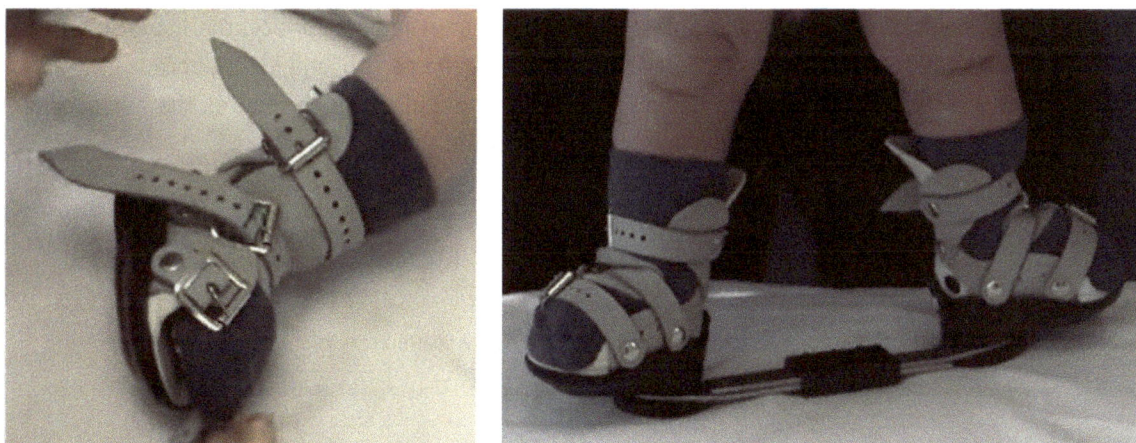

Figure 10.5   Infant's brace.

Better designed footwear, even if you are not a world-class athlete, provides benefits to all who run, hike, bike, or participate in sports for fun and recreation.

We now have the ability to record the number of steps we take each day as well as our current blood oxygen content, and to record and analyze our own golf swing and reduce our likelihood of injury while we work or play:

> The application of Biomechanical knowledge takes many forms and one, ergonomics, has combined the basic understanding of human movement, injury, and performance with other areas such as psychology, engineering, and physiology to optimize human interaction with various systems we interact with on a daily basis. "Ergonomics is the scientific discipline concerned with the understanding of interactions among humans and other elements of a system, and the profession that applies theory, principles, data and methods to design in order to optimize human well-being and overall system

performance." *International Ergonomics Association Adapted from Human Factors and Ergonomics Society, (n.d.)*

Both private and mass transportation safety have been greatly improved by studying how humans respond to crashes in cars, buses, trains, and planes. Many advances in automotive design have come about due to a better understanding of how humans respond to a crash situation. Multipoint seatbelt-restraining harnesses keep people safer by better coupling the person's inertial reaction to the sudden acceleration changes caused by a crash to that of the vehicle. A good restraint system links the person's inertia to that of the vehicle so they will respond in the same way to a change in acceleration. That means that the person will stop moving when the car stops and will not be free to fly around with the cabin of the vehicle and impact rigid structures inside the car, which could lead to injury or death.

Since a person is not a rigid structure, there will be some movement of the body, even if belted into the car properly, so to "catch" the excess body movement, airbags were invented to provide a soft surface to impact in the event of a crash. In addition to providing a softer impact surface, the increased area of impact, significantly reduces the peak pressures experienced by the person, and finally, because the airbag deflates slowly after impact, the person has a longer impact impulse, which reduces the average force applied during the impact to lessen the detrimental effects of the crash even more.

One or more interactive elements has been excluded from this version of the text. You can view them online here: https://pb.cognella.com/83647-1b/?p=58#oembed-3

Please refer to the interactive ebook in Cognella Active Learning for interactive/media content.

All of us would like to live a long healthy, active life. For that to happen, we must be aware of the possible factors that could ruin those plans. The human machine is designed to rebuild and remodel based on the stress it encounters. Regularly participating in activities such as aerobics, running, dance, tennis, or brisk walking are excellent ways for most people to generate some beneficial stress on their bodies. To keep our muscles and bones strong, resistance training has shown to be useful throughout the normal life span. Our bodies are meant to move, and we are rewarded when we do by a body that will meet most of our wishes related to movement. The types of movements that many of us enjoy occur outside in the sun. We've learned that too much sun can be damaging to our skin and can lead to skin cancer. Over 3.3 million people in the United States each year are diagnosed with skin cancer (American Cancer Society, 2023), so if you are going to be active outdoors you need to develop a plan to reduce your risk of developing skin cancer. New wearable tech, designed to monitor the damaging effects of the sun, has been incorporated into swimwear that can warn individuals when they have reached or exceeded thresholds of sun exposure that could lead to skin cancer.

Better Assessment/Tracking Across Life

For those interested in gaining or maintaining strength, there continue to be new theories and associated gadgets that will allow individuals to test themselves. VBT, velocity-based training, measurement devices that track the velocity of weight-lifting movements have proliferated recently. VBT attempts to quantify the volume and intensity of resistance training, to remove much of the subjective aspect of that activity. Portable stand-alone or smartphone app-paired systems have been created to allow individuals to accurately track the kinematics and kinetics of each lift.

Once the almost exclusive domain of men, performed in hot and smelly gyms, resistance training has become much more mainstream as its benefits for all individuals has become widely accepted. While certainly not all, much of the dialogue about the best or most correct way to weight train is still unsubstantiated or heavily influenced by hype, product marketing, and/or pseudoscience. As the various camps supporting or refuting the latest trend in weight training continue to argue, some very well-established biomechanical technologies used to determine kinematic and kinetic values are appearing in the marketplace, often with new packaging and some even tied to artificial intelligence software. These devices are based on measurement tools such as accelerometers, gyroscopes, pressure mats, videography, and computer vision. Such devices or systems are being used by average people to help them better track their weightlifting sessions. Accelerometer based units that determine velocity and force are small enough to be attached to a weight bar during exercise.

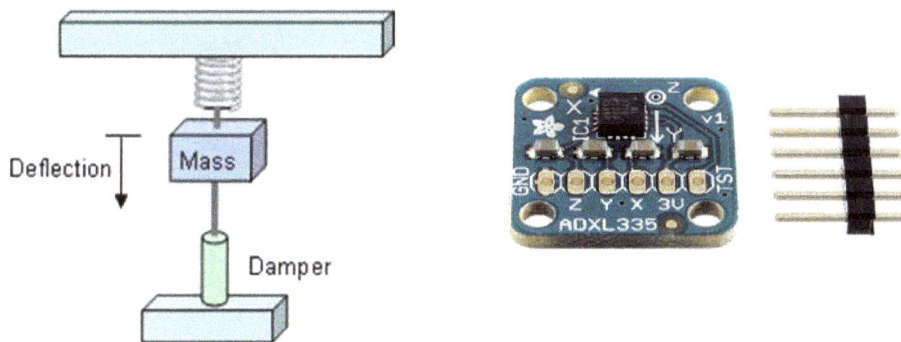

Figure 10.6   Accelerometers.

Other systems mimic the force plates found in Biomechanics labs and provide real-time force analysis during isometric and standard lifts. Others are more futuristic and bring resistance training almost into the realm of sci-fi with active motion tracking, sensor-based immediate feedback, and lifelike artificial intelligence–driven avatars acting as your personal trainer. We've come a long way from those smelly gyms!

As we move into the future, it is reasonable to assume that more and more of us will utilize knowledge and technology designed to improve our daily quality of life. From toddlers to octogenarians, we will measure, analyze, and modify our active lifestyles based on the science of biomechanics.

Advances in Medicine

Many of the advances in orthopedics are linked to an understanding and application of Biomechanics. These two fields overlap in their goals of improving/maintaining movement performance while reducing the prevalence and likelihood of injury.

Possible Future of Medicine Biomechanics

The partnership between biomechanics and the medical field is a bright one, producing advances in prediction and care for an ever-growing range of medical conditions, from the acute to chronic. Whether it is aiding those who have difficulty balancing while walking or those who never thought they would be able to walk again, the information, equipment, and understanding gained through the biomechanical analysis of the movement needs are providing breakthroughs in how the medical community treats its patients.

Even after a millennia of doctors treating patients with bone fractures, the science of bone fracture constructs is still evolving. People today have different expectations related to treatment of bone fractures compared to our predecessors. Setting a broken bone used to be a process that involved realigning the broken bone, casting, and hoping when the cast came off that the bone had set correctly, and that, after time, it would be functional again. Today, with the use of X-rays, MRIs, and other technologies, doctors have a much better understanding of the condition of the bone and surrounding tissue prior to setting the break. Casting is used more sparingly, and frequently the damaged bone is reassessed during the healing process, giving the doctor a chance to modify the bone alignment prior to the break fully healing.

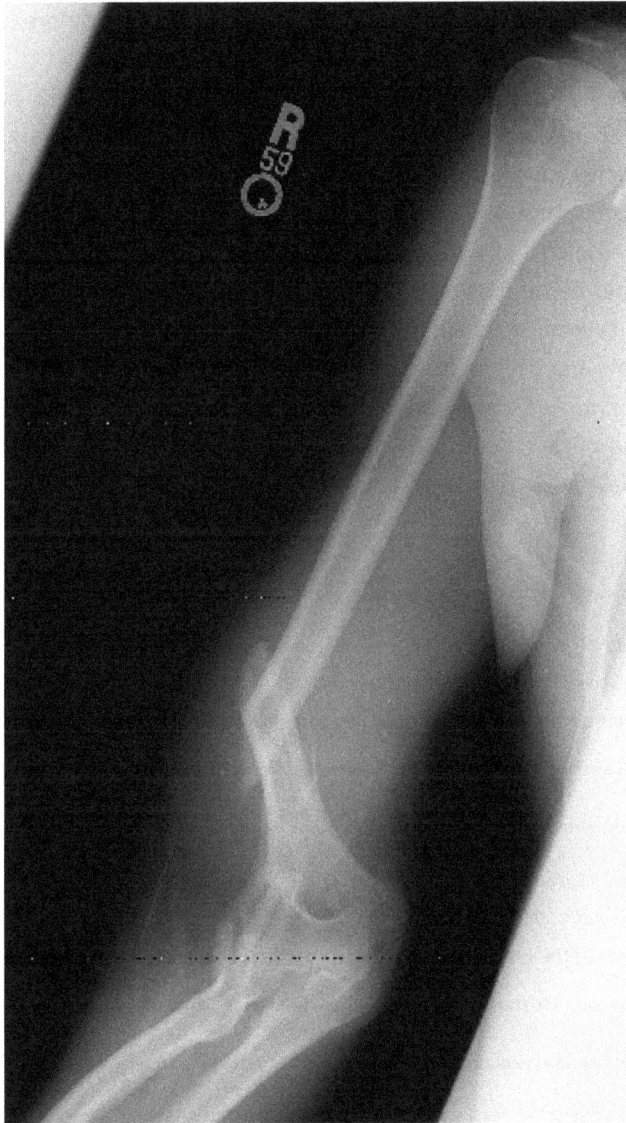

Figure 10.7   X-ray of damaged arm image.

There are programs under development designed to predict bone fatigue and failure prior to an acute break. This will never completely eliminate the accidental break as the result of a fall or car crash, but if successful will reduce the likelihood of bone fractures for individuals at risk of fracture due to participation in combat sports or those suffering from chronic disease states such as osteoporosis, or those dealing with the hostile environment of space. It has long been known that astronauts experience significant bone as the result of exposure to extended periods of low gravity. Researchers at UCSF and Baylor College of Medicine are working on a method of predicting bone fatigue and fracture for astronauts that may someday be used for those of us here on earth to accurately predict bone fracture before it happens (Science Daily, 2004).

What about other medical conditions that reduce motor function or put a person at risk of injury? Can the science of biomechanics help those with chronic diseases such as Parkinson's or diabetes? Yes! Parkinson's is a neurodegenerative disease that reduces the effect of the neural transmitter dopamine, eventually resulting in both motor and cognitive diminishment. It is also one of the, if not the, fastest growing neurological disease in the world, with more than 1 million people currently living with the disease in the United States alone (National Institute of Neurological Disorders and Stroke, n.d.) The list of life-altering symptoms caused by Parkinson's ranges from hand tremors to loss of the ability to walk. A host of biomechanical tools and treatment modalities have been and are being developed to help people afflicted with Parkinson's. From vibrating eating utensils that cancel out hand tremors to canes with lasers to help overcome freezing of gait issues, to exoskeletons designed to increase balance and assist with walking, biomechanics plays a large role in advances in improving/maintaining movement function for those with Parkinson's.

One or more interactive elements has been excluded from this version of the text. You can view them online here: https://pb.cognella.com/83647-1b/?p=58#oembed-4

Please refer to the interactive ebook in Cognella Active Learning for interactive/media content.

One or more interactive elements has been excluded from this version of the text. You can view them online here: https://pb.cognella.com/83647-1b/?p=58#oembed-5

Please refer to the interactive ebook in Cognella Active Learning for interactive/media content.

One or more interactive elements has been excluded from this version of the text. You can view them online here: https://pb.cognella.com/83647-1b/?p=58#oembed-6

Please refer to the interactive ebook in Cognella Active Learning for interactive/media content.

To combat the issues associated with diabetic foot neuropathy and its tendency to cause foot ulcerations, biomechanists have studied and developed specialized equipment to predict and pinpoint where high-pressure regions are found on the plantar surface of the diabetic foot. The insole pressure measurement systems of today lead to in-shoe exoskeletons that are designed to reduce the effects of those pressure hotspots by actively off-loading excessive pressure thereby reducing foot ulcerations (Roser et. al., 2017).

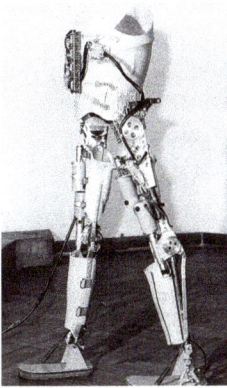

Figure 10.8   Exoskeleton.

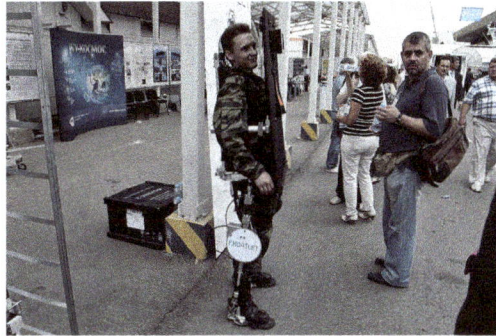

Figure 10.9   Man in an exoskeleton.

If a joint such as the hip, knee, or elbow is severely damaged as the result of an injury or aging, there are now improved medical options that may include the next generation of artificial joints coupled with improved surgical techniques used to install them. While the exact time and place of the first modern hip replacement is in some dispute, most agree that it occurred around the year 1900; the first elbow replacement surgery happened a couple decades later, and the first full knee replacement was performed in the 1960s (Learmonth et.al., 2007)

Using biomechanical knowledge of major joint functions, the medical industry continues to improve both joint replacement appliances so they function more like real biological joints. They are also improving surgical techniques to minimize collateral bone and surrounding soft tissue damage that often accompanies such procedures. These advances are making joint replacement surgery safer and better for the patient.

We are still far from creating joint replacements that are functionally as good or that will last longer than our original equipment, but huge strides have been made in the past several decades regarding joint replacement, with the expectation that even more improvements are on the horizon. It may be possible in your lifetime to have a damaged or worn-out joint medically replaced with little or no loss of mobility, function, or associated discomfort. The cyborgs are coming, and you might be one!

It is becoming more and more possible to replace a major body joint and live a healthy active life due to biomechanical and medical advances. But what about when more than just the joint has been damaged and needs replaced? Or what if part of the body, an arm or leg, is missing at birth or lost through accident or disease? Again, the teaming of biomechanics and medicine has led to the development of artificial limbs that may someday surpass those of flesh and bone.

It's one thing to replace a knee joint while all of the surrounding bone, nerves, tendons, ligaments, muscles, and so forth are intact and functioning. In the case of something like a below-the-knee running blade, the mechanism is relatively simple in design. The movement is generated by the healthy leg structures that the prosthetic is attached to, and much of the motion of the prosthetic is passive and controlled by the inertial physics of motion. The prosthetic does not need to look like a biological leg; it just needs to perform like one.

But what happens when someone loses a whole leg and wants the replacement not only to mimic the look but also the function of a normal healthy leg? Artificial legs of the future will look and feel like biological legs, and their movement will be controlled by the person in the same ways as a nonartificial leg.

Muscle activation maps, along with force, torque, and inertial properties of biological legs, will be programmed into the artificial limb, and when a signal from the brain arrives through the nervous system calling on the leg to move, it will, with the same response and outcome of a normal healthy limb. The recording of the "recipe" of biomechanical factors associated with limb movement has been being collected for years in biomechanics laboratories across the world. As medical technology increases and artificial limbs become lifelike, that recipe will be used to bring futuristic appendages to life. The result will be limbs that are difficult for anyone beyond an expert to identify as not real, and with function that will match that of living tissue.

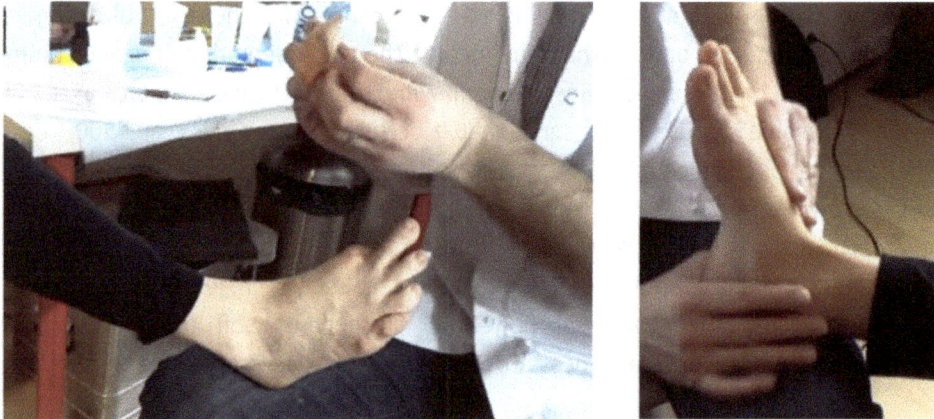

Figure 10.10   Lifelike prosthetic toe.

Summary

Biomechanics is understanding the human machine today and in the future. It helps us to appreciate our potential and our limitations. When coupled with other areas of science and medicine, it expands the possibility of being human and provides a way for us to better understand the how's and why's of movement. It provides us with a unique perspective on who we are and the life we live.

No one knows exactly what the future will bring, but if the history of biomechanics can provide us with some insight, it is likely that people will continue to want to live long and active lives. They will strive to attempt expand their ability to master whatever environment they find themselves in and push themselves to their physical limits. Biomechanists will be continue to study, analyze, and offer solutions to the types of movement problems people experience in their attempt to improve performance while doing their best to reduce the likelihood of injury and while people do what people do so well: move!

Ongoing Case Scenarios

The application of Biomechanics takes many forms. As we move into the future Biomechanics and how it is applied with continue to evolve. Creating high-speed video capture systems capable of recording images thousands of times faster than the human eye, the development of prosthetics or implants that function as well as flesh and bone, people running faster, jumping higher and lifting heavier weights than ever before used to be found only in the realm of science fiction. Today it is science fact. What will the future bring? I'm not sure but I know Biomechanics will be part of it!

How This All Works Today and, in the Future

In previous chapters, various scenarios were presented to illustrate how information from that chapter could be applied across the areas of sports, daily life, and medicine. Here, a real-life forensics case will be presented to predict how biomechanical advances in the areas of sports, daily life, and medicine could result in a much different outcome for the injured person.

In 1996 a 21-year-old man attempted to perform a shallow (10–12-degree below horizontal entry) dive in a swimming pool owned by an apartment complex. The pool depth markers near where he entered the water were incorrect and stated that the water was 4 feet deep. In reality, it was closer to 3 feet. The dive did not go as intended, and the man was severely injured when his head struck the bottom of the concrete pool. The impact fractured several of his cervical vertebra and caused a comminuted (crush) fracture of the C4 vertebra. He was left a quadriplegic. During the trial testimony experts in the area of sports (diving), daily life (the challenges of living as a quadriplegic), and medicine (descriptions of the sustained bodily damage and procedures performed in the failed attempts to return motor control to the injured) testified.

The injured man and his family brought a lawsuit against the owners of the apartment complex claiming negligence that caused the man to misinterpret the danger of diving into the pool. They claimed the mismarked depth marker was directly responsible for the injury, saying that his dive would have been safe if the water was 4 feet deep. There was no video record of the actual dive that resulted in injury.

A biomechanist was retained to provide a factual description of the actions that led to the injury. To re-create the circumstances of the dive, information related to the anatomical and athletic ability of the injured party was used, along with known information of how the spine responded to dynamic compressive loading. That information was fed into projectile motion equations that determined that the entry angle of the diver was significantly steeper (32–47 degrees) than the anticipated shallow dive angle expected (10–12 degrees). The steep entry angle, the lack of trauma to any part of the body beyond a laceration on the crown of the head, and knowledge of bone fracture mechanics proved that while he may had intended to perform a shallow dive, he most certainly did not. An analysis of the hydrodynamics of a body moving through 3 or 4 feet of water would not have appreciably changed the pool bottom impact. The bad dive mechanics caused the injury, not any other factor such as the mismarked pool depth.

The biomechanical testimony was enough to convince the jury of the circumstance surrounding the injury, and they did not find in favor of the injured man or his family, who had been seeking a substantial monetary award for damages.

Unfortunately for the young man, his life was forever changed in the ~10ms it took for the compressive load resulting from striking his head on the pool bottom to irreparably damage his spinal cord. He spent the rest of his life confined to a wheelchair, unable to speak, without the use of his arms or legs, needing 24-hour medical assistance. Today, his life after such an accident could have been very different.

If a similar injury occurred today, how could advances in biomechanics have helped this individual have lived a very different life following his accident? Provide examples in the areas of sports, daily life, and medicine.

List of Key Takeaways

- Movement sensor technology continues to improve by being able to capture more data faster and easier through a host of wearable options.
- The concept of human cyborgs is being realized today through a wide variety of implants that return and/or improve function to a growing segment of the population.
- Artificial limbs are becoming more lifelike in appearance and function and are becoming more likely to be actively controlled by the brain.
- Biomechanical advances in the areas of sports, daily life, and medicine will continue to improve human performance while striving to reduce injury, thereby improving quality of life for all.

References

American Cancer Society, (2023). Key Statistics for Basal and Squamous Cell Skin Cancers. https://www.cancer.org/cancer/types/basal-and-squamous-cell-skin-cancer/about/key-statistics.html

Bhatia, N. and El-Chami, M, (2018). Leadless pacemakers: a contemporary review. Journal of Geriatric Cardiology, 15(4), p 249-253.

Human Factors and Ergonomics Society. (n.d.) What is Human Factors and Ergonomics. https://www.hfes.org/About-HFES/What-is-Human-Factors-and-Ergonomics#:~:text=on%20their%20website%3A-,Ergonomics%20(or%20human%20factors)%20is%20the%20scientific%20discipline%20concerned%20with,overall%20system%20performance%20(definition%20adopted

Learmonth, I.D., Young, C., Rorabeck, C., (2007). The operation of the century: total hop replacement. Lancet. 370(9597), p 1508-19. doi: 10.1016/S0140-6736(07)60457-7.

National Institute on Deafness and Other Communication Disorders. (2016, statistics updated 2021). NIH Publication No. 00-4798 https://www.nidcd.nih.gov/health/cochlear-implants#:~:text=Children%20and%20adults%20who%20are,adults%20and%2065%2C000%20in%20children.

National Institute of Neurological Disorders and Stroke. (n.d.) Parkinson's Disease: Challenges, Progress, and Promise. https://www.ninds.nih.gov/current-research/focus-disorders/focus-parkinsons-disease-research/parkinsons-disease-challenges-progress-and-promise#:~:text=Approximately%20500%2C000%20Americans%20are%20diagnosed,1%20million%20Americans%20have%20PD.

Roser, M.C., Canavan, P.K., Najafi, B., Watchman, M.C., Vaishnav, K., Armstrong, D. G., (2017). Novel In-Shoe Exoskeleton for Offloading of Forefoot Pressure for Individuals with Diabetic Foot Pathology. Journal of Diabetes Science and Technology. 11(5), p 874-882. DOI: 10.1177/1932296817726349.

ScienceDaily. (2004). UCSF/Baylor Team Uses New Method to Measure Bone Loss in Astronauts Flying Long Mission. https://www.sciencedaily.com/releases/2004/03/040309072945.htm

Image Credits

Fig. 10.2: Copyright © by CSIRO (CC BY 3.0) at https://commons.wikimedia.org/wiki/File:CSIRO_ScienceImage_7664_The_wearable_bodymapping_sleeve.jpg.

Fig. 10.3: Copyright © by Ian Forsyth (CC BY 4.0) at https://commons.wikimedia.org/wiki/File:Soldier_with_Prosthetic_Limb_at_the_Personnel_Recovery_Centre_in_Edinburgh_MOD_45152289.jpg.

Fig. 10.4: Source: https://www.youtube.com/watch?v=kG4eMZqppT4.

Fig. 10.5a: Source: https://www.youtube.com/watch?v=6JJQYc8HqVk.

Fig. 10.5b: Source: https://www.youtube.com/watch?v=6JJQYc8HqVk.

Fig. 10.6a: Source: https://commons.wikimedia.org/wiki/File:Pendular_acceleration.jpg.

Fig. 10.6b: Copyright © by oomlout (CC BY-SA 2.0) at https://commons.wikimedia.org/wiki/File:Adafruit_ADXL335_triple-axis_accelerometer_module.jpg.

Fig. 10.7: Copyright © by Chrisnorlin (CC BY-SA 3.0) at https://commons.wikimedia.org/wiki/File:Arm-Wrestle-Xray.jpg.

Fig. 10.8: Copyright © by (CC BY-SA 3.0) at https://commons.wikimedia.org/wiki/File:Aktivni_egzoskelet_02,_1974._godina.jpg.

Fig. 10.9: Copyright © by Vitaly V. Kuzmin (CC BY-SA 4.0) at https://commons.wikimedia.org/wiki/File:ExoAtlet_P-1_-_InnovationDay2013part1-59.jpg.

Fig. 10.10a: Source: https://www.youtube.com/watch?v=2jSt0t2War4.

Fig. 10.10b: Source: https://www.youtube.com/watch?v=2jSt0t2War4.

www.ingramcontent.com/pod-product-compliance
Lightning Source LLC
Chambersburg PA
CBHW061347210326
41598CB00035B/5911

* 9 7 8 1 7 9 3 5 6 5 7 6 1 *